PREHOSPITAL
EMERGENCY
MEDICINE

SECRETS

T0195203

PREHOSPITAL EMERGENCY MEDICINE

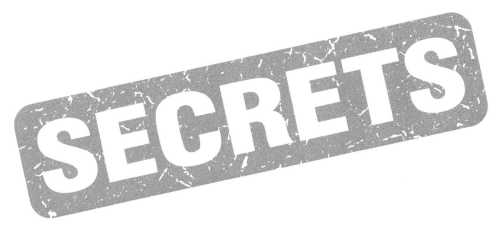

SECRETS

ROBERT P. OLYMPIA, MD
Professor, Departments of Emergency
Medicine and Pediatrics
Penn State College of Medicine;
Assistant Director of Research,
Department of Emergency Medicine
Attending Physician, Department of
Emergency Medicine
Penn State Health Milton S. Hershey
Medical Center/Penn State Children's
Hospital
Hershey, Pennsylvania

JEFFREY S. LUBIN, MD, MPH
Professor, Departments of Emergency
Medicine and Public Health Sciences
Program Director, Combined MD/MPH
Dual Degree Program
Penn State College of Medicine;
Vice Chair of Research, Department of
Emergency Medicine
Attending Physician, Department of
Emergency Medicine
Penn State Health Milton S. Hershey
Medical Center
Hershey, Pennsylvania

ELSEVIER

Elsevier
1600 John F. Kennedy Blvd.
Ste 1800
Philadelphia, PA 19103-2899

PREHOSPITAL EMERGENCY MEDICINE SECRETS   ISBN: 978-0-323-72266-7

Library of Congress Control Number: 2021943966

Senior Content Strategist: Marybeth Thiel
Director, Content Development: Ellen Wurm-Cutter
Content Development Manager: Meghan Andress
Content Development Specialists: Angie Breckon and Beth LoGiudice
Publishing Services Manager: Shereen Jameel
Project Manager: Rukmani Krishnan and Manikandan Chandrasekaran
Designer: Bridget Hoette

Printed in The United States of America.

Last digit is the print number: 9 8 7 6 5 4 3 2 1

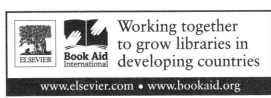

To my wife, Jodi, for supporting me with unconditional love and allowing me to pursue my professional and personal dreams. Any success in my life is because of you, and your belief in me has allowed me to soar. "Love is putting someone else's needs before yours." Olaf, *Frozen*

To my children, Abigail and Madelyn. I am so lucky and blessed to be your daddy. You inspire me every day to be the best person I can be. My world is complete because you are part of my life. "You are my greatest adventure." Mr. Incredible, *The Incredibles*

To my grandparents (Manuel, Avelina, Teofilo, Gliceria), my parents (Manuel and Delia), Coco, my sisters (Patricia and Catherine), my brothers (Rob and Mark), Grant, Isabel, and Gracie, the Brady and Cruzan families, and extended family from all over the world, thank you for your love and support and for being amazing role models. I hope I have made you proud. "Ohana means family. Family means nobody gets left behind." Lilo, *Lilo & Stitch*

To my mentors, Drs. Magdy Attia, Steven Selbst, Waseem Hafeez, and Jeff Avner, thank you for believing in me. "All it takes is faith and trust." Peter Pan

And lastly, to all of the emergency department and prehospital care staff that I have worked with over my 25-year career, at the DuPont Hospital for Children, Christiana Care Hospital, Children's Hospital at Montefiore, Newark Beth Israel Medical Center, and Penn State Health Milton S. Hershey Medical Center. I am the physician I am today because of the compassion, dedication, hard work, and selflessness that I have learned from each and every one of you. We make an amazing team. "The flower that blooms in adversity is the most rare and beautiful of all." The Emperor, *Mulan*

"All our dreams can come true, if we have the courage to pursue them."
"It's kind of fun to do the impossible" Walt Disney
Robert P. Olympia

To my wife, Jill, and my children, who put up with my crazy schedule, nonstop desire to get to the "next step," and my irresistible reflex to look up when I hear a siren going by or a helicopter overhead. Thank you for supporting me in all of the ways that you do.

To my many mentors, from Emergency Medicine, EMS Medicine, and other fields. I am inspired to do more and be more because of the great people who surround and support me.

And, of course, to all of the emergency and prehospital providers that I have been fortunate enough to work with over the past 30 years. It takes a special kind of person to do what you do, helping strangers during some of the most traumatic and horrific moments of their lives. I am honored to be a part of an amazing Emergency Medicine/EMS family.
Jeffrey S. Lubin

SECTION EDITORS

Michelle A. Fischer, MD, MPH
Residency Program Director
Associate Professor, Department of Emergency Medicine
Penn State College of Medicine;
Penn State Health Milton S. Hershey Medical Center
Hershey, Pennsylvania

Joseph Grover, MD
Clinical Assistant Professor, Department of Emergency
    Medicine
University of North Carolina School of Medicine
Chapel Hill, North Carolina

Jeffrey H. Luk, MD, MS, FACEP, FAEMS
Associate Professor, Department of Emergency Medicine
Case Western Reserve University School of Medicine;
Director, Prehospital and Disaster Medicine
Department of Emergency Medicine
University Hospitals Cleveland Medical Center
Cleveland, Ohio

Jessica Mann, MD, MS
Assistant Professor, Department of Emergency Medicine
Penn State College of Medicine;
Medical Director, Life Lion EMS
Penn State Health Milton S. Hershey Medical Center
Hershey, Pennsylvania

Diane L. Miller, MD, MS
Clinical Assistant Professor, Department of Emergency
    Medicine
University of North Carolina School of Medicine
Chapel Hill, North Carolina;
Medical Director, North Carolina State Highway Patrol
Raleigh, North Carolina

Chadd E. Nesbit, MD, PhD, FACEP, FAEMS
System EMS Medical Director, Allegheny Health Network
Pittsburgh, Pennsylvania;
Assistant Professor, Department of Emergency Medicine
Penn State College of Medicine
Penn State Health Milton S. Hershey Medical Center
Hershey, Pennsylvania

Robert P. Olympia, MD
Professor, Departments of Emergency Medicine and
    Pediatrics
Penn State College of Medicine;
Assistant Director of Research, Department of Emergency
    Medicine
Attending Physician, Department of Emergency Medicine
Penn State Health Milton S. Hershey Medical Center/Penn
    State Children's Hospital
Hershey, Pennsylvania

CONTRIBUTORS

Krystal Baciak, MD
Attending Physician, Emergency Department
Swedish Medical Center
Seattle, Washington

Erica Bates, MD
Assistant Professor, Departments of Emergency Medicine
and Internal Medicine
Penn State College of Medicine;
Attending Physician, Emergency Medicine
Penn State Health Milton S. Hershey Medical Center
Hershey, Pennsylvania

Marina Boushra, MD
Assistant Professor, Emergency Medicine
East Carolina University
Greenville, North Carolina

Michael J. Burla, DO
Clinical Faculty, Emergency Medicine
Maine Health;
Assistant Professor, Emergency Medicine
Tufts University School of Medicine
Biddeford, Maine;
Instructor, Emergency Medicine
Oakland University William Beaumont School of Medicine
Royal Oak, Michigan

Derya Caglar, MD
Associate Professor, Pediatrics
University of Washington;
Fellowship Director
Pediatric Emergency Medicine
Seattle Children's Hospital
Seattle, Washington

Brett Campbell, MD
Resident Physician, Orthopaedic Surgery
Penn State Health Milton S. Hershey Medical Center
Hershey, Pennsylvania

Angelica Mazzarini, MD
Fellow, Pediatric Emergency Medicine
UPMC Children's Hospital of Pittsburgh
Pittsburgh, Pennsylvania

Bradley Chappell, DO, MHA, FACOEP
Medical Director, Emergency Department
Harbor-UCLA Medical Center
Torrance, California;
Assistant Professor, Emergency Medicine
David Geffen School of Medicine at UCLA
Los Angeles, California

Remle Crowe, PhD, NREMT
Research Scientist and Performance Improvement Manager
ESO
Austin, Texas

Matthew Cully, DO
Fellow, Emergency Medicine
Nemours Alfred I. duPont Hospital for Children
Wilmington, Delaware

Christopher Davis, MD
Assistant Professor, Emergency Medicine
Wake Forest School of Medicine
Winston-Salem, North Carolina

Joshua J. Davis, MD
Clinical Instructor, Department of Emergency Medicine
University of Kansas School of Medicine
Attending Physician, Emergency Medicine
Vituity
Wichita, Kansas

Kaynan Doctor, MD, MBBS, BSc
Attending Physician, Pediatric Emergency Medicine
Division of Emergency Medicine
Nemours/Alfred I. duPont Hospital for Children
Wilmington, Delaware;
Assistant Professor, Pediatrics
The Sidney Kimmel Medical College at Thomas Jefferson
University
Philadelphia, Pennsylvania

Eleanor Dunham, MD, MBA, FACEP
Assistant Professor, Department of Emergency Medicine
Penn State College of Medicine;
Penn State Health Milton S. Hershey Medical Center
Hershey, Pennsylvania

Jennifer Dunnick, MD, MPH
Assistant Professor, Pediatrics
Division of Emergency Medicine
UPMC Children's Hospital of Pittsburgh
Pittsburgh, Pennsylvania

Daniel M. Fein, MD
Associate Professor of Pediatrics
Albert Einstein College of Medicine
Interim Division Chief
Division of Pediatric Emergency Medicine
Children's Hospital at Montefiore
Bronx, New York

William C. Ferguson, Jr., MD, FACEP, FAEMS
Medical Director
Birmingham Regional Emergency Medical Services;
Associate Professor, Emergency Medicine
University of Alabama at Birmingham
Birmingham, Alabama

Michelle A. Fischer, MD, MPH
Residency Program Director
Associate Professor, Department of Emergency Medicine
Penn State College of Medicine;
Penn State Health Milton S. Hershey Medical Center
Hershey, Pennsylvania

Walker Foland, DO, FACEP
Physician, Emergency Medicine
Covenant HealthCare,
Grand Blanc, Michigan;
Special Deputy, Emergency Services Team (SWAT)
Saginaw County Sheriff's Office,
Saginaw, Michigan;
Professional Member, Disciplinary Subcommittee
Michigan Board of Osteopathic Medicine and Surgery,
Lansing, Michigan

Robert N.E. French, MD
Physician, Emergency Department
Banner University Medical Center;
Medical Toxicologist
Arizona Poison and Drug Information Center
Tucson, Arizona

Matthew R. Garner, MD
Associate Professor, Department of Orthopaedics and
Rehabilitation
Penn State School of Medicine
Penn State Health Milton S. Hershey Medical Center
Hershey, Pennsylvania

Sarah A. Gibson, MPAS, PAC
Physician Assistant, Emergency Medicine
Penn State Health Milton S. Hershey Medical Center
Hershey, Pennsylvania

John Gonzales, AAS, BAAS
Commander, Clinical Practices
Williamson County EMS
Georgetown, Texas

Joseph Grover, MD
Clinical Assistant Professor, Department of Emergency
Medicine
University of North Carolina School of Medicine
Chapel Hill, North Carolina

Puneet Gupta, MD, FACEP
Assistant Medical Director, Los Angeles County Fire
Department
Physician, Department of Emergency Medicine
Harbor-UCLA Medical Center
Torrance, California

Selena Hariharan, MD, MHSA
Professor, Department of Pediatrics
University of Cincinnati College of Medicine;
Physician, Emergency Medicine
Cincinnati Children's Hospital Medical Center
Cincinnati, Ohio

Emily Hegamyer, MD, MPH
Attending Physician, Pediatric Emergency Medicine
Inova Children's Hospital
Falls Church, Virginia

Alexander P. Isakov, MD, MPH, FAEMS
Professor, Department of Emergency Medicine
Director, Section of Prehospital and Disaster Medicine
Emory University School of Medicine
Atlanta, Georgia

Jeffrey L. Jarvis, MD, MS, EMT-P, FACEP, FAEMS
Medical Director
Williamson County EMS
Emergency Medical Services Williamson County
Georgetown, Texas;
EMS Medical Director, Marble Falls Area EMS
Marble Falls, Texas;
Physician, Emergency Medicine
Baylor Scott and White Healthcare
Round Rock, Texas

Jason Jones, MD
Assistant Professor, Department of Emergency Medicine,
University of Florida;
Medical Director, Alachua County Fire Rescue
Gainesville, Florida

Leah Kaye, BA, MD
Instructor, Section of Emergency Medicine/Network of
Care
University of Colorado, Children's Hospital Colorado
Aurora, Colorado

Ryan Kelly, MSN, RN, CRNP, FNP-C, ENP-C, CEN, WEMT-B
Assistant Director, Advanced Practice Emergency
Medicine Fellowship Program
Nurse Practitioner
Emergency Department
Penn State Health Milton S. Hershey Medical Center
Hershey, Pennsylvania;
Operations Flight Commander
459th Aeromedical Evacuation Squadron
United States Air Force, Joint Base Andrews
Camp Springs, Maryland

Josh Knapp, MD
Associate EMS Medical Director, Geisinger EMS
Attending Physician, Department of Emergency
Medicine
Geisinger Holy Spirit Hospital
Camp Hill, Pennsylvania

Melissa D. Kohn, MD, MS, FACEP, EMT-PHP
Attending Physician, Emergency Medicine/EMS
Director, EMS Resident Education
Department of Emergency Medicine
Einstein Medical Center Philadelphia;
Clinical Instructor of Emergency Medicine
SKMC of Thomas Jefferson University
Philadelphia, Pennsylvania

Andrew T. Krack, MD, MS
Clinical Instructor, Department of Pediatrics
University of Colorado School of Medicine
Physician, Emergency Medicine
Children's Hospital Colorado
Aurora, Colorado

Lekshmi Kumar, MD, MPH, FAEMS
Associate Professor, Department of Emergency Medicine
Section of Prehospital and Disaster Medicine
Emory University School of Medicine
Atlanta, Georgia

Karen Y. Kwan, MD
Assistant Professor of Clinical Pediatrics
Keck School of Medicine/University of Southern California;
Attending Physician, Children's Hospital Los Angeles;
Emergency Medicine Resident and Medical Student Director
Division of Emergency and Transport Medicine
Director of CHLA Virtual Urgent Care
Los Angeles, California

Richard Kwun, MD
Attending Physician, Department of Emergency Medicine
Swedish Medical Center
Issaquah, Washington

Stephanie Lareau, MD
Associate Professor, Emergency Medicine
Wilderness Medicine Fellowship Director
Virginia Tech—Carilion Clinic
Roanoke, Virginia

Sarah K. Lewis, BS, BA, MHS, PA-C
Assistant Professor, Departments of Emergency Medicine
    and Physician Assistant Studies
Penn State School of Medicine
Hershey, Pennsylvania

Jeffrey S. Lubin, MD, MPH
Professor, Departments of Emergency Medicine and
    Public Health Sciences
Program Director, Combined MD/MPH Dual Degree Program
Penn State College of Medicine;
Vice Chair of Research, Department of Emergency Medicine
Attending Physician, Department of Emergency Medicine
Penn State Health Milton S. Hershey Medical Center
Hershey, Pennsylvania

Jessica Mann, MD, MS
Assistant Professor, Department of Emergency Medicine
Penn State College of Medicine;
Medical Director, Life Lion EMS
Penn State Health Milton S. Hershey Medical Center
Hershey, Pennsylvania

Johannah K. Merrill, BS, MD
Physician and EMS Medical Director Lawrence General
    Hospital
Lawrence, Massachusetts

Brendan Mulcahy, DO, MPAS
EMS Medical Director
AHN Wexford Hospital
Wexford, Pennsylvania

Philip S. Nawrocki, MD
Physician, Department of Emergency Medicine
EMS Medical Director
Allegheny General Hospital
Pittsburgh, Pennsylvania

Chadd E. Nesbit, MD, PhD, FACEP, FAEMS
System EMS Medical Director, Allegheny Health Network
Pittsburgh, Pennsylvania;
Assistant Professor, Department of Emergency Medicine
Penn State College of Medicine
Penn State Health Milton S. Hershey Medical Center
Hershey, Pennsylvania

J. Elizabeth Neuman, DO, FACEP
Assistant Professor, Department of Emergency Medicine
Penn State School of Medicine;
Attending Physician, Department of Emergency Medicine
Penn State Hershey Medical Center
Hershey, Pennsylvania

Robert P. Olympia, MD
Professor, Departments of Emergency Medicine and Pediatrics
Penn State College of Medicine;
Assistant Director of Research, Department of Emergency
    Medicine
Attending Physician, Department of Emergency Medicine
Penn State Health Milton S. Hershey Medical Center/Penn
    State Children's Hospital
Hershey, Pennsylvania

John Park, MD
Attending Physician, Pediatric Emergency Medicine
Westchester Medical Center
Valhalla, New York

James F. Parker, MD, FAAP
Medical Director
PM Pediatrics;
Associate Professor, Pediatric Emergency Medicine
    University of Connecticut School of Medicine Farmington
Manchester, Connecticut

Carolina Pereira, MD, FACEP, FAEMS
Assistant Professor, Emergency Medicine and EMS
UF Health Jacksonville
Jacksonville, Florida

Matthew Poremba, DO
Physician, Department of Emergency Medicine
Medical Director, LIfeFlight
Allegheny General Hospital
Pittsburgh, Pennsylvania

Kian Preston-Suni, MD, MPH
Assistant Chief, Emergency Medicine
Greater Los Angeles VA Medical Center
Assistant Clinical Professor, Emergency Medicine
David Geffen School of Medicine at UCLA;
Los Angeles, California

Susan B. Promes, MD, MBA, FACEP
Professor and Chair, Emergency Medicine
Penn State College of Medicine
Hershey, Pennsylvania

Colby Redfield, BS, MD
Assistant Medical Director, Emergency Services
Tallahassee Memorial Hospital
Tallahassee, Florida;
Medical Director, Gadsden County Emergency Medical
    Services
Quincy, Florida;
Medical Director of Emergency Medical Services
Healthcare Professions
Tallahassee Community College
Tallahassee, Florida

Abagayle E. Renko, MD, NREMT-B
Resident Physician, Department of Emergency Medicine
Cooper University Hospital
Camden, New Jersey

Lilia Reyes, MD, FAAP
Assistant Professor, Departments of Emergency Medicine
  and Pediatrics
Penn State College of Medicine;
Attending Physician, Department of Emergency Medicine
Penn State Health Milton S. Hershey Medical Center
Hershey, Pennsylvania

Munaza Batool Rizvi, MD
Instructor of Pediatric Emergency Medicine
Pediatric Emergency Ultrasound Fellow
Department of Emergency Medicine
Columbia University, Vagelos College of Physicians and
  Surgeons
New York, New York

Dorothy Rocourt, MD
Associate Professor, Department of Surgery and Pediatrics
Penn State College of Medicine;
Penn State Cancer Institute;
Attending Physician, Penn State Children's Hospital
Hershey, Pennsylvania

Ellen Beth Rodman, DO, FACOP, FACOEP
Attending Physician, Pediatric Emergency Department
Sunrise Children's Hospital
Las Vegas, Nevada

Rohit B. Sangal, MD, MBA
Assistant Professor, Department of Emergency Medicine
Yale University School of Medicine;
Associate Medical Director, Department of Emergency
  Medicine
Yale New Haven Hospital
New Haven, Connecticut

Jordan B. Schooler, MD, PhD, NRP, FACEP
Assistant Professor, Department of Emergency Medicine
Assistant Professor, Heart and Vascular Institute
Penn State College of Medicine;
Attending Physician, Emergency Medicine
Penn State Health Milton S. Hershey Medical Center
Hershey, Pennsylvania

Michael Shukis, MD, MS
Assistant Professor of Emergency Medicine
West Virginia University School of Medicine
Morgantown, West Virginia

Duane D. Siberski, DO, FACOEP-D, FACEP, PHP
EMS Medical Director, Emergency Department
Penn State Health—St. Joseph Medical Center
Reading, Pennsylvania;
Regional Medical Director
Eastern Pennsylvania Regional EMS Council
Orefield, Pennsylvania

Erica M. Simon, DO, MPH, MHA
Staff Physician, Emergency Medicine
San Antonio Uniformed Services Health Education
  Consortium
San Antonio, Texas

Bryan Sloane, MD
EMS Fellow, Emergency Medicine
Stanford University Medical Center
Palo Alto, California

Kayla Stiffler, BS, MPAS
Physician Assistant, Emergency Department
Penn State Health Milton S. Hershey Medical Center
Hershey, Pennsylvania

Matthew J. Streitz, MD
Assistant Professor, Military and Emergency Medicine
Uniformed Services University of the Health Sciences
San Antonio, Texas

Christopher Tems, MD, FACEP, FAWM
Attending Physician, Department of Emergency
  Medicine
The Medical Center of Aurora
Aurora, Colorado

Anthony Tsai, MD
Assistant Professor, Department of Surgery
Penn State College of Medicine;
Attending Physician, Department of Surgery
Penn State Health Milton S. Hershey Medical Center
Hershey, Pennsylvania

Brandon Wattai, BS
Program Supervisor, Life Lion EMS Community
  Paramedicine
Emergency Medicine
Penn State Health Milton S. Hershey Medical Center
Hershey, Pennsylvania

Elizabeth Barrall Werley, MD
Assistant Professor, Department of Emergency Medicine
Penn State College of Medicine;
Attending Physician, Emergency Medicine
Penn State Health Milton S. Hershey Medical Center
Hershey, Pennsylvania

Kelsey Wilhelm, MD
EMS and Disaster Fellow, Los Angeles County EMS
  Agency
Physician, Department of Emergency Medicine
Harbor-UCLA Medical Center
Torrance, California

Ethan J. Young, DO, NRP, FAAEM
Staff Emergency Physician
EMS Medical Director
Sacred Heart Hospital Hospital
Eau Claire, Wisconsin

Lydia R. Younger, BS, MSPAS
Physician Assistant, Departments of Emergency Medicine
  and Pediatric Hospital Medicine
Penn State Health Milton S. Hershey Medical Center
Hershey, Pennsylvania

PREFACE

I have been a fan of the *Secrets Series* since medical school. I love the simplicity of the question-and-answer format and value the depth of medical knowledge that each page holds. I remember using each of the *Secrets Series* specialty books during every rotation of medical school, helping me to answer questions while on rounds, to research the diagnosis of the undifferentiated patient, or to prepare for in-training and board examinations. Throughout my career, the *Secret Series* has been a large part of my professional life. I was blessed to be involved with the first, and subsequent, editions of *Pediatric Emergency Medicine Secrets* and, more recently, was editor, along with Drs. Rory M. O'Neill and Matthew L. Silvis, of the first edition of *Urgent Care Medicine Secrets* (2017). Our department at Penn State Hershey Medical Center uses both the *Emergency Medicine Secrets* and *Pediatric Emergency Medicine Secrets* books as required reading for the medical student rotations.

The advancement of the field of Prehospital Emergency Medicine during the past few decades, along with my affinity for the *Secret Series*, fueled my desire to resuscitate the previously published *Prehospital Emergency Care Secrets*, published in 1998 by editors Peter T. Pons and Vincent J. Markovchick. I was blessed to embark on this journey with my colleague Dr. Jeffrey Lubin, an emergency medicine physician with specialized training in prehospital and EMS care.

Jeff and I felt it was important to create a book that focused on evidence-based medicine, targeted toward prehospital and emergency medicine care providers from different levels of experience (graduate-level students to experienced providers) and different specialty backgrounds (medical, nursing, nurse practitioners and physician assistants, EMT and paramedics). We searched far and wide for contributors who have demonstrated scholarship in their careers and are experts in their fields. Our contributors represent varied backgrounds, including emergency medicine, pediatrics, prehospital medicine, and surgery.

We hope that *Prehospital Emergency Medicine Secrets* will provide a valuable tool for the prehospital emergency medicine care provider and subsequently improves the care of critically ill and injured pediatric and adult patients. Our book is divided into nine sections. Section 1 focuses on EMS operations. Sections 2 and 3 focus on adult medicine and trauma care, while sections 4 and 5 focus on pediatric medicine and trauma care. Disaster and Multiple Casualty Incidents and Wilderness EMS and Austere Medicine are covered in sections 6 and 7, respectively. Section 8 covers special prehospital situations, including transport, bariatric and geriatric emergencies, community paramedicine, and end-of-life issues. Lastly, section 9 focuses on prehospital skills and procedures.

Robert P. Olympia
July 2021

CONTENTS

3 ADULT TRAUMA CARE

4 PEDIATRIC MEDICAL CARE

TOP 100 SECRETS

(associated chapter number in parentheses)

1. Emergency medical services (EMS) are believed to have existed since the time of Caesar and were founded because of a need noted during military conflicts. (1)
2. Some patients present with disease processes requiring transport to specialty centers; determining where to transport a patient is a critical element of prehospital care. (2)
3. There are four nationally recognized levels of EMS providers, and each EMS system utilizes the deployment of these levels as it best fits their community. (3)
4. There are two main systems for EMS communications: land mobile radio and telephone communications. Having both systems creates the optimal redundancy to ensure appropriate communication capabilities. (3)
5. Having a designated public information officer for your department can ensure that there is only one message being communicated. (4)
6. The capacity to make medical decisions is situation specific and is determined by a patient's ability to understand the acute condition, the benefits of the recommended treatment or transport, and the risks of refusal of these recommendations. (5)
7. The EMS system plays a significant role in the prevention, detection, and intervention in public health emergencies. (6)
8. Quality improvement and research both rely heavily on measurement. While quality improvement aims to improve a process toward a known standard of care, research seeks to answer a question and enhance knowledge. (7)
9. Situational awareness is crucial to ensuring safety; throughout every call, EMS providers need to continuously reassess the scene and try to predict active threats. (8)
10. Extra caution should be used at scenes of roadway accidents and at scenes with patients under the influence of drugs and alcohol or with psychiatric diseases. (8)
11. When physically restraining a patient, a team approach should be taken, with at least one person per extremity, staying off the chest and protecting the head and airway. This should typically be followed by some form of chemical restraint. (8)
12. Over time, the approach to managing psychological stress for EMS workers has changed, with a new emphasis on individualized response to traumatic events, implementing wellness initiatives, and taking a less structured approach to debriefings. (9)
13. The most commonly encountered occupational hazards for EMS providers are injuries related to environmental and patient hazards, ambulance/transport crashes, and repetitive stress injuries such as lifting a patient and mechanical slips, trips, or falls. (9)
14. Rapid physical assessment is essential in determining the need for life-saving and primary exam stabilizing maneuvers. (10)
15. Vital signs can provide objective evaluation of vital organ function and must be interpreted in a clinical context. (10)
16. Nearly all of those who survive out of hospital cardiac arrest have return of spontaneous circulation in the field. (11)
17. The definition of undifferentiated shock is inadequate tissue perfusion. Hypotension and hypoxia from inadequate tissue perfusion may result in unmet metabolic demands. (12)
18. Shock is differentiated into four categories: cardiogenic, hypovolemic, distributive, and obstructive. Treatment is based on determining the underlying cause. (12)
19. All patients with altered mental status should be assessed for rapidly correctable etiologies, such as hypoglycemia, and treated accordingly. (13)
20. If the patient can provide little or no history, it is important to get as much historical information from the persons with the patient and environmental cues. (13)
21. Treatment of arrhythmias in the prehospital setting should be based on whether the patient is symptomatic or unstable. (14)
22. The "serious 6" concerning etiologies for chest pain are tension pneumothorax, pulmonary embolism, ruptured esophagus, cardiac tamponade, aortic dissection, and acute coronary syndrome. (15)
23. In patients with an implanted defibrillator or pacemaker, consider that the device may be malfunctioning and firing more than it should or not firing when it should be. (16)
24. Providing analgesia for severe abdominal pain does not prevent adequate diagnosis at the hospital. (17)
25. Glucose levels need to be closely managed in patients with a stroke or with seizures. The brain is very sensitive to low or high glucose. (18)

26. EMS professionals are in a unique position to initiate early intervention for septic patients, with some literature suggesting improved survival when sepsis is identified by EMS personnel rather than identified later by the emergency department. (19)
27. Transport to predetermined hospitals, identified by the EMS medical director, for an obviously pregnant patient can expedite care. (20)
28. The similarities of chronic obstructive pulmonary disease (COPD) and congestive heart failure (CHF) can make it difficult to differentiate the two in the field. Capnography may be a helpful tool in distinguishing them. (21)
29. Evaluation of a seizure patient should include evaluation for trauma, hypoxia, and hypoglycemia. (22)
30. For patients with suspected cerebrovascular accidents, obtain a fingerstick blood glucose, obtain the patient's last known normal neurologic status, and notify the receiving hospital to ensure that appropriate resources are available upon arrival. (23)
31. Seizures, preceding head trauma, neurologic deficits, or persistent symptoms such as confusion, chest pain, or dyspnea exclude a diagnosis of syncope and should raise concern for more dangerous etiologies. (24)
32. Knowing the mechanism of injury and the kinetics of the injury can provide valuable insight into the injuries that the patient has sustained. (25)
33. Take photos of trauma scenes when possible. (25)
34. Avoiding hypoxemia and hypotension is a critical action to help mitigate secondary brain injury in patients with head trauma. (26)
35. Blunt trauma patients who are ambulatory at the scene should still have spinal motion restriction if they fulfill appropriate criteria. (27)
36. If a patient with pneumothorax requires emergent airway management, a needle decompression of the pneumothorax should be performed *prior* to intubation. (28)
37. Pelvic binding using either a wrapped sheet with towel clamps or a commercially available pelvic binder can be effective in reducing pelvic volume in the setting of certain pelvic fractures for patients showing signs of shock. (28)
38. Tourniquets can be a very effective method for achieving hemostasis in trauma patients but are not without risk; it is important to know when and how to properly use them to avoid unnecessary complications. (29)
39. Inhalation injury can be associated with upper airway structures, lower airway structures, or both. If there is any clinical concern for airway involvement, it is better to secure the airway via intubation early. (30)
40. Prior to releasing a crushed/entrapped limb, consider applying a tourniquet to limit the rapid systemic release of toxins. The patient should have continuous cardiac monitoring, and consideration should be given to the administration of calcium and bicarbonate immediately before freeing the crushed limb to prevent decompensation from hyperkalemia. (31)
41. Your initial impression of a pediatric patient should include the patient's appearance (tone, ability to interact, consolability, look/gaze, speech/cry), circulation (skin color, pallor, mottling, cyanosis), and work of breathing (abnormal breath sounds, abnormal positioning, retractions, nasal flaring). This is otherwise known as the Pediatric Assessment Triangle. (32)
42. Cardiac arrest in children is most often due to respiratory failure. (33)
43. Signs of compensated shock in children include tachycardia for age, cool extremities, and increased capillary refill time. Of note, initially, tachycardia may be the only finding in compensated shock in pediatric patients. (34)
44. A method to quickly assess the mental status of a pediatric patient: AVPU (alert, responsive to verbal stimuli, responsive to painful stimuli, unresponsive). (35)
45. Chest pain in the pediatric population is usually benign, with chest wall pain/costochondritis being the most common cause. (36)
46. The most common cause of syncope in children is a vasovagal response, which can have several triggers. (36)
47. In children with respiratory distress, keep them in a position of comfort, provide supplemental oxygen as needed, and minimize agitation as you determine the underlying cause of their respiratory compromise. (37)
48. If aggressive anticonvulsant treatment is indicated in a child with seizures, look out for respiratory depression and apnea. (38)
49. Cushing's triad is a triad of hypertension, bradycardia, and irregular decreased respiration that occurs in the setting of increased intracranial pressure. Be aware in children with head trauma or ventriculoperitoneal shunts. (39)
50. While the prevalence of blunt pediatric injuries varies by geography and region, blunt injury accounts for approximately 90% of all pediatric trauma. (40)
51. For brief transport times in children with head injury, survival rates are the same with endotracheal intubation versus effective bag-mask ventilation. (41)
52. Physiologic and anatomic differences of the pediatric spine must be taken into account when evaluating these patients for spine injury. Pediatric injury patterns differ significantly from those of their adult counterparts. (42)
53. Predictors of intrathoracic injuries in children include low systolic blood pressure, elevated age-adjusted respiratory rate, abnormal results on thorax physical exam, abnormal chest auscultation findings, femur fracture, and Glasgow Coma Scale (GCS) score <15. (43)

54. Predictors of intra-abdominal injuries in children include evidence of abdominal wall trauma or seatbelt sign, GCS score <14, abdominal tenderness, evidence of thoracic wall trauma, complaints of abdominal pain, decreased breath sounds, and vomiting. (43)
55. Fractures or dislocations with neurovascular compromise, compartment syndrome, and open fractures require immediate emergency and orthopedic intervention. (44)
56. A child's palm equals 1% of their total body surface area (TBSA) when dealing with burns. (45)
57. Oxygen by nonrebreather should be given to all patients exposed to flame or smoke. (45)
58. A comprehensive approach to a mass casualty incident is using the National Incident Management System. (46)
59. There are multiple triage systems that are available to use for a mass casualty incident, with the most popular being START. (47)
60. Organizing traffic flow, evaluating need of medical professionals, and identifying landing zones are all imperative to the implementation of patient evacuation during a mass casualty incident. (48)
61. Red flags to identify biological terrorism include off-season flu symptoms, unexpected antibiotic resistance, large numbers of patients presenting simultaneously with similar complaints, localization of outbreaks, infected animal populations, and excessive morbidity and mortality. (49)
62. Red flags to identify chemical terrorism include explosions and/or large numbers of patients presenting simultaneously with similar complaints. (49)
63. Becoming symptomatic within 1 hour of radiation exposure is a very bad sign and the person will likely die. (50)
64. Most initial survivors of blasts will have injuries familiar to prehospital personnel. Some initial survivors may have injuries caused by primary blast injury. These may have delayed presentation and often require specialized care. (51)
65. Use the Emergency Response Guide (ERG) and other available resources to help identify hazardous substances, guide incident response, and optimize patient management. (52)
66. Tactical EMS (TEMS) increases survivability by 44%, and the first step of the Tactical Primary Survey is always security. (53)
67. Search and rescue is a specialized function that requires special training, equipment, and personnel to perform. (54)
68. Education to the community by EMS can involve instructing people on not only what resources are available but also how they can personally prepare for a disaster. (55)
69. One of the concepts commonly used in patient assessment in wilderness medicine is MARCH, where M is massive hemorrhage, A is airway, R is respiration, C is circulation, and H is hypothermia (hyperthermia/hike/helicopter). (56)
70. Many bites or stings can result in or mimic allergic reactions or anaphylaxis. Prioritize on stabilizing the airway, breathing and circulation with oxygen, an artificial airway (if needed), intravenous (IV) fluids, epinephrine, diphenhydramine, and analgesia. (57)
71. Determining the onset of patient symptoms will aid in the development of a differential diagnosis and allow you to identify dysbarisms, which require urgent transportation for treatment. (58)
72. In patients with heat-related illnesses, dopamine and dobutamine are the vasopressors of choice for refractory hypotension. (59)
73. In mild hypothermia, focus on active external rewarming efforts on the trunk to avoid core after-drop (e.g., sudden peripheral vasodilation that shunts cold blood to the core). Core after-drop may result in hypotension and cardiovascular collapse. (59)
74. Injury from electricity is related to exposure time, so even a low-voltage exposure can cause significant injury. (60)
75. As cardiac arrest in drowning is due to profound hypoxia from respiratory impairment, focus should be on establishing an airway and providing oxygen. Unlike the current layperson cardiopulmonary resuscitation (CPR) guidelines, which focus on hands-only CPR, rescue breaths and establishing an airway are of utmost priority in the drowning patient. (61)
76. Successful interfacility transport depends on thorough patient preparation and planning, including a contingency plan for unexpected clinically significant events. (62)
77. Obesity causes significant alterations to anatomy and physiology that can impact healthcare needs and hinder typical resuscitative interventions. (63)
78. Unless there is a time-sensitive emergency such as acute stoke, ST-elevation myocardial infarction (STEMI), or trauma, sometimes it is reasonable to manage the obese patient on scene and stabilize the ABCs before initiating transport. (63)
79. Baseline vital signs will typically look different in the geriatric population and may not be a reliable indicator of underlying pathology or worsening disease process. (64)
80. While there are far fewer accidents involving aeromedical services than ground vehicles, aircraft accidents have a higher likelihood of fatalities. (65)
81. Patient condition, weather, terrain, and medical personnel capabilities all factor into the decision to transport a patient by air. (65)

82. Community paramedics should assess both a patient's clinical and social condition. Multidisciplinary collaboration is critical to community paramedicine services and patient care. (66)
83. EMS providers must know their local regulations and resources with regard to intimate partner violence, sexual assault, and child abuse. (67)
84. A do-not-resuscitate (DNR) or advanced directive may limit the types of care that a patient or their proxy would like them to receive at the end of their life. (68)
85. Overdose of commonly available, over-the-counter medications can cause life-threatening toxicity. (69)
86. If providers are going to intubate, they should pay close attention to physiologic optimization of oxygen saturation and blood pressure before, during, and after the intubation, as well as avoiding overventilation. (70)
87. Airway management should never interrupt chest compressions or delay defibrillation in cardiac arrest. (70)
88. Opioids have been traditionally first line for pain management due to many desirable properties that they have. Alternatives to opioid medications include ketamine, nonsteroidal anti-inflammatory drugs (NSAIDs), acetaminophen, and nitrous oxide. All of them have been used in the prehospital setting and have proven safety profiles. (71)
89. Approach suicidal patients with a calm, courteous, and empathic manner in order to establish rapport and trust. (72)
90. Uninterrupted, high-quality compressions and early defibrillation are the keys to increasing your patient's chance of survival. (73)
91. While automated compression devices can be useful in certain scenarios, they do not provide any survival benefit to patients when compared with conventional, manual compressions. (73)
92. The most common indication for a field amputation is when the patient either cannot be extricated, or the time to extricate the patient will be too lengthy given the extent of the patient's injuries. Another indication is the patient has life-threatening injury to an area of the body that cannot be accessed due to the manner in which the patient is entrapped. (74)
93. Tranexamic acid (TXA) has been shown to decrease mortality when given within 3 hours of injury associated with massive hemorrhage. (75)
94. Humoral intraosseous (IO) access allows much higher flow rates compared to the proximal tibia. (76)
95. Perimortem caesarian section increases maternal cardiac output and reduces circulatory demand and may improve the chance of survival for both the mother and the fetus. (77)
96. The medical literature does not clearly support the utility of prehospital troponin and lactate measurement. (78)
97. Early application of a pelvic binder in a suspected open-book pelvic fracture is critical to prevent life-threatening hemorrhage. (79)
98. The decision to perform a cricothyrotomy should be made early. The procedure is designed for a patient who cannot be intubated and cannot be ventilated. (79)
99. Telemedicine use has increased significantly over the last decades. With increasing technological advancements, it will be a bigger part of medicine and prehospital care. (80)
100. As a commitment to safe practice, out-of-hospital healthcare workers need to be educated about infectious pathogens, signs and symptoms of illness, modes of transmission, incubation periods, available treatments and vaccines, and general management of the patient. Training should also include appropriate indications for use of personal protective equipment. (81)

1 EMERGENCY MEDICAL SERVICES OPERATIONS

CHAPTER 1

HISTORY OF EMERGENCY MEDICAL SERVICES

Melissa D. Kohn

QUESTIONS AND ANSWERS

1. When did emergency medical services originate?

   There are reports from biblical times where care was performed outside of places for healing. The Edwin Smith Papyrus and Babylonian Code of Hammurabi detailed early treatment and transport protocols. The Good Samaritan parable tells the story of a man who remedied travelers' wounds with oil and wine on the roadways. The man also helped care for an injured man and assisted in transporting him to an inn to receive further treatment. However, many concepts in emergency medical services (EMS) were actually developed in the battlefield and were later transitioned to civilian EMS.

2. Who created the first ambulances?

   Spain is attributed with first using ambulances, which were more like battlefield hospitals. Initiated by Queen Isabella of Spain during the 1487 siege of Malaga these treatment areas developed. The royalty felt the need to care for the injured members of their troops, further encouraging the usage of medical and surgical supplies on the battlefields. That said, some artwork also exists that suggests the use of battlefield medical transport by Caesar. The first transports were thought to have been by the Anglo-Saxon hammock around CE 900. The hammock was fitted with wheels, which had chains that were held by other attendants in order to prevent it from gaining speed going downhill. A few hundred years later during the Norman conquest of England, horses were employed in transporting patients. A covered bed attached to poles was carried between horses to aid in a more comfortable journey.

3. How did Napoleon's troops utilize ambulances?

   Dominique-Jean Larrey, who went on to become Napoleon's surgeon, noted injured troops during the Prussian wars remaining on the battlefield until the fighting had ceased, thus receiving no treatment until they could be extracted. He developed ambulances for the Army of the Rhine in 1793, which then got him noticed and he was sent to join Napoleon's Army of Italy. With his partner Baron Percy, they established two-wheeled and four-wheeled ambulances that were lightweight and easily mobile. These ambulances allowed a surgeon to potentially treat a soldier in the field with early amputations of limbs to prevent gangrene, or they could be utilized to transport soldiers to hospital instead.

4. When did EMS get started in the United States?

   Soldiers in the Civil War learned from European troops and established a medical service within the Union Army. The service performed field evacuations and created a uniform army ambulance service. The Rucker ambulance, a covered wagon on wheels that could be pulled by horses, was a more advanced and much safer version of the two-wheeled ambulances in European wars. Military forces also adapted steamships and railway cars so they could be used to transport patients longer distances to receive prolonged care.

5. When did civilian EMS get its start in the United States?

   Hospital-based ambulances in Cincinnati and New York were the beginning of civilian EMS programs. Horse-drawn ambulances were stocked with medical equipment of the time, such as bandages, splints, surgical sponges, brandy, and even handcuffs and straitjackets. On occasion, a nurse would staff the ambulance with a driver, but this was less common. Motorized vehicles were used once they became more commonplace. The staffing of the ambulance also changed as private ambulance companies joined in, some of which were operated by funeral homes. In fact, before 1966, half of all ambulance services in the United States were run by funeral homes.

6. When did aeromedical services first develop?

   During the Prussian siege of Paris, hot air balloons were used to transport wounded soldiers. Reports state that approximately 160 injured soldiers were transported in this manner. In World War I, both French and American forces adapted airplanes to transport patients. Eventually around 1929, airplanes were designed for medical transport of injured troops. Helicopters were initially used in the Korean War. With the Vietnam War, rotor wing medical transport became the typical mode of care. Because of the rapid advancement in prehospital military transport, it was believed that injured soldiers in a war zone had a better chance of survival than the victim in a domestic motor vehicle accident.

7. What is the history of modern EMS?

Mobile coronary care units were established in Belfast, Ireland, in 1964 and were shown to reduce mortality of acute myocardial infarction patients by providing some prehospital care. Attempts were made to reproduce these results in the United States but were costly due to the use of physicians in the field. As a result, prehospital care developed into EKG interpretation, intubation, defibrillation, and medication administration being performed by the first paramedics. The National Academy of Sciences published a statement in 1967 showing that the prehospital treatments were inadequate for the needs of an advancing population. Because of this statement, the National Highway Traffic Safety Administration (NHTSA) was established under the Department of Transportation (DOT). The training curricula for all prehospital treatment providers is developed and standardized by the NHTSA. Funding under the NHTSA has provided opportunities for program development and system improvements.

8. Who were Johnny and Roy from Rescue 51 out of Rampart General?

The two characters were paramedics on a popular TV show from the 1970s called "Emergency!". The show brought prehospital systems and prehospital providers into the public eye. Thus educated on what prehospital medical care could be provided, the public pleaded for these services to be made available in their respective areas.

9. How was the demand for EMS realized?

Some of the public awareness from the TV show drove the need for EMS. The "Emergency Medical Services Act of 1973" provided the funding to establish more than 300 regional EMS systems throughout the United States. EMS programs and systems were cultivated with the idea of creating standards for system-based prehospital care. The funding helped to develop training centers, purchase equipment, and cover administrative expenses. The federal funding had a limit and was exhausted after approximately 8 years. But once the basic structure and facilities had been initiated, many organizations found new funding sources and were able to remain in service.

10. How has the role of physicians in prehospital care changed over time?

Physicians' roles vary regionally and over time. Early in prehospital care in the United States, physicians rode in the ambulances with a driver to the patients' homes and provided definitive care when possible. In some areas of the world EMS physicians continue to respond to some calls. However, physicians generally spend more effort on helping to create protocols, reviewing calls for quality improvement, helping to develop education plans, and offering on-line medical oversight.

11. How has EMS changed in the past 30 years?

A host of national and international agencies have been a part of the evolution of EMS care. In 1996, on the 30th anniversary of "Accidental Death and Disability" (white paper published by the National Academy of Sciences in 1973. The research in the report revealed the ignorance of the volume of accidental deaths and injuries annually. The report included how ill-prepared ambulances and EMS staff were to handle these situations). The EMS Agenda for the Future was released and renewed the focus on prehospital care. EMS-provider education became the emphasis when the "EMS Education Agenda" portion was written in 2000, intending to create the "National EMS Scope of Practice and Education Standards." The Department of Transportation, along with multiple EMS-focused organizations, continue to update and attempt to standardize the curriculum for the various levels of prehospital providers. New levels of providers are being considered and work is being done to develop the respective educational materials. The Commission on Accreditation of Ambulance Services has improved standards for ambulance agencies to attain in order to continue quality care throughout the country. Additionally, in 2013 EMS was declared a subspecialty by the American Board of Emergency Medicine (ABEM). Fellowship programs in EMS have been established throughout the country based on requirements created by ABEM.

12. What plans are in place to help advance EMS beyond current practices?

Multiple programs and committees focused on the advancement of EMS practices have been developed. The "Emergency Medical Services for Children Program" by the Health Resources and Services Administration continues to provide the funding necessary for research, training, and injury-prevention programs aimed at the care of children. As technology continues to advance, EMS systems have become a part of the "National EMS Information System" (NEMSIS). NEMSIS allows EMS data to be shared and analyzed to help research and performance improvement. The National EMS Advisory Council, staffed with both EMS representatives and EMS consumers, currently advises DOT and the Federal Interagency Committee on EMS (FICEMS) on topics in order to advance EMS in ways beneficial to everyone. Revisions of education standards and materials continue to work on the advancement of quality providers and services available.

KEY POINTS

- Emergency Medical Services are believed to have existed since the time of Caesar.
- The basis of EMS was founded because of a need noted during military conflicts.
- Civilian EMS initially was based out of hospitals but has since expanded to include municipal and private agencies.
- EMS education and standards were created by the Department of Transportation and are continuously evolving.

BIBLIOGRAPHY

1. 50 Years of Helping EMS Systems Improve. https://www.ems.gov/OEMShistory.html.
2. Major R. *A History of Medicine*. Springfield, IL: C. Thomas Charles; 1954.
3. National Association of EMS Physicians. *Prehospital Systems and Medical Oversight*, Vol. 1. Atlanta, GA: Kendall Hunt Publishing Company; 2002.
4. National Highway Traffic Safety Administration. *Emergency Medical Services Agenda for the Future*. Washington, DC: United States Department of Transportation; 1996.
5. National Highway Traffic Safety Administration. *Emergency Medical Services Agenda for the Future 2050*. Washington, DC: United States Department of Transportation; 2019.
6. Shah MN. The formation of the emergency medical services system. *Am J Public Health*. 2006;96(3):414–423.

CHAPTER 2

DESTINATION GUIDELINES AND HOSPITAL DESIGNATION

Johannah K. Merrill and Joseph Grover

QUESTIONS AND ANSWERS

1. Are there other important determinants of patient outcome besides assessment and treatment of a patient?
   While prehospital assessment and interventions are important to patient care, the determination of where to transport is also critical. If there is only one available hospital, the choice is easy. However, if there are multiple potential facilities, the decision must be based on the patient's medical needs. When a patient has a condition requiring treatment at a specialty receiving center (e.g., trauma, stroke, and ST-elevation myocardial infarction [STEMI]), it is important that providers recognize the condition and transport to the appropriate center. Similarly, prenotification to a receiving facility reduces in-hospital intervention times and may improve patient outcomes.[1,2]

2. How do I know which hospital to go to?
   This decision must be made on an individual basis. While some patients are appropriate for transport to the closest hospital, others will present with conditions requiring services provided by specialty centers, such as burns, STEMI, trauma, and stroke. Consequently, it becomes necessary to bypass the closest hospital in favor of a hospital meeting with specific capabilities. State, regional, or local destination protocols may provide guidance.

3. Are there national guidelines to help identify the correct hospital?
   There are several organizations, including the American Burn Association, American Heart Association, American College of Surgeons, and American Stroke Association, which determine criteria required for hospitals to provide optimal care to specific patient groups (burns, STEMI, trauma, and stroke, respectively).[3-5] In conjunction with the Joint Commission, these organizations ensure that hospitals with specialty designations remain prepared to provide care to these patients.

4. What factors determine whether a trauma patient should be transported emergently to a trauma center?
   The Centers for Disease Control has developed guidelines to determine which patients require transport to a trauma center. These guidelines, entitled "Guidelines for Field Triage of Injured Patients," direct the care of individual patients as well as establishment of trauma criteria by trauma centers.[6] The criteria are divided into four categories: physiologic, anatomic, mechanism of injury, and special considerations.

5. What is a level I trauma center and how does it differ from level II, III, and IV trauma centers?
   Trauma center designation criteria vary based on state; however, there are several common elements. A level I trauma center is capable of providing care for every aspect of patient injury, requiring 24-hour coverage by trauma surgeons and all surgical and medical subspecialty services.[5] Level II centers have fewer subspecialties available, although they retain 24-hour coverage by the majority of services.[5] Level III centers are capable of 24-hour care by emergency medicine, general surgery, and anesthesia.[5] Level IV centers can provide Adult Trauma Life Support care to trauma patients prior to transfer to a facility with greater trauma capabilities.[5]

6. How does trauma care differ in rural versus urban areas?
   Rural traumas provide unique challenges due to their distance from definitive care, difficult patient access, and the potential for prolonged time until patient encounter. These patients require prolonged transport and potentially additional manpower or interventions exceeding what is dictated for urban traumas. In addition, given the longer distance to trauma centers, rotor or fixed wing transport is used more often.

7. Do pediatric traumas require special considerations?
   Not all adult trauma centers retain pediatric trauma capabilities. Pediatric trauma centers must possess adult-level trauma designation as well as pediatric-specific services. These services include a pediatric trauma program directed by a pediatric surgeon, separate pediatric emergency department, pediatric intensive care unit, pediatric specialists in multiple subspecialties, and trauma surgeons credentialed for pediatric care.[7]

8. What is a primary stroke center (PSC)? How does it differ from a comprehensive stroke center (CSC)?
   A PSC is a hospital with a specialty certification in the care of stroke victims. Certification requires 24-hour coverage by an acute stroke team (includes at least one nurse, physician assistant, or nurse practitioner and

physician who have had specific training in acute stroke care), neurologist, designated stroke beds, and the ability to provide intravenous thrombolytics.[4] A CSC is able to care for the most complex stroke patients, possessing the previous qualifications as well as a neurointensive care unit with neurospecialist coverage, 24-hour neurosurgical capabilities, and the ability to care for two complex stroke patients at once.[4] These facilities are capable of treating aneurysms and using embolectomy to treat large vessel occlusion (LVO) stroke.

9. Does every patient presenting with stroke symptoms require transport to a PSC?

Any patient presenting with stroke symptoms should be taken to the facility with the greatest capacity to care for strokes if it is the closest facility. If a CSC is not immediately available, suspected stroke patients must be assessed based on individual need. When patients within the treatment window for embolectomy or tissue plasminogen activator (tPA) present with symptoms of an LVO, they may require transport to a designated CSC if one can be reached in a timely manner (<25 additional minutes), even if this means bypassing a PSC.[3] If they display symptoms of a small vessel stroke and may require only tPA, transport to a PSC is preferable if it is closer. If no stroke center is within >30 minutes of transport, the patient should be taken to the nearest hospital capable of providing care.[2]

10. How can an emergency medical service (EMS) provider determine which patient would benefit from a PSC and which requires a CSC?

There are several screening tools that can be used in the prehospital setting to diagnose a potential LVO and determine appropriate patient destination (e.g., Los Angeles Motor Scale, Cincinnati Prehospital Stroke Severity Scale, Rapid Arterial Occlusion Evaluation, Field Assessment Stroke Triage for Emergency Destination, and National Institute for Health Stroke Scale).[8] No one scale is recommended over another, so it is up to the individual EMS system which scale is the easiest to use for rapid prehospital evaluation while maintaining high interprovider reliability. Use of these tools may be dictated by protocol at the local, regional, and/or state level.

11. Are there special considerations when dealing with patients whose electrocardiograms (EKGs) are consistent with STEMI?

Patients who meet criteria for a STEMI on prehospital EKG should be rapidly transported to the nearest hospital with percutaneous intervention (PCI) capabilities. EMS should bypass non-PCI centers in favor of an institution with PCI capabilities if one is available within 120 minutes.[1] Prearrival notification is essential and decreases door-to-balloon time.[1]

12. When should aeromedical transport be considered?

Helicopters and fixed-wing planes can shorten patient transport time, rapidly delivering them to a facility capable of providing definitive care. However, aeromedical transport has its own associated risks, requiring EMS providers to think carefully before requesting helicopter dispatch. Patients meeting criteria for trauma or burns who are unable to reach an appropriate center in a timely manner (>30-minute transport) or those presenting with stroke symptoms or STEMI without access to a specialty center should be considered for air transport.[9]

13. How is transport designated during mass casualty incidents (MCIs)?

The role of EMS during an MCI is to provide the best healthcare with limited resources to the largest number of people. High-acuity patients (triaged red, followed by yellow) should be transported first to the closest hospital with the ability to provide appropriate care.[10] If there are multiple capable hospitals, the patients should be divided based on each hospital's resources. Patients triaged green should be transported to a facility farthest from the area of the MCI to lessen the burden on closer hospitals.[10]

14. When should burn patients be transported to a burn center?

The American Burn Association recommends the following criteria to determine need for burn center care[3]:
- Partial-thickness burns >10% total body surface area (BSA)
- Face, hands, feet, genitalia, perineum, or major joint burns
- Third-degree, electrical, chemical, or inhalational burns
- Burns in patients with preexisting complicating medical disorders
- Patients with concomitant trauma in which the burn is the major injury

15. What are the guidelines for transport of patients with medical emergencies?

Patients with medical emergencies, including those in cardiac arrest, should be taken to the closest hospital, unless they have time-sensitive conditions best treated at specialty centers. Nonemergent medical patients may be taken to the hospital of their choosing as long as the EMS agency is capable of honoring their request.

16. When should a patient be taken to a hospital with a hyperbaric oxygen chamber?

Hyperbaric oxygen chambers are the required therapy for victims of diving accidents concerning for decompression illness or embolism as well as patients with severe carbon monoxide poisoning presenting with seizures, dysrhythmias, or altered mental status.

17. What should I do if a hospital is on diversion status?

Diversion rules vary widely and are made at a local level. EMS should attempt to honor when a hospital is on diversion status unless one of the following criteria is present:

- Unable to intubate or ventilate
- Recent discharge (<1 week) with related condition
- Specialty designation centers
- Patient demanding transport to that hospital
- MCIs
- Provider judgment

EMS providers should be aware that diversion has not been shown to improve patient outcome or alleviate ED overcrowding.[11]

KEY POINTS

- Determining where to transport a patient is a critical element of prehospital care.
- Some patients present with disease processes requiring transport to specialty centers.
- EMS providers should transport to the closest facility capable of providing definitive care for the patient.

REFERENCES

1. Steg G, James SK, Atar D, et al. ESC guidelines for the management of acute myocardial infarction in patients presenting with ST-segment elevation: the Task Force on the Management of ST-segment Elevation Acute Myocardial Infarction of the European Society of Cardiology (ESC). *Eur Heart J.* 2012;33(20):2569-2619.
2. Xu Y, Parikh NS, Jiao B, Willey JZ, Boehme AK, Elkind M. Decision analysis model for prehospital triage of patients with acute stroke. *Stroke.* 2019;50(4):970-977.
3. American Burn Association. Guidelines for the operation of burn centers. In: *Resources for Optimal Care of the Injured Patient.* 2007:79-86.
4. Stroke Certification. https://www.jointcommission.org/assets/1/6/TJC-Stroke-brochure-vfinal-low-rez1.PDF.
5. Trauma Center Levels Explained. Designation vs. verification. https://www.amtrauma.org/page/traumalevels?
6. Sasser SM, Hunt RC, Faul M, et al. Guidelines for field triage of injured patients: Recommendations of the National Expert Panel on field triage, 2011. *CDC Recommendations and Reports.* 2012;61:1-20.
7. Wesson DE, Coselli JS. Pediatric trauma centers: coming of age. *Tex Heart Instr J.* 2012;39:871-873.
8. American Heart Association, American Stroke Association. Stroke screenings and severity tools for large vessel occlusions. https://www.stroke.org/-/media/stroke-files/ischemic-stroke-professional-materials/stroke-screening-and-severity-tools-for-lvo-ucm_492585.pdf.
9. Butler DP, Anwar I, Willett K. Is it the H or the EMS in HEMS that has an impact on trauma patient mortality? A systematic review of the evidence. *Emerg Med J.* 2010;27(9):692-701.
10. Lerner EB, Schwartz RB, Coule PL, et al. Mass casualty triage: an evaluation of the data and development of a proposed national guideline. *Disaster Med Public Health Preparedness.* 2008;2:525-534.
11. Burke LG, Joyce N, Baker WE, et al. The effect of an ambulance diversion ban on emergency department length of stay and ambulance turnaround time. *Ann Emerg Med.* 2013;61(3):303-311.

CHAPTER 3

EMERGENCY VEHICLE OPERATION, EMS SYSTEM DESIGN, AND PREHOSPITAL COMMUNICATIONS

Krystal Baciak

QUESTIONS AND ANSWERS

1. What types of vehicles are used by emergency medical services (EMS) systems?

   There are multiple types of vehicles employed in emergency services response, with the most common being an ambulance. Other vehicle types like helicopters, airplanes, four-wheel all-terrain vehicles, snowmobiles, and boats or nontransport vehicles like bicycles and fire engines may also be utilized. Vehicle choice is dependent on multiple factors including, but not exclusive of, the geography of the area, the type of event, available staffing, and budget.

2. Why do different services have different sized ambulances?

   As a general rule, there are three different types of ambulance designs for ground transport. Type 1 is built on a truck chassis and has separate cab and patient compartments. This allows for refurbishing of the patient compartment on a new cab rather than replacement of the entire ambulance. They tend to be heavier and less fuel efficient but last longer. Type 2 ambulances are built on a van chassis and tend to be smaller than type 1 ambulances. They are more fuel-efficient and can more easily navigate smaller areas but have a shorter lifespan than type 1. Type 3 ambulances are also built on a van chassis but have a separate cab and patient compartment.

3. Why do some ambulances use lights and sirens during vehicle operations and some do not?

   The use of lights and sirens after initial dispatch and during patient transport depends on the medical guidelines and standard operating procedures of each company, department, or municipality. Studies have shown that the use of lights and sirens saves approximately 3 minutes; however, it is associated with a higher number of fatal ambulance accidents. Given the minimal time savings, lack of clinical benefit, risk of fatal accidents, and liability, more systems are moving toward significantly decreasing the use of lights and sirens during response and transport.

4. What are the different types of EMS systems worldwide?

   There are two predominant EMS "models" used around the world: the Anglo-American system and the Franco-German system. The paradigm in the Anglo-American model is to bring the patient to the physician. Thus, the system is designed with prehospital providers who are dispatched, provide specific treatments according to their protocols, and then transport the patient to the hospital. The paradigm in the Franco-German model is to bring the physician to the patient. This system provides for a much more robust prehospital physician presence in addition to the other prehospital care providers. It also allows more on-scene care and in certain instances can treat and release patients more easily due to the prehospital physician presence.

5. What are the main EMS system designs within the United States?

   There are multiple different EMS system designs including fire department–based EMS systems, municipal EMS systems, and private EMS providers.

6. What are differences in the types of EMS systems in the United States?

   Many urban areas with career fire departments incorporate EMS services into their departments. Because of National Fire Protection Association (NFPA) 1710 standards, fire departments are required to respond to structure fires within 6 minutes 90% of the time. This requirement makes for an easy transition to providing timely EMS services. Additionally, they typically have sufficient personnel as well as the building infrastructure in all the communities in their response area to house an ambulance and additional crew members. However, the cost of ambulances, training, and medical supplies can be high, as they are not typically used for fire suppression activities. Furthermore, fire-based systems typically do not use system status management to optimize the availability of ambulances to call volume, making these systems slightly less efficient than other types of systems.

   Municipal EMS services are most common in suburban and urban areas and have previously been referred to as a third service model. This setup allows the service to focus on one mission, which is the provision of prehospital care without competing interests. The service can hire employees and managers who are uniquely interested only in the provision of medical care. However, the greatest disadvantage is the potential cost of running a separate city service rather than integrating it into the fire service.

Private EMS has many variations that include private ambulances companies, hospital-based ambulance services, volunteer ambulances services, and nontransport rescue squads. There are many ways to integrate private EMS providers into the EMS system of a community, including a public utility model. This model designates a single ambulance company to provide EMS services to a community while the governmental entity does the billing and may own the capital equipment.

7. Why might a fire truck respond to a medical call?

In a tiered system, different apparatus or agencies may be dispatched to the same call with the goal of providing time-critical medical care prior to ambulance arrival. This usually involves sending a fire apparatus or a law enforcement officer in addition to the patient transport vehicle. The premise of this type of dispatch is that the ambulances are usually one of the busiest apparatus in the system and the patient may require care prior to ambulance arrival; fire apparatus or law enforcement may arrive sooner as they often have more units available at any given time. Many regions require a minimum level of certification to be an Emergency Medical Responder (EMR) for these first responders, and some areas require Emergency Medical Technician (EMT) certification. By having fire or law enforcement units arrive first, time-sensitive, lifesaving interventions can be initiated. The advantages of a tiered system are best exemplified for cardiac arrest care. The best outcomes from cardiac arrest are when the patient receives early cardiopulmonary resuscitation and defibrillation, which can be provided by the closest trained first responder. In these situations, sending the closest first responder in addition to the ambulance improves patient care. The disadvantage of a tiered system is using crews and apparatus for lower-acuity calls where they add little value but can add considerable expense to the operating budget.

8. What are the different national certification levels of EMS provider and what are the educational hours required for each certification?

While each state may offer different licensure levels, there are currently four nationally recognized certification levels for EMS providers: EMR, which requires at least 40 hours of instruction; EMT-Basic, which requires approximately 144 hours; Advanced EMT (AEMT), which requires roughly 400 hours; and Paramedic (EMT-Paramedic), which requires a minimum of 1000–1200 hours. There is a difference between licensure and certification. While certification shows that you have met an entry-level competency standard, state licensure gives you the right to work in a particular capacity. For example, nationally certified EMS providers who are not state licensed cannot practice.

9. What types of crew configurations are used by EMS systems?

The appropriate complement of the EMS crew has been debated since the very beginning of modern-day EMS. Numerous models exist, differing in both the number of practitioners that compose a crew and the levels of training each possesses. Some areas utilize all advanced life support (ALS) ambulances (medic-medic) in a single-tier system, while others use separate response ALS units (with partial or all-ALS crews, which may or may not use transport-capable vehicles) and basic life support (BLS) ambulances, dispatched together and converging on the scene. Other areas use BLS ambulances (EMT-EMT or EMR-EMT) and are sent without ALS units on cases considered less serious or non-life-threatening. The only standard that appears universal is that a minimum of two crew members is necessary to staff the unit that transports a patient to definitive care.

10. Is an all-ALS system better than a BLS system?

Historically, ALS units were the only units who could provide defibrillation and life-saving medications; however, as the scope of practice of BLS providers has increased, the need for an ALS-only service has decreased. Despite this trend, one of the advantages of an ALS system is the ability to provide any level of service that is required by the call with one apparatus. The cost of upgrading a BLS ambulance to an ALS ambulance in terms of supplies is minimal if that system already has ALS providers. However, the cost of training and quality control can be significantly more in an ALS system. Additionally, the more ALS providers a system has, the more challenging skill retention becomes for high risk, low frequency skills such as endotracheal intubation. While there are EMS calls that do not require an ALS provider, at this time there is insufficient literature to suggest which system is the best for providing care to a specific community.

11. What are the different components of EMS communications infrastructure?

The major components currently in use in EMS communications are land mobile radio systems, and telephone systems. The land mobile radio systems (LMRSs) consist of the traditional very-high-frequency (VHF) and ultra-high-frequency (UFH) radio systems as well as the newer 700 MHz and 800 MHz public safety truncated systems. There are many new communication systems currently under development, including the multiband radio and software-defined radio, as well as FirstNet.

12. What are the differences in the types of LMRS?

The different LMRSs encompass the majority of EMS communication applications, including dispatch-to-vehicle, vehicle-to-vehicle, vehicle-to-hospital, and hospital-to-hospital communications. VHF and UHF radio frequencies have been in use since the 1970s. VHF communications are best suited for long-range transmission and are used commonly in suburban, rural, and frontier environments for communication. VHF is frequently used for dispatch and, occasionally, ambulance-to-hospital communications. UHF radio frequencies encompass the 10 "MED" channels. These are much shorter range, but better penetrate buildings. The "MED" channels are predominantly used for ambulance-to-hospital communications, including voice transmission and telemetry data such as electrocardiograms. The Federal Communications Commission (FCC) has redesignated the 700 MHz and 800 MHz frequencies for public safety use to reduce interference from wireless communications. In truncated systems, the radio transmission automatically searches for the available frequency so the user does not need to choose a channel. However, the 800 MHz frequencies have a limited range and require many more antennas than are required for a VHF or UHF system.

13. How are telephone systems being used in EMS communications?

EMS has historically used telephones from patient homes and other sites to convey information to the hospital or their medical direction. With the introduction of mobile phones, this mode of communication is becoming commonplace. The advantages of cell phone use include increased patient privacy, ability to send pictures of crash scenes, ability to use in places where the radio has dead zones, and ease of use. However, in a disaster situation, wireless networks can become overloaded or unreliable. While cell phones are a vital component to EMS communications, due to these limitations, they should not be the sole method of communication available to EMS providers.

KEY POINTS

- Regional EMS systems utilize different types of vehicles, provider levels, and system designs to best fit the needs of their communities.
- There are many different models of EMS systems throughout the world; no one system is the "right system" for all communities.
- There are four nationally recognized levels of EMS providers, and each EMS system utilizes the deployment of these levels as it best fits their community.
- There are two main systems for EMS communications, land mobile radio and telephone communications. Having both systems creates the optimal redundancy to ensure appropriate communication capabilities.

BIBLIOGRAPHY

1. Gunderson M. Principles of EMS system design. In: Cone D, ed. *Emergency Medical Services Clinical Practices and Systems Oversight*, Vol 2. Singapore: John Wiley & Sons; 2015:3-16.
2. Ho J, Casey B. Time saved with use of emergency warning lights and sirens during response to requests for emergency medical aid in an urban environment. *Ann Emerg Med.* 1998;32(5):585.
3. Kahn C, Pirralo R, Kuhn E. Characteristics of fatal ambulance crashes in the United States: an 11-year retrospective analysis. *Prehosp Emerg Care.* 2001;5(3):216.
4. in press Lights And Sirens Use by Emergency Medical Services (EMS): Above All Do No Harm. https://www.ems.gov/pdf/Lights_and_Sirens_Use_by_EMS_May_2017.pdf.
5. McGinnis K, Communications. Cone D, ed. *Emergency Medical Services Clinical Practices and Systems Oversight*, Vol 2. Singapore: John Wiley & Sons; 2015:113-122.
6. Murray B, Kue R. The use of emergency lights and sirens by ambulances and their effect on patient outcomes and public safety: a comprehensive review of the literature. *Prehosp Disaster Med.* 2017;32(2):209.
7. National Emergency Medical Services Education Standards. https://www.ems.gov/pdf/National-EMS-Education-Standards-FINAL-Jan-2009.pdf.

CHAPTER 4

MEDIA AND PUBLIC RELATIONS

Eleanor Dunham

QUESTIONS AND ANSWERS

1. What is the role of a public information officer (PIO)?

   PIOs are the relay between the organization/department and the public/media. They serve as the spokespersons providing information as necessary to the media.[1] Having a designated spokesperson for your department who works with the marketing/public relations team before and when addressing the media will ensure that there is only one message being communicated.

2. What types of interactions may a prehospital provider have with the media?

   A prehospital provider can have different interactions with the media as there are different formats that can be used to deliver information to the public. There can be press releases, interviews either live or prerecorded, letters to the editor/op-eds, audio news releases, press conferences, television, radio, website media, and social media such as Facebook, Twitter, and YouTube.[2]

3. Should I wait for the media to call me for information on a story?

   Whether the focus is on a community outreach project, a high-profile patient, or a poor patient outcome, an EMS agency should be proactive about reaching out to the media. The only way to ensure that your agency's message is clearly and accurately shared with the community is by providing the media with that information.[3] It is easy for the media to focus on "bad news" because it has easier access to that information. For example, the media is more likely to write about citations from the Department of Health because that information is on public record. However, so many great events take place that the community never hears about. Make note of the wins—handling a response to a traumatic accident or a live-saving story that may stand out to you—anything that would be seen as "good news."[3]

4. How does the Health Insurance Portability and Accountability Act (HIPAA) apply to media reports?

   HIPAA does apply in that health care providers cannot invite or allow media personnel, including film crews, into treatment or other areas of their facilities where patients' public health information (PHI) will be accessible in any form or without prior written authorization from each individual whose PHI might be accessible.[4] When speaking to the media, full disclosure is not always necessary especially in the era of HIPAA.[5]

5. What are some tips for speaking with reporters?

   Depending on the medium, the way you speak with reporters may be different. Print media generally have more allowance for longer quotes, and responses to questions can be a bit on the longer side.

   Television and radio interviews target specific "soundbites." While you may be interviewed for 10 minutes, only a brief section—12–15 seconds—of the interview will be aired. Consequently, it is important to provide clear and concise answers.

   Whether providing information to the print media, television, or radio, make sure to speak in layman's terms. Avoid complicated medical terminology and keep in mind that the target audience for the media is at the sixth-grade reading level.

   Realize that anything said to a reporter is "on the record." This rule applies to time before and after the official interview takes place.

   When you are interacting with the media, be professional at all times. You are representing your organization, so physical appearance is just as important as what you say. Avoid acting in a casual manner and avoid foul language or extreme facial expressions.

   Sometimes, a reporter may make a statement, rather than ask a question, and then be silent, in hopes of provoking an emotional soundbite from a source. For example, they might say something like, "Wow that sounds really terrible," "That must have been painful," "How sad for the family," or "Sounds like your regulating bodies are really asking a lot of you." Be comfortable with the silence and do not feel obligated to respond to anything that is not a question. Instead, pause and answer with a genuine, positive, yet sincere message.

6. What should I be aware of and always doing during an interview?

   Remember that everything is on the record—even when the camera is off.

   Relax, be conversational.

   If possible, reach out to the public relations representative for your agency ahead of your interview. The representative can ensure that you have the most current information and help to polish your answers.

Typically, interviews will not be live. They will be taped and edited to air later. You can take your time and be thoughtful about how you will respond. Do not be afraid to stop mid-response and start over if you feel like you are stumbling or misspeaking. The media want their product to look good, too.

For filmed interviews, look directly at the interviewer, not the camera.

Do not be afraid to say "I don't know" or "I cannot recall" if you do not have the answer to a question. You can always work with a media liaison to get any outstanding questions answered by media's deadline.

Speak in layman's terms.

Be direct and tell the truth.

Remember that you are the subject matter expert, but you should not give your personal opinion on almost anything—unless it is something very obvious as it relates to public health.

KEY POINTS

- Be proactive with releasing information to the media.
- Remember HIPAA when dealing with the media.
- It is OK not to answer every single question asked.
- Do not give your personal opinion. Give the facts in simple layman's terms.
- Remember that you are always "ON" with the media, even when the cameras are off.

REFERENCES

1. Pons PT, Markovchick VJ. *Prehospital Emergency Care Secrets*. 1st ed. XV Medial and Public Relations. Philadelphia, PA: Hanley & Belfus; 1998, 279.
2. Section 18—media relations. July 2007. https://www.ACEP.org.
3. Schindo B. Media Relations Specialist. Penn State Health Communications. October 2019.
4. US Department of Health & Human Services. https://www.hhs.gov/hipaa/for-professionals/faq/2023/film-and-media/index.html.
5. Bass RR, Lauvner B, Lee D, Nable JV. *Emergency Medical Services: Clinical Practice and Systems Oversight—2nd Volume*. In: Cone D, Brice JH, Delbridge TR, Myers JB, eds. *Medical Oversight*. United Kingdom: John Wiley and Sons, Ltd 2009:Chapter 10, 134–150.

CHAPTER 5

MEDICAL DIRECTION AND MEDICOLEGAL ISSUES

Rohit B. Sangal

QUESTIONS AND ANSWERS

1. What is direct medical oversight?

    While state specific, emergency medical services (EMS) agencies have providers (typically physicians or advanced practice providers) on standby to provide direct medical oversight. Direct medical oversight, also referred to as online medical control, medical command, or online medical direction, refers to orders given by a physician or designee to the prehospital provider either in person or via telephone or radio. Direct medical oversight is utilized when interventions required are outside the scope of protocols as well as for high-risk refusals, termination of resuscitation, and other complex situations.

2. What is indirect medical oversight?

    Indirect medical oversight, also known as offline medical control, refers to treatment protocols, policies, procedures, and standing orders that have been preapproved by a medical director. These interventions may be utilized by a prehospital provider without the need for a direct order from a physician.

3. Do physicians receive training in direct medical oversight?

    States differ in their requirements; however, all emergency medicine residency trained physicians receive some form of EMS education. Oftentimes, these physicians-in-training do ride-alongs with EMS providers to gain a basic understanding of the circumstances faced by first responders. They may also take a base station course and provide direct medical oversight under the supervision of a trained physician.

4. Do physicians ever go to the scene?

    Some medical centers have physician teams that can be dispatched to the scene. This is more common in European EMS models. In-person physician oversight is seen most often in cases of severe trauma, cardiac arrest, or mass casualty incidents to aid in complex, unusual patient care or scene logistics. It is more common for physicians to have a role in EMS education, quality assurance, and protocol development.[1] However, on-scene presence allows for on-scene quality management, bedside teaching approving paramedic training, and occasionally facilitating patient care.

5. When should you call for direct medical oversight?

    State and local protocols differ in their guidelines. In general, direct medical oversight should be utilized for consultation on complex or critically ill patients or for approval of medication administration or procedures outside the scope of protocols. Direct medical oversight can also be a useful resource for high-risk refusals. Additionally, specialized resources, such as cardiac catheterization, stroke, and trauma evaluations, can be activated or requested after EMS consultation with the designated provider. In some systems, prehospital providers are required to contact medical oversight to request aeromedical dispatch. Be mindful that depending on your agency, the provider giving medical oversight may not be at the receiving hospital or may not have experience in EMS.

6. How should you present the information on the phone?

    When contacting direct medical oversight, identify yourself and unit number. Provide a brief description of the patient's condition, including vital signs, pertinent patient history and exam findings, and treatments administered. Clearly state your request and reasoning for this request. Document the physician name and recommendation or approved intervention. If given orders, use closed-loop communication by repeating back the orders to the physician for confirmation.

7. Who can refuse treatment?

    Any person who is above the age of consent (state specific), is an emancipated minor, and has medical decision-making capacity can refuse treatment or transport. An emancipated minor is a minor who is married, has a child, is a member of the military, or is living independently of parental financial support. Refusal protocols vary by agency, but often, indirect medical oversight includes protocols for patient refusals. Certain situations such as hypoglycemia correction or opioid overdose reversal have data demonstrating that refusal can be safe.[2,3] Fundamentally, refusal forms often contain checklists that if the patient does not meet criteria, then direct medical oversight is required, or by EMS provider request.

8. If a patient refuses treatment or transport, what do you do?

For high-risk refusals, consider additional resources. You may enlist the help of family or friends, the patient's personal physician, your supervisor, and direct medical oversight. Some studies have shown that nearly half the time, speaking with direct medical oversight can result in a patient agreeing to come to the hospital.[4,5]

9. How do you determine if a patient has capacity to make medical decisions?

To refuse treatment or transport, a patient must demonstrate medical decision-making capacity. Capacity is situation specific and is determined by a patient's ability to understand the acute condition, the benefits of the recommended treatment or transport, and the risks of refusal of these recommendations.[6] Factors that can affect a patient's capacity include intoxication, delirium or dementia, intellectual disability, and head injury or other medical condition. This is different from *competence*, which is a legal definition determined by a judge.

10. What can be done to reduce my chance of being involved in litigation?

Avoiding the potential for a lawsuit involves careful attention to detail and adherence to good patient care and treatment guidelines, but that alone cannot guarantee protection. A major step you can take to avoid a lawsuit is being compassionate and professional and communicating effectively with the patient and family, especially in highly emotionally charged situations like cardiac arrest and trauma. In addition, proper documentation can serve you well if litigation moves forward, including showing effort to obtain history, perform a physical exam, and follow indirect medical oversight.[7]

11. What is being determined in civil litigation?

Attorneys will try to establish that medical negligence was committed or that the provider deviated beyond the accepted standard of care. The merits of a civil lawsuit are based on a legal duty to care for a patient, a breach of that duty, and harm caused by that breach of duty. Unlike a criminal proceeding, the burden of proof is not beyond a reasonable doubt.

12. When does my legal duty begin?

Generally speaking, legal duty to the patient begins when the patient accepts healthcare services from a provider (i.e., you).

13. What is "standard of care?"

Standard of care is based on what a reasonable healthcare provider would do if placed in similar circumstances. It is often based on the practice patterns in the region. Therefore, the standard of care in two states may be different. This underscores the importance of documentation to show what care you provided.

14. What is informed consent?

Informed consent refers to the patient's ability and right to make decisions. For the patient to make an informed decision, they must be counseled on the suspected medical condition, the proposed treatment, treatment alternatives, and the risks and benefits associated with treatment versus no treatment.

15. What if the patient is unresponsive or otherwise unable to signal consent?

Implied consent is an assumption that the patient, if not suffering from a medical condition or disability preventing consent, would normally consent to treatment if able to communicate.[8] If EMS is unable to obtain consent, due to patient unresponsiveness, impairment, or other cause for lack of capacity, implied consent can be considered.

16. What are the different forms and abbreviations that you may encounter for patient preferences or end-of-life care?

While recommended for all patients, EMS may encounter some patients with an advanced directive. An advanced directive is a legal document that gives general guidance about a patient's treatment wishes when the patient is unable to express those wishes. A patient may also designate a surrogate as a healthcare power of attorney in situations when the patient cannot advocate for themselves.

Provider orders for life sustaining treatment (POLST) or medical orders for scope of treatment (MOST) are just two broad abbreviations (vary by state) of forms you may encounter outlining what patient preferences are during a medical emergency.[9] EMS providers will find patients who have do not resuscitate (DNR) or do not intubate (DNI) preferences. DNRs refer to not performing cardiopulmonary resuscitation (CPR), while DNI specifically refers to not placing an advanced airway. Patients can request one or both of these options at any given time. Prehospital providers should make a good faith effort to inspect a document if told of its existence before withholding care. POLST forms represent the most current description of the patient's wishes and should be followed. If there is contradiction or disagreement between a power of attorney, next of kin, and advanced directive, then direct medical oversight can help assist with navigation of the situation. If a signed advanced directive is not available, providers should operate under the assumption that the patient would want all life-saving measures performed.

17. What is the responsibility of EMS to maintain patient privacy?

EMS providers should take reasonable steps to protect patient physical privacy such as moving patients from public to private areas or creating space from bystanders. Additionally, EMS providers have an obligation to maintain the privacy of patient information. The Health Insurance Portability and Accountability Act (HIPAA) established the protection of protected health information (PHI), which is patient information that is individually identifiable. A specific exception within HIPAA allows EMS to disclose PHI for the purposes of treatment such as communicating with healthcare facilities.[6]

18. What is EMTALA and how does it affect me?

The Emergency Medical Treatment and Active Labor Act (EMTALA), briefly, requires medical screening of all patients and stabilization of any emergent medical condition prior to transfer to the most appropriate facility. This act was created to prevent the diversion of uninsured or underinsured patients away from a hospital.[10]

For hospital-owned EMS crews, the ambulance is an extension of the emergency department, and patients should be transported to that hospital unless another more appropriate facility is justified, such as a trauma, stroke, or ST-elevation myocardial infarction (STEMI) center.[11]

19. How is my practice affected by Good Samaritan laws?

Good Samaritan laws have been enacted to limit liability to individuals who volunteer to help others in an emergency situation. Such laws are state specific but generally apply to anyone who provides aid and does not have a duty to treat the patient.[12] Therefore, if you are off duty and provide aid within your training and experience, you may be protected under such laws. The exception is that Good Samaritan laws protect against ordinary negligence which is based on how a reasonable person would behave in a similar situation. Gross negligence, or simply stated, reckless care, is not protected.

KEY POINTS

- Direct medical oversight refers to orders given by a provider to a prehospital team and is utilized when patient care dictates, such as high-risk refusals and termination of resuscitation.
- When calling, your concern or question should be clearly stated, along with pertinent information related to the patient.
- Patients are allowed to refuse transport if they demonstrate decision-making capacity.
- As the population ages, more patients have advanced directives and orders for life-sustaining treatment, so prehospital providers should understand their state regulations pertaining to such documents.

REFERENCES

1. Benitez FL, Pepe PE. Role of the physician in prehospital management of trauma: North American perspective. *Curr Opin Crit Care*. 2002;8:551-558.
2. Socransky SJ, Pirrallo RG, Rubin JM. Out-of-hospital treatment of hypoglycemia: refusal of transport and patient outcome. *Acad Emerg Med*. 1998;5:1080-1085.
3. Wampler DA, Molina DK, McManus J, Laws P, Manifold CA. No deaths associated with patient refusal of transport after naloxone-reversed opioid overdose. *Prehosp Emerg Care*. 2011;15:320-324.
4. Alicandro J, Hollander JE, Henry MC, Sciammarella J, Stapleton E, Gentile D. Impact of interventions for patients refusing emergency medical services transport. *Acad Emerg Med*. 1995;2:480-485.
5. Burstein JL, Hollander JE, Delagi R, Gold M, Henry MC, Alicandro JM. Refusal of out-of-hospital medical care: effect of medical-control physician assertiveness on transport rate. *Acad Emerg Med*. 1998;5:4-8.
6. Brenner JM, Aswegan AL, Vearrier LE, Basford JB, Iserson KV. The ethics of real-time EMS Direction: suggested curricular content. *Prehosp Disaster Med*. 2018;33:201-212.
7. Selden BS, Schnitzer PG, Nolan FX. Medicolegal documentation of prehospital triage. *Ann Emerg Med*. 1990;19:547-551.
8. Easton RB, Graber MA, Monnahan J, Hughes J. Defining the scope of implied consent in the emergency department. *Am J Bioethics*. 2007;7:35-38.
9. POLST N. POLST & advance directives. Available from: https://polst.org/polst-and-advance-directives/. [Accessed April, 2020]
10. Bitterman RA. Emergency Medical Treatment and Active Labor Act and medicolegal issues. In: Walls RM, Hockberger RS, Gausche-Hill M, eds. *Rosen's Emergency Medicine: Concepts and Clinical Practice*. Philadelphia, PA: Elsevier; 2018:119-135.
11. Testa PA, Gang M, Triage. EMTALA, consultations, and prehospital medical control. *Emerg Med Clin N Am*. 2009;27:627-640. viii-ix.
12. Stewart PH, Agin WS, Douglas SP. What does the law say to Good Samaritans?: a review of Good Samaritan statutes in 50 states and on US airlines. *Chest*. 2013;143:1774-1783.

CHAPTER 6

PUBLIC HEALTH AND EMS

Melissa D. Kohn

QUESTIONS AND ANSWERS

1. What is public health?

   Public health can be a very wide-ranging field that can include injury prevention, disease surveillance, and management of underserved populations. The American Public Health Association is a group based in Washington, DC, that advocates for and promotes the topic of public health. The group currently has 34 topics listed on their website, of which they are currently focused. The subjects affecting public health are constantly evolving based on the needs of the population. Some topics that are constant, such as public health accreditation and standards, and other topics are directly related to current affairs. At the time of this publication, relevant issues listed include pandemic infectious disease, immigrant health, gun violence, and prescription drug overdose. Emergency medical services (EMS) and emergency care are areas that are typically a constant in the whole of public health.

2. How is public health related to EMS?

   Because emergency services are the initial access to care in certain situations, EMS is often the face of public health on a day-to-day basis. The state and city health departments can also serve as the regulatory organization for EMS providers and their respective agencies. States will typically have minimum standards designated by the state EMS offices for the systems within their area. The state EMS offices are then responsible to address issues or complaints regarding the established standards.

3. Describe the types of prevention that public health workers manage.

   The goal of primary prevention is to intervene on a public health issue before it has a chance to develop. Examples of primary prevention are vaccinations, working to address risky behaviors such as smoking, or prohibiting substances known to cause harm. Secondary prevention is the concept of screening during the early phases of a disease outbreak, ideally before any signs or symptoms are noted. Treatments or behavior modifications are initiated in order to prevent the disease from progressing to more morbid stages. Public health assessments under secondary prevention would include blood pressure measurements for hypertension, mammograms for breast cancer, or blood testing for prostate cancer. Tertiary prevention moves into the treatment phase, attempting to limit further progression once the disease is already known to be present. Examples of tertiary prevention are rehabilitation from damage that the illness has already caused and screening for the potential future problems from the known disease, such as cardiac or stroke rehabilitation programs.

4. What disease outbreaks has EMS played a role in?

   Diseases are typically classified as infectious or noninfectious. Infectious diseases include influenza, measles, malaria, Zika, Ebola, and COVID-19. Noninfectious diseases are characteristically long-term disease processes such as asthma, heart disease, or diabetes. Trauma is a less commonly thought of as a disease but is still a public health issue where EMS is likely to be involved. Some diseases processes such as hepatitis can cross over both categories as it has an acute infectious phase as well as long-term effects.

5. How does public health cross over into emergency preparedness and response?

   Since EMS providers are often the first contact with the public, they are in a prime position to act as surveillance for diseases that would potentially have effects on the general population. They may also participate in epidemiological responses, which evaluate the distribution and patterns of diseases in the public. In the 2015 Ebola outbreak, EMS was involved in the planning, monitoring, and treatment of potentially exposed patients. Along with public health officials and local hospitals, they developed plans to triage and transport high-risk patients to the appropriate facilities while minimizing exposure risks to the community. In addition, EMS is part of mitigation, preparation, response, and recovery of natural and manmade disasters. EMS members are commonly part of specialized groups such as Search and Rescue Units, Disaster Medical Assistance Teams, or State Medical Assistance Teams.

6. Explain a public health assessment and how EMS would be involved.

   An assessment is done as part of planning and preparedness. Public health officials will contact public health agencies in the area, including EMS. The assessment will evaluate the regional public health risks and the assets available to intervene. EMS can contribute by gathering information about the population and the resources. Reassessments should occur on a regular basis in order to update plans, adding or removing resources.

7. During a disaster, how might EMS be integrated with the public health program?

Ideally, EMS agencies and the public health departments have an established relationship and participate in regular tabletop exercises in preparation for mass casualty incidents. Through these relationships, EMS agencies and public health departments pool resources including manpower, equipment, funding, and data. They may also recruit additional resources from local hospitals, state medical assistance teams, disaster medical assistance teams, nongovernmental organizations, and other volunteer agencies.

8. What are other examples of partnerships between public health and EMS?

If an incident or a disaster causes mass fatalities, EMS will likely be called upon as the first responders and assist in coordinating the initial operational period. EMS will already have an established relationship with the medical examiner/coroner given the need for interactions on a routine basis. EMS and the health department will then work together to establish the next steps and decide what other groups will need to be involved for the following operational periods. As previously noted, during a disaster, the public health department can provide additional supplies to EMS if needed. For example, during an influenza pandemic, EMS could be requested to assist with mass vaccination clinics. In situations like the Ebola epidemic, EMS may be involved in the coordination of transportation of potentially infectious patients to specially designated treatment facilities.

9. How are EMS data being used to help public health programs?

In the early 2000s, the National Highway Traffic Safety Administration began developing a plan to collect data from EMS agencies. Over the last two decades, the National Emergency Medical Services Information System (NEMSIS) was developed and now receives data input from 49 states and US territories. More than 50 studies have been published using data gathered by this system. States EMS officials can pull data to assess performance and success rates of interventions and perform cost-benefit analysis on established standards. Current public health projects involve the topics of opioid overdoses and trauma care for traffic crash injuries.

10. Describe the developing field of community paramedicine.

Community paramedicine is a relatively new concept. There is a wide variety in the roles of community paramedics. Areas of focus for these programs can include reduction of medically unnecessary transports to emergency department through alternative destination protocols; access to public assistance programs like home medication delivery; and disease prevention programs like fall risk assessments and vaccination programs. These programs are intended to improve the overall health and wellness of a community, as well as improve access to care and reduce the burden on healthcare system resources.

11. What are some of the challenges to the integration of EMS and public health?

There are several challenges to the integration of EMS, specifically the need for additional education of providers, development of new policies and procedures, financial support for implementation of new programs, and support from regional, state, and federal legislative bodies. In addition, as with any change, barriers may exist in the development of new roles and relationships between EMS and public health agencies.

12. Where is the future of public health and EMS headed?

Most states have a Department of Health that is responsible for establishing the regulations for EMS in their state. Because of this assignment, there is a guaranteed long-term relationship for the future. EMS will also continue to be intertwined with public health since they are the frontline providers. Since EMS is often the primary point of contact with the public, they can often recognize new disease patterns in the community.

KEY POINTS

- The EMS system plays a significant role in the prevention, detection and intervention in public health emergencies.
- Prehospital providers can help to identify disease patterns in their region.
- During a disaster, EMS is often the frontline resource for the public health system.
- Integration of EMS and public health continues to develop through emergency preparedness and community paramedicine programs.

BIBLIOGRAPHY

Addressing public health issues with EMS Data. Office of EMS: Addressing Public Health Issues with EMS Data. National Highway Traffic Safety Administration. https://www.ems.gov/projects/addressing-public-health-issues-ems-data.html.

American Public Health Association. Topics & issues. https://www.apha.org/topics-and-issues.

Barishansky R. The intersection of public health and EMS. *EMS World.* July 2012.

Beitsch LM, Brooks RG, Glasser JH, Coble YD. The medicine and public health initiative. *Am J Prev Med.* 2005;29(2):149-153.

Caffrey S. What EMS leaders need to know about public health. *EMS1*, Praetorian Digital. December 7, 2016. https://www.ems1.com/ems-management/articles/what-ems-leaders-need-to-know-about-public-health-IOKjSWsmoXXyA4rv/.

Cone DC, Brice JH, Delbridge TR, Myers JB. *Emergency Medical Services: Clinical Practice and Systems Oversight.* Hoboken, NJ: John Wiley & Sons Inc; 2015. 00

History of NEMSIS. NEMSIS. https://nemsis.org/what-is-nemsis/history-of-nemsis/.

National Association of County and City Health Officials. Public health infrastructure and systems. https://www.naccho.org/programs/public-health-infrastructure.

Reiser SJ. Topics for our times: the medicine/public health initiative. *Am J Public Health.* 1997;87(7):1098-1099.

United States Congress. Prevention. Picture of America: Our Health and Environment. April 6, 2017. https://www.cdc.gov/pictureofamerica/pdfs/picture_of_america_prevention.pdf.

CHAPTER 7

PREHOSPITAL EMERGENCY CARE SECRETS—QUALITY IMPROVEMENT AND RESEARCH

Remle Crowe and Jeffrey L. Jarvis

QUESTIONS AND ANSWERS

1. What is the difference between *quality assurance* and *quality improvement*?

   Sometimes used synonymously, the terms *quality assurance* (QA) and *quality improvement* (QI) refer to distinct processes with different goals. The goal of QA is to monitor and measure compliance against a standard. In this way, QA is a reactive process that detects errors after they have occurred. On the other hand, the goal of QI is to improve systems. QA is a proactive process that seeks to improve performance or prevent errors from occurring.

2. What is the difference between QI and research?

   While QI and research both rely heavily on measurement, the goals and requirements differ. QI aims to improve a process toward a known standard of care. Meanwhile, research seeks to answer a question, often by testing a hypothesis, and enhance knowledge. The approach to data collection also differs. QI uses rapid cycles of testing to generate learning and create sustained improvement. Research relies on larger sample sizes and longer periods of observation.

3. Is there an established QI methodology?

   Yes, there are several popular QI methodologies. The Institute for Healthcare Improvement uses the Model for Improvement as a framework for projects. This model has been used in many countries and in various healthcare settings, including EMS, to successfully improve quality of care and patient safety. The model consists of three fundamental questions and rapid plan-do-study-act cycles.

   The three fundamental questions are as follows:

   1. **What are we trying to accomplish?**

      The aim of an improvement project is a specific, measurable, time-specific statement that describes the process to be improved and what improvement is expected in a specified time frame. The aim should be aligned with the overall vision of the organization and should be meaningful. It should be clearly worded in an unambiguous manner.

   2. **How will we know that a change is an improvement?**

      Defining a "family of measures" to determine if a change has led to an improvement is critical to the success of any improvement project. There are three types of measures in a family of measures: process (reflect the things being done and how systems are operating), outcome (demonstrate the end result of doing things), and balancing (measuring whether unintended consequences have been introduced elsewhere in the system). Each measure must have a clear definition of both the numerator and denominator to allow for consistent comparisons across time.

   3. **What change can we make that will result in improvement?**

      Ideas for change, also called change theories, may be generated from those who work in the system or from other successful improvement projects. Brainstorming can be structured using tools like Driver Diagrams or Cause-and-Effect Diagrams. Additionally, baseline data grouped into a Pareto chart can provide meaningful insight into where to start testing change ideas.

      With the answers to these three questions in hand, small, rapid *tests of change* are undertaken. Tests of change involve using multiple sequential plan-do-study-act (PDSA) cycles. PDSA cycles should start on a small scale (think one crew at one station on one shift for one day) rather than implementing a change idea across the entire system. Starting small prevents wasting time and resources on an intervention that does not result in meaningful change. At the end of each PDSA cycle, data are analyzed, and project leaders decide whether to adopt the intervention outright, adapt the intervention by making adjustments and test again, or abandon the intervention and move on to testing the next change idea.

4. How should data for improvement be analyzed and displayed?

   Summary measures like averages and percentages hide important information regarding variation in a process. Plotting data over time provides much more information.

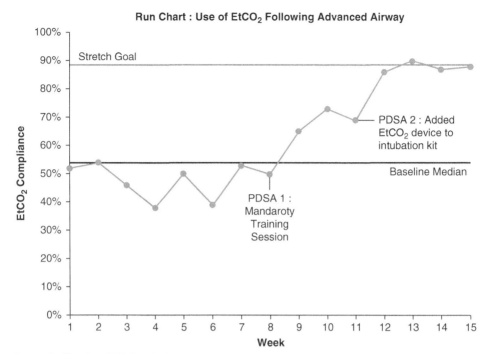

Fig. 7.1. Run Chart: Use of $EtCO_2$ Following Advanced Airway.

A *run chart* is a simple graph of data over time. Time is on the X axis and the measure you are trying to improve is on the Y axis. The median is drawn as a horizontal line. Annotations are made as PDSA cycles are undertaken to help assess their impact on the measure. Ideally, you should have 10–15 data points before constructing a run chart (see Fig. 7.1).

5. What are the types of variation?
   All processes vary over time. Some variations are expected, while others are not.
   Common cause variation is the inherent change in a system over time and arises due to random chance. It is important to not overreact to this type of random movement on your run chart. Ups and downs of this type are due to chance and do not reflect improvement or lack of improvement.
   Special cause variation, on the other hand, is not part of the system and arises because of specific circumstances. This type of variation can signal when a change has resulted in a true improvement.

6. How can special cause variation be identified?
   A *control chart* takes the analysis of data over time one step further and helps distinguish between common cause variation and special cause variation. In addition to a central line for the average, control charts have upper and lower control limits. These limits are determined from historical data and the variation present in the data. There are many types of control charts. Selecting the appropriate control chart will depend on the type of data and sampling strategy.
   In addition to helping teams identify when a change has resulted in improvement, these charts can be used to monitor a process for sustained improvement. A control chart should be used when there are at least 15 data points (see Fig. 7.2).

7. What are the common types of research studies?
   Research studies can be divided into experimental and observational designs. In an experimental design, the researcher controls or intervenes upon the independent variable (treatment). In an observational study, the researcher does not manipulate the independent variable, but rather compares groups with different levels of the independent variable.
   Experimental Study Designs
   Controlled trials—Participants are assigned to an experimental group or a control group. The experimental group receives the study intervention while the control group receives either a placebo (inert ingredient) or the

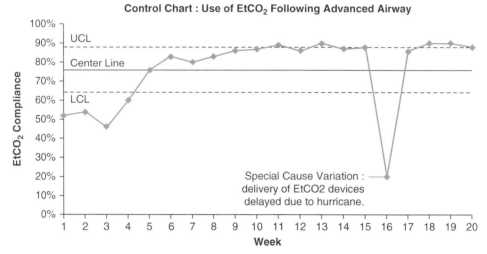

Fig. 7.2. Control Chart: Use of EtCO$_2$ Following Advanced Airway (*UCL*, Upper Control Limit; *LCL*, Lower Control Limit).

standard of care. Often, this assignment is done using randomization, in which case the design is a randomized controlled trial. Good randomization helps ensure that the two groups are similar in terms of all characteristics other than the intervention being tested.

Blinding is a process used in controlled trials to reduce bias. A participant's compliance with the trial, or their perception of benefit or harm from the intervention, may be influenced if they know they have been assigned to a particular arm of the trial. Similarly, the investigator's assessment of outcome may also be influenced if they know the participant's group assignment. If both the participant and investigator are blinded to the assignment, this bias can be reduced.

Observational Study Designs
a. *Case study and case series.* A case study is an in-depth description of a single individual, group, or event, while a case series reports on a collection of similar individuals, groups, or events.
b. *Cross-sectional study.* This type of study analyzes data from a group at a specific point in time and describes the frequency of a condition and the characteristics of a population. These studies can be used to estimate the prevalence of a condition or explore associations between a risk factor and an outcome.
c. *Cohort study.* This longitudinal study design involves a group of people who share a defining characteristic and a comparison group that does not possess that characteristic. The incidence of the outcome is then compared between groups. Cohort studies can be either prospective or retrospective.
d. *Case-control study.* At the beginning of a case-control study, subjects are identified based on outcome status. Once subjects who have the outcome are selected (cases), subjects who do not have the outcome (controls) are selected from the same source population. Case-control studies can be matched or unmatched. This type of study is well suited for investigations involving rare outcomes or outcomes with a long latency period.
e. *Systematic review.* Systematic methods are used to identify, critically appraise, and synthesize all relevant studies on a particular topic qualitatively.
f. *Meta-analysis.* A meta-analysis takes the data collected in a systematic review and, if the studies are similar enough, pools the data. Statistical techniques are used to analyze all of the pooled data as a group providing an increased sample size and greater power to detect differences than each individual study.

8. What are the typical parts of a research paper?
Different scientific disciplines use different formats, but the following are the traditional sections of a clinical research paper:
a. *Abstract.* This is a brief summary of the paper.
b. *Introduction.* This section provides background information on the topic and describes why the topic is impor-tant. This section should also briefly discuss what is already known and what gaps in knowledge remain. The introduction typically ends by stating the clearly worded research question or objective.
c. *Methods.* This section should clearly describe how the study was designed, conducted, and analyzed. Key components of a methods section include a description of the study design, participants, measures in terms of independent and dependent variables, data collection instruments or procedures, and analysis. A well-written methods section will allow other researchers to reproduce the study.
d. *Results.* This section describes the findings of the study in an orderly and logical sequence.

e. *Discussion.* The goal of this section is to interpret the results. Findings should be placed into context in comparison to previous studies. New understanding and implications based on the results of the study should also be presented. Areas where additional work is needed may also be highlighted.

f. *Limitations.* All studies have limitations in their ability to answer the research question. Limitations can be characteristics related to the study design or methodology that may influence the generalizability, application, or utility of the findings presented.

g. *Conclusions.* A research paper should end with a very brief restatement of the primary outcome and most important findings. Conclusions must be supported by the study findings and not extend beyond what was explored in the study.

9. **Where can I find interesting research?**

In the past, the only way to find the latest research was to subscribe to journals or go to a library and browse their journal stacks. Most people read journal articles online now. Fortunately, search engines and websites have been developed to help make the latest studies more accessible. Here are some of the most common and helpful resources:

- PubMed (https://www.ncbi.nlm.nih.gov/pubmed/): This is the indexed search engine of clinical and biomedical research. Consider it the Google of research papers.
- Read by QxMD (https://read.qxmd.com): This is a free app that helps you find papers of interest. You describe the topics you are interested in and you get emails alerting you to new papers.
- FOAMEd (Free Open Access Medical Education): There are many free websites, blogs, and podcasts dedicated to finding, reviewing, and discussing clinical research.
- Medical Associations: Most medical professional associations provide access to their journals as well as various blogs/pods to discuss the results of papers published in them.

KEY POINTS

- Three types of quality improvement measurements are: process, outcome, and balancing.
- Balancing measures are important to watch for unintended consequences of improvement efforts.
- "Tests of change" should be small and include well-defined measures of success. They can involve multiple "Plan-Do-Study-Act" (PDSA) cycles.
- Common cause and special cause are two types of process variation. Common cause is inherent to a system and special cause arises because of specific circumstances and can indicate that change has occurred.
- Randomization in research helps to ensure that two groups (experimental and control) are as similar as possible.

BIBLIOGRAPHY

Babbs CF, Tacker MM. Writing a scientific paper prior to the research. *Am J Emerg Med.* 1985;3:360-363.
Bastian H. 5 Tips for avoiding *P*-value potholes. PLOS Blogs. 2016.
Crowl A, Sharma A, Sorge L, Sorensen T. Accelerating quality improvement within your organization: applying the model for improvement. *J Am Pharm Assoc (2003).* 2015 Jul-Aug;55:e364-e374.
Gilbert EH, Lowenstein SR, Koziol McLain J, Barta DC, Steiner J. Chart reviews in emergency medicine research: where are the methods? *Ann Emerg Med.* 1996;27:305-308.
Kaji AH, Schriger D, Green S. Looking through the retrospectoscope: reducing bias in emergency medicine chart review studies. *Ann Emerg Med.* 2014;64:292-298.
Kelly AM. The minimum clinically significant difference in visual analogue scale pain score does not differ with severity of pain. *Emerg Med J.* 2001 May;18:205-207.
Krousel-Wood MA, Chambers RB, Muntner P. Clinicians guide to statistics for medical practice and research: part I. *Ochsner J.* 2006;6:68-83.
Institute for Healthcare Improvement. *Quality Improvement Toolkit.* Boston, MA: Institute for Healthcare Improvement. http://www.ihi.org/resources/Pages/Tools/Quality-Improvement-Essentials-Toolkit.aspx.
Lewis RJ, Angus DC. Time for clinicians to embrace their inner Bayesian?: reanalysis of results of a clinical trial of extracorporeal membrane oxygenation. *JAMA.* 2018;320:2208-2210.
Lincoln EW, Reed-Schrader E, Jarvis JL. *EMS, quality improvement programs.* StatPearls; 2019.
McAlister FA. The "number needed to treat" turns 20—and continues to be used and misused. *CMAJ.* 2008;179:549-553.
Myers JB, Slovis CM, Eckstein M, et al. Evidence-based performance measures for emergency medical services systems: a model for expanded EMS benchmarking. *Prehosp Emerg Care.* 2008 Apr-Jun;12:141-151.
Nuzzo R. Statistical errors. *Nature.* 2014;506:50-152.
Perla RJ, Provost LP, Murray SK. The run chart: a simple analytical tool for learning from variation in healthcare processes. *BMJ Qual Saf.* 2011;20(1):46-51.
Purugganan M, Hewitt J. How to Read a Scientific Article. Rice University.2004. Accessed Aug 2021.
Ranstam J. Why the *P*-value culture is bad and confidence intervals a better alternative. *Osteoarthritis Cartilage.* 2012 Aug;20:805-808.
Schechtman E, Odds ratio. relative risk, absolute risk, and the number needed to treat—which of these should we use? *Value Health.* 2002;5:431-436.
Singer AJ, Hollander JE. How to write a manuscript. *J Emerg Med.* 2009 Jan;36:89-93.
Siriwardena AN, Shaw D, Donohoe R, Black S, Stephenson J. National Ambulance Clinical Audit Steering G. Development and pilot of clinical performance indicators for English ambulance services. *Emerg Med J.* 2010 Apr;27:327-331.
Siriwardena AN, Donohoe R, Stephenson J, Phillips P. Supporting research and development in ambulance services: research for better health care in prehospital settings. *Emerg Med J.* 2010 Apr;27:324-326.

CHAPTER 8

SCENE SAFETY

Bryan Sloane and Bradley Chappell

QUESTIONS AND ANSWERS

1. What is scene safety and how does it affect emergency medical service (EMS) providers?

   Scene safety is the general principle of keeping safe from all hazards while working as an EMS provider. Scene safety is critical to all emergency responders and starts the moment they receive a call. Providers face risks, including traffic accidents, infectious disease exposures, and violence. While some events cannot be avoided, having a better understanding of your surroundings is paramount to staying safe while on scene as well as during patient transport.

   EMS providers need to know their surroundings, plan a route of egress, and understand the emotional atmosphere of their environment. Throughout every call, they must continuously reassess the scene around them and try to predict active threats. They must see the big picture and avoid the tendency to have tunnel vision while providing direct patient care. Providers are wholly responsible for their own well-being, and the principle of scene safety must be taken into account on every call, no matter the circumstances or situation.[1]

2. Is scene safety something that will affect day-to-day activities?

   Scene safety affects all EMS providers. EMS providers have higher-than-average rates of workplace-related fatalities than all other professions, and the majority of EMS providers will experience violence in the workplace. Roadway accidents are a leading cause of fatalities among EMS providers, with ambulance crashes being responsible for the majority of these fatalities. Even during the most well-controlled call, EMS providers are at risk of injury and must constantly be alert.[2]

3. What can EMS providers do to keep safe on scene?

   When first arriving to an emergency scene, responders must take a moment to review the area around them, identifying any clear threats. This may include things such as fuel spills, fires, fast moving traffic, armed people, unruly crowds, or any other situations that may provide a direct threat. They should use this time to call for backup, discuss the potential threats with their partner, plan their approach, and identify an egress route. An extra few moments before exiting their vehicle can help formulate a plan to keep them safe. If there is an immediate threat, EMS providers should not get out of their vehicle but instead call for backup and retreat to a staging area. Even when police are present, it is never safe to assume that a scene is clear. They must communicate with the local authorities and use their own judgment regarding the safety and stability of a scene.

4. How should hazardous material (HAZMAT) calls be handled?

   When encountering a HAZMAT scene, EMS providers should always park upwind and uphill while maintaining clear communication with incident command. The Emergency Response Guidebook, a reference developed by the Department of Transportation, is a resource that provides first responders with a go-to manual to help deal with HAZMAT transportation accidents during the critical first 30 minutes.

5. What are the greatest threats to prehospital personnel?

   EMS providers are most vulnerable to infectious diseases, including blood-borne pathogens like hepatitis B or infections spread by respiratory droplets such as COVID-19, influenza, or meningitis. Standard precautions are the best defense against the spread of potentially contagious diseases. Disease-specific precautions, including contact, airborne, and droplet, should also be considered based on patient history and presentation.

6. How do EMS providers approach a high-risk scene?

   Many patient encounters including mental health crisis, domestic violence, and mass gatherings have the potential to be high risk. To minimize risk to the prehospital provider, it may be prudent to turn off lights and sirens prior to arrival, allowing providers to survey the scene prior to approaching. They should approach buildings and doors from the side, not directly in front, while also scanning for signs of danger and listening for sounds of violence. Responders should always wait for police to clear a potentially violent scene, but caution must be used with routine calls as they can rapidly deteriorate. If something does not feel right, they should trust their instincts. If at any point, responders feel they are losing control of the scene, they should quickly secure and transport the patient.

7. How do EMS providers approach an active shooter situation?

   EMS providers should not approach the scene of a shooting or stabbing until cleared by law enforcement. They should stage their vehicle at a safe location away from the scene and wait for orders to approach for patient care. If law enforcement is not yet present, EMS should consider leaving the area and staging at a safe distance until the police arrive. For an active shooter situation, they should not enter the area until cleared. Law enforcement will be responding en masse and is tasked with neutralizing the threat. Some EMS providers are part of Rescue Task Forces and may enter the warm zone. However, this is high-risk and requires additional training and specialized equipment to do so.

8. What is tactical EMS?

Tactical EMS is an emerging field where EMS providers work side by side with law enforcement to provide aid to victims of violence while they are still under direct threat. The amount of involvement that a tactical EMT has is based on local policies and procedures. Tactical medical care has been well-developed by the US military during conflicts, and strong guidelines have been established.

9. What are best practices to stay safe on the roadside?

Patient care on or alongside roadways can prove extremely hazardous to first responders. As a result, first responders are struck by passing vehicles many times every year. A helmet and reflective vest are important tools to increase visibility and reduce injuries. Additionally, use of a heavy fire vehicle as a barrier may also decrease risks of injury and death.

10. How can EMS providers keep safe while transporting patients?

Whenever in a moving ambulance, it is important to use the restraint system. In ambulance crashes, occupants of patient care compartments have greater morbidity and mortality. Equipment should be secured to the greatest extent possible as it can cause severe damage when flying about a patient compartment during a crash.[3] Vehicle drivers should also never be distracted by phones, electronic devices, radios, or food.[4]

11. What are the risks and benefits of lights and sirens?

The use of lights and sirens has been shown to significantly increase the rate of ambulance crashes.[5] This risk becomes amplified during emergency transport of patients to the hospital. For many patients, the risks of lights and sirens may outweigh the benefits. However, certain medical conditions are time sensitive and life threatening and may potentially benefit from expedited transport. Providers should use caution and be judicious with the use of lights and sirens.

12. Can EMS providers be held liable for an ambulance crash?

While rare, some prehospital providers have been found personally liable for ambulance crashes, and others have faced criminal charges and jail time. It is important to always follow local policies, stay alert, and be cautious when using lights and sirens and interrupting normal traffic patterns.[4]

13. What is workplace violence and are EMS providers at risk?

Workplace violence is any act or threat of physical violence, harassment, intimidation, or other threatening disruptive behavior that occurs at the work site. Prehospital providers are at risk not only from coworkers but also from patients and bystanders. While underacknowledged in the past, multiple states are passing or considering legislation to include special protections for public service workers against workplace violence.[6]

14. How common is workplace violence in the prehospital environment?

Studies vary; however, it is estimated that between 50% and 80% of prehospital providers have experienced some form of workplace violence. Additionally, there is an average of one to two homicides of prehospital providers every year.[7]

15. What can be done to reduce the risk of workplace violence?

In potentially hostile or unsafe situations, EMS providers should maintain physical distance and request backup. At every call, they should identify an exit route and keep themselves between the patient and this egress route. With agitated patients, if verbal de-escalation techniques fail, the police may need to assist in physically restraining the patient. When physically restraining a patient, a team approach should be taken with at least one person per extremity. Patients should never be placed in the prone position due to the risk for positional asphyxia. Chemical restraints may also be indicated to ensure the safety of the patient and EMS crew during transport. Local protocols or on-line medical oversight may provide further guidance on sedation of the agitated patient.

16. What are some of the long-term effects of workplace violence on EMS personnel?

Long-term disability, increased stress, workplace dissatisfaction, increased burnout, anxiety, and poor effect on personal relationships are all by-products of workplace violence.[8]

17. What should be done if a provider does not feel comfortable transporting or not transporting a patient from the field?

When in doubt, EMS providers should call for backup. Having more providers and law enforcement on scene can help maintain safety and avoid a possibly dangerous situation. EMS providers are often instructed to not transport traumatic or medical cardiac arrest patients. However, these scenes can be particularly sensitive and family or bystanders may become aggressive or violent if they perceive no treatment is being provided to a loved one. If providers feel like they might be in danger, they should transport the patient. Even if the patient is clearly deceased, EMS should not be faulted for transporting a body if their safety is at risk.

KEY POINTS

- Situational awareness is paramount to ensuring your own safety. Throughout every call, continuously reassess the scene and try to predict active threats.
- Extra caution should be used at the scenes of roadway accidents due to associated hazards, as well as calls related to patients under the influence of drugs and alcohol or with psychiatric diseases, as the behavior of the patients, family, and bystanders is often unpredictable.
- Always wear appropriate personal protective equipment (gloves, eye protection, mask, and/or gown).
- When physically restraining a patient, a team approach should be taken with at least one person per extremity, staying off the chest and protecting the head and airway. This should typically be followed by some form of chemical restraint.
- Judicious use of lights and sirens is recommended.

REFERENCES

1. Koser BW, Lee BH. EMS, Care in a hostile environment. StatPearls. Treasure Island, FL: StatPearls Publishing; 2019. http://www.ncbi. nlm.nih.gov/books/NBK537217/.
2. Maguire BJ, Smith S. Injuries and fatalities among emergency medical technicians and paramedics in the United States. *Prehosp Disaster Med.* 2013;28(4):376-382.
3. Fournier M, Chenaitia H, Masson C, Michelet P, Behr M, Auffray J-P. Crew and patient safety in ambulances: results of a personnel survey and experimental side impact crash test. *Prehosp Disaster Med.* 2013;28(4):370-375.
4. Friese G. How to avoid, survive an ambulance crash. EMS1. https://www.ems1.com/ems-products/ambulance-safety/articles/how-to-avoid-survive-an-ambulance-collision-ZK7cK8nqbdUQkqOR/.
5. Watanabe BL, Patterson GS, Kempema JM, Magallanes O, Brown LH. Is use of warning lights and sirens associated with increased risk of ambulance crashes? A Contemporary analysis using National EMS Information System (NEMSIS) data. *Ann Emerg Med.* 2019;74(1):101-109.
6. Occupational Safety and Health Administration. Safety and health topics: workplace violence. https://www.osha.gov/SLTC/workplaceviolence/.
7. Maguire BJ, O'Meara P, O'Neill BJ, Brightwell R. Violence against emergency medical services personnel: a systematic review of the literature. *Am J Ind Med.* 2018;61(2):167-180.
8. Richards J. *Management of Workplace Violence Victims.* Geneva, Switzerland: Joint Programme on Workplace Violence in the Health Sector; 2003.

CRITICAL INCIDENT STRESS AND OCCUPATIONAL HEALTH ISSUES IN EMS

Kelsey Wilhelm and Puneet Gupta

CHAPTER 9

QUESTIONS AND ANSWERS

CRITICAL INCIDENT STRESS

1. What is a critical incident?

   A critical or incident is defined as a powerful or emotionally provoking event experienced by the EMS provider. This stressor typically overwhelms the person's normal coping mechanisms and significantly differs from the ordinary events experienced on the job. Incidents such as line-of-duty death or critical injury, death of child, severe child abuse case, mass casualty or disaster event, injury to a known victim such as family or friend, or acts of workplace violence are examples of possible critical incidents.

2. What is critical incident stress?

   Critical incident stress is a term used to describe the human emotional response to a critical or traumatic incident. Some providers will experience symptoms immediately, while others will have symptoms develop gradually. The symptoms of critical incident stress can vary significantly between providers, even if they have experienced the same traumatic incident. The reaction can be subjective, so we must ask, "Does the provider consider this significant?".

3. Why is critical incident stress an important topic for prehospital providers?

   Psychologically stressful events are an inherent part of a career in EMS. Critical incidents differ from the daily stressors experienced by providers and can be a matter of life and death. A 2016 national survey found a rate of 5.2% for deaths by suicide among EMTs, paramedics, and firefighters. This rate exceeds the rate of deaths by suicides for non-EMS professionals by 3%.[1] Maintaining the health, safety, and success of EMS providers is critical to the profession and to patient care.

4. What types of "stress" are experienced by prehospital providers?

   The job of an EMS provider is spontaneous, unpredictable, and potentially dangerous. Providers assist the sick and dying as well as the traumatic and dramatic. There is a constant struggle to cope with the stressors of the job in healthy ways. Reactions to events often stem from an individual's experiences, values, and stressors at the time. The stressors of the job can permeate the lives of providers and their families, contributing to negative habits. Intrinsically, the unpredictable nature of EMS work poses a unique challenge for work site wellness program implementation and maintenance.

5. How has managing critical incident stress changed in recent years?

   Over the past 30 years, programs built around critical incident stress management (CISM) and its signature intervention, "critical incident stress debriefing" (CISD), have become popular.[2] CISD consists of nonevaluative discussion between members of the CISM team and the EMS providers about their reactions to the incident. CISM was meant to be a comprehensive service that provides support and crisis intervention resources to EMS providers.[3]

   In the early 2000s, a review article by Bledsoe challenged the concept that CISM decreased the risk of posttraumatic stress disorder (PTSD).[4] Several studies included in Bledsoe's review article found possible worsening of symptoms in persons who received CISM services. As a result of the findings of this article, there has been a transition away from mandatory debriefings and toward a less structured approach and recognizing the need for ongoing care for some providers.

   Psychological first aid is a new paradigm that was developed to be a method for addressing the immediate, acute mental stress response following crisis. Key concepts in this model involve promoting calm, safety, connectedness, self-efficacy, and help.[5] More open team communication and the institution of wellness initiatives have bolstered the new comprehensive approach to psychological stress care.

6. What warning signs should I look for in myself or my colleagues with regard to depression or suicide risk?

   The Combat and Operational Stress Guide (US Navy and Marine Corps) is a model to identify high-risk features and warning signs in oneself and others (Fig. 9.1).[6] This model proposes a spectrum of risk based on the symptoms and actions of providers to help identify providers at high risk.

READY (Green Zone)	REACTING (Yellow Zone)	INJURED (Orange Zone)	ILL (Red Zone)
Definition - Adaptive coping and mastery - Optimal functioning - Wellness **Features** - Well trained and prepared - Fit and focused - In control - Optimally effective - Behaving ethically - Having fun	**Definition** - Mild and transient distress or loss of optimal functioning - Always goes away - Low risk for illness **Features** - Irritable, angry - Anxious or depressed - Physically too pumped up or tired - Loss of complete self-control - Poor focus - Poor sleep - Not having fun	**Definition** - More severe and persistent distress or loss of function - Leaves a "scar" - Higher risk for illness **Causes** - Life threat - Loss - Inner conflict - Wear and tear **Features** - Panic or rage - Loss of control of body or mind - Can't sleep - Recurrent nightmares or bad memories - Persistent shame, guilt, or blame - Loss of moral values and beliefs	**Definition** - Persistent and disabling distress or loss of function - Clinical mental disorders - Unhealed stress injuries **Types** - PTSD - Depression - Anxiety - Substance abuse **Features** - Symptoms and disability persist over many weeks - Symptoms and disability get worse over time
Unit Leader Responsibility	**Individual, Peer, Family Responsibility**		**Caregiver Responsibility**

Fig. 9.1. Combat and Operational Stress Continuum Model. *(From US Navy and Marine Corps, Combat and Operational Stress Continuum Model. Combat and Operational Stress Control 2010. Table 1-2. https://www.marines.mil/Portals/1/Publications/MCTP%203-30E%20 Formerly%20MCRP%206-11C.pdf?ver=2017-09-28-081327-517)*

OCCUPATIONAL HEALTH ISSUES IN EMS

1. What are common job hazards that EMS personnel face? How often are they being injured?
   According to the National Institute for Occupational Safety and Health surveillance tool (NEISS-Work), in 2017, there were approximately 21,000 injuries sustained by EMS providers in the United States.[7] The most common injuries include sprains and strains, and the most common locations involve the neck and back. Common hazards include repetitive stress injuries such as lifting patients and equipment, treating patients with infectious diseases, being exposed to hazardous chemicals and bodily substances, and participating in the emergency transport of patients in ground and air vehicles.[8,9]

2. What are some ways to prevent injury or pathogen transmission on the job?
   Standard precautions to prevent the transmission of infectious agents should be taken for each healthcare encounter. Standard precautions include hand hygiene after touching blood, body fluids, secretions, excretions, contaminated items, or equipment and between each patient contact.[9] Personal protective equipment including gloves, gowns, masks, and eye protection should also be used as appropriate. Safe handling and disposing of needles and other sharp instruments and the use of devices with safety features reduce the likelihood of injury or transmission of disease. Protocols for cleaning surfaces, textiles, and equipment should be followed and respiratory hygiene and cough etiquette should always be followed.[10]
   Assessment of scene safety before approaching a patient is critical to reduce the risk of injuries. Downed power lines, active shootings, falling debris, moving vehicles, unstable structures, and combative patients all put the provider at increased risk for injury.
   Wearing slip-resistant footwear may prevent slips and falls. Education and training on repetitive stress injuries and proper lifting and transferring of patients reduce injury to both the providers and patients. When it comes to slips, trips, and falls, up to 40% occur while going up or down steps or a curb. Other injuries were attributed to getting in or out of an ambulance or slipping on wet or slick surfaces. Nearly half of slips, trips, and falls occurred while a provider was pushing, pulling, lifting, or carrying a patient or equipment.[9]

Table 9.1. Isolation Precautions

DISEASE/ SYNDROME	POTENTIAL PATHOGENS	EMPIRIC PRECAUTIONS (ALWAYS INCLUDES STANDARD PRECAUTIONS)
Acute diarrhea	Enteric pathogens	Contact precautions (pediatrics and adult)
Meningitis	*Neisseria meningitidis*	Droplet precautions for the first 24 hours of antimicrobial therapy; mask and face protection for intubation
	Enteroviruses	Contact precautions for infants and children
	Mycobacterium tuberculosis	Airborne precautions if pulmonary infiltrate Airborne precautions plus contact precautions if potentially infectious draining body fluid present
Viral hemorrhagic fever + history of travel to area with outbreak in 10 days before onset of fever	Ebola, Lassa, Marburg viruses	Droplet precautions plus contact precautions, with face/eye protection, emphasizing safety sharps and barrier precautions when blood exposure likely. Use N95 or higher respiratory protection when aerosol-generating procedure performed.
Vesicular rash	Varicella-zoster, *herpes simplex*, variola (smallpox), vaccinia viruses	Airborne plus contact precautions; contact precautions only if herpes simplex, localized zoster in an immunocompetent host, or vaccinia viruses most likely
Maculopapular rash with cough, coryza, and fever	Rubeola (measles) virus	Airborne precautions
Respiratory infections	*M. tuberculosis*, Respiratory viruses, *Streptococcus pneumoniae*, *Staphylococcus aureus* (MSSA or MRSA)	Airborne precautions plus contact precautions Use eye/face protection if aerosol-generating procedure performed or contact with respiratory secretions anticipated.
	M. tuberculosis, severe acute respiratory syndrome virus (SARS-CoV), avian influenza	Airborne plus contact precautions plus eye protection If SARS and tuberculosis unlikely, use droplet precautions instead of airborne precautions
Viral respiratory infections	Respiratory syncytial virus, parainfluenza virus, adenovirus, influenza virus, *Human metapneumovirus*	Contact plus droplet precautions
Skin or wound infection involving abscess that cannot be covered	*S. aureus* (MSSA or MRSA), group A streptococcus	Contact precautions Add droplet precautions for the first 24 hours of appropriate antimicrobial therapy if invasive Group A streptococcal disease is suspected

MRSA, Methicillin-resistant *Staphylococcus aureus*; MSSA, methicillin-sensitive *Staphylococcus aureus*.
Modified from Siegel JD, Rhinehart E, Jackson M, Chiarello L and the Healthcare Infection Control Practices Advisory Committee. 2007 Guideline for Isolation Precautions: Preventing Transmission of Infectious Agents in Healthcare Settings. https://www.cdc.gov/ncidod/dhqp/pdf/isolation2007.pdf

Reducing injuries involves the joint commitment of EMS personnel and employers to cultivate a culture of safety that empowers team members, improves the safety knowledge, and creates an open environment to encourage reporting of near-misses.[9]

3. What precautions should I take for specific pathogen transmission?
Standard precautions should be utilized in every patient encounter, regardless of the perceived risk.[10] Table 9.1 is a summary of the Centers for Disease Control and Prevention's recommendations for isolation precautions for specific pathogens.[11]

4. If I have a needlestick, what do I need to do? What are the risks of disease transmission?
If a needlestick exposure occurs, immediately secure the instrument that caused the injury and place it in a safe location. Next, copiously irrigate the site with water or normal saline. Notify your supervisor, per protocol, and seek immediate medical attention. The medical provider or infection control officer should assist in obtaining testing for the source, if possible, and guide further management with regard to postexposure prophylaxis (Table 9.2).[2]

Table 9.2. Risks of Seroconversion after Clinical Meaningful Bodily Fluid Exposure[2]

	SEROCONVERSION AFTER PERCUTANEOUS EXPOSURE[a]	PROPHYLAXIS	POSTEXPOSURE PROPHYLAXIS (PEP)
Hepatitis C	1.8%	None	None
Hepatitis B	Unvaccinated: 6%–30% Vaccinated with serum anti-HBs <10 mIU/mL): virtually no risk	Hepatitis B series vaccine	Hepatitis B vaccine + HBIg depending on source patient status
HIV	0.3% after percutaneous exposure 0.09% after splash exposure	None for health-care workers	If source positive or unknown, likely start PEP (raltegravir plus the combination drug Truvada [tenofovir and emtricitabine])

[a]Percutaneous exposure as defined by single needlestick or cut exposure to a positive source patient. Higher risk for infectivity based on viral load of the patient and exact mechanism of transmission (deep injury, hollow-bore, visible blood on needle, etc.). Splash injuries are very low risk but nonzero.
HB, Hepatitis B; *HBIg,* hepatitis B immune globulin.

5. What immunizations are recommended for EMS personnel?
   EMS personnel should be offered hepatitis B series vaccine, MMR (measles/mumps/rubella) vaccine, varicella vaccine (if not immune), tuberculin (TB) skin testing in accordance with TB risk assessment, and annual influenza vaccinations. Other vaccines can be obtained as necessary depending on endemic disease in their area (i.e., hepatitis A, meningitis). Additionally, Tdap (combination tetanus + diphtheria + acellular pertussis) is recommended for those with direct patient contact.[2]

KEY POINTS

- A critical or "traumatic" incident is defined as a powerful or emotionally provoking event experienced by the EMS provider. This stressor typically overwhelms the person's normal coping mechanisms and significantly differs from the normal events experienced on the job.
- Over time, the approach to managing psychological stress for EMS workers has changed, with a new emphasis on individualized response to traumatic events, implementing wellness initiatives, and taking a less structured approach to debriefings.
- The most commonly encountered occupational hazards that EMS providers are exposed to include injuries related to environmental scene and patient hazards, ambulance/transport crashes, repetitive stress injuries such as lifting a patient and mechanical slips, trips, or falls.
- HIV, hepatitis C, and hepatitis B are three blood-borne diseases transmissible by splashes, needlesticks, or other percutaneous injuries.
- Ambulance transport and aircraft crashes are the most common causes of work-related EMS fatalities.

REFERENCES

1. Vigil NH, Grant AR, Perez O, et al. Death by suicide—the EMS profession compared to the general public. *Prehosp Emerg Care.* 2019;23(3):340-345. doi: 10.1080/10903127.2018.1514090. https://www.ncbi.nlm.nih.gov/pubmed/30136908.
2. Cone D, Brice JH, Delbridge TR, Myers JB. *Emergency Medical Services: Clinical Practice and Systems Oversight. 2nd ed. Volume 2: Medical Oversight of EMS.* United Kingdom: John Wiley & Sons; 2015. www.wiley.com\go\cone\naemsp.
3. Pons P, Markovchick VJ. *Prehospital Emergency Care Secrets.* Amsterdam, The Netherlands: Elsevier; 1998:35-42.
4. Bledsoe B. Critical incident stress management (CISM): benefit or risk for emergency services. *Prehosp Emerge Care.* 2003;7(2):272-279.
5. United States Department of Health and Human Surfaces. Psychological First Aid for First Responders Tips for Emergency and Disaster Response Workers. 2005. https://store.samhsa.gov/product/Psychological-First-Aid-for-First-Responders/NMH05-0210.
6. US Navy and Marine Corps. Combat and Operational Stress Continuum Model: Combat and Operational Stress Control. 2010. Table 1-2. P 1-8. https://www.marines.mil/Portals/1/Publications/MCTP%203-30E%20Formerly%20MCRP%206-11C.pdf?ver=2017-09-28-081327-517.
7. The National Institute for Occupational Safety and Health (NIOSH). Workplace safety & health topics. https://www.cdc.gov/niosh/topics/ems/default.html.
8. The National Institute for Occupational Safety and Health (NIOSH). EMS workers injury data. https://www.cdc.gov/niosh/topics/ems/data.html.
9. Reichard A, Wijetunge GU, Marsh SM, Konda S. 5 Causes of high injury rate in EMS providers: NIOSH and NHTSA collaborated to use emergency department visit data to identify the five primary types of injury events experienced by EMS providers. November 6, 2017. https://www.ems1.com/paramedic-chief/articles/5-causes-of-high-injury-rate-in-ems-providers-I6dHrLcjldehcxZe/.
10. Centers for Diseases Control and Prevention. Recommendations for application of standard precautions for the care of all patients in all healthcare settings: guideline for isolation precautions: preventing transmission of infectious agents in healthcare settings (2007). Appendix A, Table 4. https://www.cdc.gov/infectioncontrol/guidelines/isolation/appendix/standard-precautions.html.
11. Centers for Disease Control and Prevention. Clinical syndromes or conditions warranting empiric transmission-based precautions in addition to standard precautions: guideline for isolation precautions: preventing transmission of infectious agents in healthcare settings (2007). Appendix A, Table 2. https://www.cdc.gov/infectioncontrol/guidelines/isolation/appendix/transmission-precautions.html.

PREHOSPITAL PHYSICAL ASSESSMENT AND CRITICAL INTERPRETATION OF VITAL SIGNS

William C. Ferguson, Jr.

CHAPTER 10

QUESTIONS AND ANSWERS

Case: You arrive on scene at a high school football game to find an adult male lying under the bleachers with first responders on scene. He has an abrasion to his forehead and there is emesis on his shirt. The EMT on the scene turns to you as you approach and your partner yells, "What are his vitals?"

1. How do you rapidly determine airway patency?

   Airway assessment is a primary component of any patient assessment. Patients without airways require immediate intervention to prevent death. Airway assessment can be started as you approach your patient on scene, looking for clues as to mental status. A patient who is upright and talking has a stable airway at least long enough for you to complete the primary exam. As you approach the patient, ask them a question. The goal is to elicit a verbal response. If there is a verbal response, then next ask yourself, do you hear any upper airway noises? Stridor, a muffled voice, and dysarthria are all clues that the airway is patent but may be tenuous.

   Nonverbal patients require early hands-on assessment, potentially jaw thrust to reposition the airway as looking for obstructions, the tongue, edema, vomitus, or airway trauma. Then suctioning or clearing the airway as needed while assessing for breathing, and potentially placing an Oropharyngeal airway (OPA) or nasopharyngeal airway (NPA) simultaneously. In the verbal patient with concerns for partial airway obstructions, look for angioedema, consider racemic epinephrine, or potentially prepare for a surgical airway. Stridor would also suggest upper airway edema, from allergic reactions, infections, or foreign body (FB) obstruction. Dysarthria may indicate cerebrovascular accidents (CVA), requiring the patient to be repositioned to maintain an airway and prevent aspiration.

2. How do you assess respiratory rate and overall breathing status?

   Assessment and intervention of breathing are also not performed in a vacuum; it is the second step in the process but is performed almost simultaneously as determining airway patency. Across-the-room assessment of respiratory status is an important skill for EMS providers to learn. The actual counting of respiratory rate (RR) has been found to be problematic for all providers. There seems to be variability in both the way providers count the rate and the answer obtained. The real question is, does the rate matter? Obviously, at the extremes, it does. Rates <8 per min or >26 per min in adults are very concerning for respiratory distress and impending doom. But is there a significant difference in the adult with a rate of 12 versus 16? Work of breathing, end organ perfusion, and oxygenation and ventilation assessment are much more important. A patient with an RR of 12 and lying in bed with complaints of chest pain is in less distress than the adult with a RR of 12 sitting up, leaning forward, and using accessory muscles. So, the vital sign of RR must be used in the context of the clinical situation. Patients with impaired ventilation due to trauma or obstruction will show increased accessory muscle use. End organ oxygenation can be assessed in some by skin color. Oxygen saturation is a useful tool in patients with adequate skin perfusion and blood pressure. However, the best determination of end organ oxygenation and ventilation is mental status. Patients who are significantly hypoxic are altered. With impaired gas exchange and either low or impaired ventilation, carbon dioxide is retained (hypercapnia) and leads to altered mental status and worsening ventilations and potentially loss of airway. If alterations in work of breathing, mental status, or extremes in the RR are noted in your initial across-the-room assessment, a hands-on primary assessment can lead you to the underlying problem that needs to be addressed.

   The chest should be exposed, and auscultation of lung fields and hands-on assessment for asymmetric chest movement, crepitus, tenderness, and soft tissue trauma should be carried out. Even though some environments yield difficulty in auscultation of lung fields, it is still a valuable tool in determining the cause of breathing disturbances. Auscultate to determine symmetry and presence of adventitious sounds. Wheezing may indicate a reactive airway such as in asthma or chronic obstructive pulmonary disease (COPD), which may require nebulized medications. Rales or crackles may be indicative of pulmonary edema, which would require appropriate patient positioning, preload reductions, and positive pressure ventilation (continuous positive airway pressure [CPAP]/

bilevel positive airway pressure [BiPAP]). Diminished breath sounds or asymmetry could be due to pneumonia or in the setting of trauma could be a pulmonary contusion or pneumothorax.

3. How do you rapidly assess circulation to detect life threats and confirm adequate end organ perfusion and does their pulse rate and blood pressure matter?

Pulse rates hint at cardiac output and give some information on patient status as there are some rates at the extremes that need to be addressed in the primary exam. Rates <50 or >150 are concerning for impending cardiovascular collapse. However, the goal of the pulse rate assessment is to look at overall perfusion and determine "sick" or "not sick." The across-the-room assessment as mentioned earlier can ascertain if the patient is verbal and alert, giving you data that the AB and now C of the primary exam are stable enough to continue with your ongoing assessment. As appropriate, mental status implies good perfusion, and good perfusion implies that the patient has an airway and is breathing. A quick hand on the pulse can give the rate, determining if it is "too fast," "too slow," or relatively "ok." It can also determine regularity and gives you an idea if the skin is warm, cool, moist, or dry. These additional findings can give you clues as to overall perfusion. If there is a sympathetic response ongoing, they may be diaphoretic. Maybe they are cool due to cardiogenic shock or hot secondary to a fever.

A global approach to a patient's cardiovascular status in the unstable patient would be rapid exposure for life-threatening bleeding while assessing central and peripheral pulses. Heart sounds have routinely been taught as a cardiac assessment tool, but in reality, they only give you data that are emergently needed for a few situations. A significant murmur in the setting of syncope would lead you to be concerned for aortic stenosis, which requires surgical intervention. Murmurs in the setting of an ST-elevation myocardial infarction (STEMI) and cardiogenic shock hint at papillary muscle rupture and the need for a cardiothoracic surgeon and not just a catheterization lab. And in a patient who appears septic, it would hint of endocarditis.

Blood pressure evaluation in the critically ill patients can be obtained but should not delay treatment in an unstable patient with signs of cardiovascular compromise. Current trends in therapy for trauma patients are permissive hypotension, limiting isotonic fluids and their diluting effects on blood. However, if there is a concurrent head injury, even a few minutes of hypotension can worsen secondary brain injury. In medical patients with hypotension, considerations for sepsis, hypovolemia, or cardiogenic shock, trending of blood pressure, are valuable as one lone blood pressure without clinical context has limited value. With hypertension, current emergency medicine literature is conservative on aggressive blood pressure control unless we see signs of end organ perfusion or blood pressures greater than 220/110. Obviously, some clinical scenarios would require addressing of hypertension before that, as in hemorrhagic strokes or hypertensive emergency with severe chest pain or alterations in mental status.

4. Is the patient alert?

The across-the-room assessment can also be a tool for a rapid determination of mental status changes. A nonverbal, nonalert patient can be critically ill, with serious alterations in potentially multiple portions of the primary exam, and may need emergent maneuvers to stabilize the ABCs and Ds. If the ABCs are relatively stable, the next question is why their mental status is altered. Assess for conditions we can fix first. A rapid blood glucose evaluation is paramount. Brain cells die without glucose, altered hypoglycemic patients not treated can have significant morbidity and mortality, and there is no reason not to correct this as it is readily diagnosable. Use the other clues readily available to you to help determine other causes of altered mental status (AMS). The environment, bystanders, physical and exam findings can all help you reasonably make a list of potential causes.

CASE PROGRESSION

First responders are establishing an IV and obtaining a glucose level as you approach and notice the patient is unresponsive. Respirations are slow and labored. You perform a jaw thrust, note secretions in his oral pharynx, and rapidly suction the airway. Respiratory effort improves, your partner is quickly exposing the chest and applying the monitor as you lay hands on their chest and note chest wall crepitus with decreased breath sounds on the left. His radial pulse is fast but strong, and you see no obvious uncontrolled external hemorrhage. Vitals are noted; heart rate is 124, RR is 10+ with significant accessory muscle use, and SpO_2 is 91%. Glucose was 116. Blood pressure is 142/68, supplemental O_2 is applied, and rapid transport is initiated. During transport, the patient's respirations become agonal and the pulse rate rapidly declines. On reassessment, he has no breath sounds on the left and no longer has a radial pulse. Chest decompression is performed with immediate change of heart rate back to 116 and a palpable pulse. You arrive at the trauma center and the first question asked by the trauma team is "what are his vitals?"

KEY POINTS

- Rapid physical assessment is paramount in determining the need for life-saving and primary exam stabilizing maneuvers. Assessment should be done simultaneously with a focused history and hands-on interventions. The ABCD approach is not linear, but rather a global approach to assessment with interventions made as deficiencies are noted.
- Vital signs are vital not because of the number they provide but in their ability to sometimes provide objective value to vital organ function, and they must be interpreted in a clinical context.

BIBLIOGRAPHY

Birmingham Regional Emergency Medical Services System. Alabama EMS Challenge, core content. 2019. http://www.bremss.org/alabama-ems-challenge/.

Horeczko T, Eriquez B, McGrath NE, Gausche-Hill M, Lewis RJ. The Pediatric Assessment Triangle: accuracy of its application by nurses in the triage of children. *J Emerg Nurs.* 2013;39(2):182-189.

Raja A, Zane RD. Initial management of trauma in adults. *Up-to-Date.* Sept 2019.

Smith I, Mackay J, Fahrid N, Kruchek D. Respiratory rate measurement: a comparison of methods. *Br J Healthc Assistants.* 2011;5(1.)doi: 10.12968/bjha.2011.5.1.18.

Trauma Nursing Core Curriculum Provider Manual. 8th ed. Jones and Bartlett Publisher, Emergency Nurses Association; 2019.

CHAPTER 11

CARDIAC ARREST AND ECMO

Jordan B. Schooler and Joshua J. Davis

QUESTIONS AND ANSWERS

1. You arrive on the scene at a local restaurant to find a 65-year-old gentleman who reportedly had a witnessed cardiac arrest. Cardiopulmonary resuscitation (CPR) was started by bystanders. How common is out-of-hospital cardiac arrest?

   350,000 patients suffer an out-of-hospital cardiac arrest annually in the United States, and the overall fatality rate is over 90%.

2. After you stabilize your patient, what is important information to gather at the scene?

   It is useful prognostically to determine whether the cardiac arrest was witnessed or unwitnessed, as well as the duration of time before CPR and duration of bystander CPR. Of course, obtaining any preceding symptoms, relevant medical history, medications, allergies, and trauma sustained during the arrest is also important.

3. How often do people survive out-of-hospital cardiac arrest?

   Overall, about 25%–30% of patients survive to hospital admission, and just under 10% survive to hospital discharge. The highest survival rate, with 30% discharged from the hospital alive, is in witnessed arrests with shockable initial rhythm and immediate bystander CPR. Asystole as the initial rhythm carries the worst prognosis, likely because it often signifies extended downtime. Unwitnessed arrest has a survival to hospital discharge of about 4%. Cardiac arrest witnessed by a 911 responder leads to about 18%–20% survival to hospital discharge on average.

4. What are the priorities in prehospital care for cardiac arrest?

   The interventions that have been shown to have the greatest impact on survival remain high-quality CPR—including adequate depth, rate, and recoil with minimal interruptions—and defibrillation in patients with a shockable rhythm. Effective oxygenation and ventilation increases in importance as the duration of the arrest becomes longer, and may be the most important factor in selected patients with a respiratory cause for their arrest. It remains controversial whether mask ventilation, supraglottic airway, or endotracheal intubation has any relative survival benefit; whichever is chosen, the effectiveness should be monitored by waveform capnography. Treatment of reversible causes of arrest is important, although many of these are difficult to identify in the prehospital setting. Chest compressions and airway management generally should take priority over vascular access and medication administration.

5. CPR was started by an unrelated bystander. How many patients receive bystander CPR?

   Recent data suggest that about 50% of witnessed cardiac arrest patients receive CPR prior to 911 responder arrival. Fewer than 5% of those eligible receive treatment with an automatic external defibrillator (AED). Dispatcher-assisted CPR (DA-CPR) has been shown to have similar survival benefits as bystander CPR when coupled with earlier recognition of cardiac arrest and is an extremely important component of emergency medical dispatching (EMD). High-functioning systems should monitor the time it takes for DA-CPR instructions to be given to reduce the time it takes to begin bystander CPR in cardiac arrest.

6. What are common causes of out-of-hospital cardiac arrest?

   Myocardial infarction is likely the most common cause, although high-quality modern data are lacking. Respiratory decompensation and sepsis likely account for a substantial proportion. A search for causes using H's and T's is commonly taught as a mnemonic for reversible causes of cardiac arrest (Table 11.1), although some of these are either routinely addressed by standard care (hypoxia), difficult to diagnose and treat in the field (thrombosis), or quite rare (tamponade, isolated hypoglycemia).

7. What is "pit crew CPR," how is it performed, and does it improve outcomes?

   Pit crew CPR is named after Formula One pit crews, who use a highly choreographed approach to task completion. During a resuscitation, this approach assigns crew members to discrete tasks that are performed without specific direction from a team leader. They include airway management, CPR delivery, monitoring and defibrillation, medication administration, and documentation. Positions are assigned before scene arrival and a prespecified location at the side of the victim is identified for each crew member. There is some research to suggest that this approach may improve outcomes.

Table 11.1. H's and T's Mnemonic for Reversible Causes of Cardiac Arrest

POTENTIAL CAUSE	KEYS TO DIAGNOSIS	POTENTIAL TREATMENT(S)
Hypovolemia	Tachycardia, recent illness with dehydration, trauma	Infusion of IV crystalloids or occasionally blood
Hypoxia	Slow heart rate, cyanosis	Airway management, oxygenation
H+ (acidosis)	Recent illness, prolonged downtime, possibly severe hyperglycemia	Correct underlying cause, sodium bicarbonate, hyperventilation
Hypokalemia	U waves, flat T waves, prolonged QTc, GI losses, or diuretic use	IV potassium (slow), IV magnesium (rapid)
Hyperkalemia	Bradycardia, junctional rhythm, peaked T waves, wide QRS, "sine wave" pattern, history of renal failure	Calcium chloride, sodium bicarbonate (if acidotic), insulin (with glucose if needed), high-dose albuterol
Hypothermia	Found outside or in cold environment, cool/cold to touch	Rapid rewarming, do not cease resuscitative efforts until core temperature >35 °C
Hypoglycemia	Low bedside glucose testing, history of diabetes	IV dextrose
Toxins	Depends on toxin, possibly prolonged QTc, history of suicide attempt or ingestion, history of drug abuse	Based on the specific toxin
Thrombosis (pulmonary embolus)	History of leg pain, swelling, dyspnea, sinus tachycardia	Thrombolysis, anticoagulation, surgical intervention
Thrombosis (myocardial infarction)	ECG with signs of ischemia (ST elevation, depression, T-wave inversion), history of coronary disease or risk factors (hypertension, diabetes, high cholesterol, smoking, obesity)	Antiplatelet agents (e.g., aspirin), thrombolysis, percutaneous coronary intervention
Tension pneumothorax	Preceding shortness of breath, trauma, absent breath sounds on one side	Thoracostomy (chest tube) or needle decompression
Tamponade	Tachycardia, electrical alternans on EKG, trauma	Pericardiocentesis, thoracotomy

EKG, Electrocardiogram; *GI,* gastrointestinal; *IV,* intravenous.

8. As you continue CPR, you consider medications for cardiac arrest. What medications are commonly administered in cardiac arrest and for what reason?
   The mainstay of cardiac arrest is high-quality CPR and treating reversible causes. No medication has been shown to increase the rate of neurologically intact survival in cardiac arrest, although there may be benefit in selected patients. Epinephrine is recommended by advanced cardiac life support (ACLS) guidelines, although it has only been shown to increase return of spontaneous circulation and possibly survival with unfavorable neurologic outcome. Antiarrhythmics are recommended for shockable rhythms, but amiodarone and lidocaine do not appear to improve survival to hospital discharge.

9. Should my service invest in a mechanical CPR device?
   To date, the evidence suggests no survival benefit for mechanical CPR in place of traditional manual CPR. Systems might consider the utilization of a mechanical CPR device when they do not have adequate responders to perform good-quality CPR or in select circumstances if it becomes necessary to transport a patient in cardiac arrest for more definitive care such as initiation of extracorporeal membrane oxygenation (ECMO) or cardiac catheterization.

10. When should I discontinue CPR in the field?
    This should be guided by local protocol. However, multiple studies have shown that it is possible to predict that certain groups of patients are extremely unlikely to survive, and it is reasonable to stop resuscitative efforts without transporting to a hospital. The most commonly used criteria include unwitnessed arrest without bystander CPR, nonshockable rhythm, lack of return of spontaneous circulation in the field, and persistent end-tidal CO_2 less than 10. There may be situations when such patients should still be transported, for example, if grieving bystanders pose a threat to the safety of EMS personnel.

11. What are ECMO, ECLS, and ECPR?

ECMO is a technology that can artificially replace the function of the heart and lungs. ECLS (extracorporeal life support) is a term that is used synonymously with ECMO. ECPR, or extracorporeal CPR, refers to the use of ECMO in a cardiac arrest patient. Large bore cannulae are placed in the femoral artery and vein, and these are connected to a machine that pumps the blood out, oxygenates it and removes carbon dioxide, and returns it to the body. This can completely replace the function of the heart and lungs, even in patients who have not had return of spontaneous circulation. However, this is only temporary. To be discharged alive, the patient must either have cardiac recovery, perhaps after treatment of a reversible injury such as an ST-elevation myocardial infarction (STEMI), or undergo left ventricular assist device (LVAD) implantation or transplant. Also, ECMO cannot reverse damage to organs such as the brain, liver, and kidneys from the initial arrest.

12. How might ECMO impact prehospital cardiac arrest care?

Nearly all of those who survive out-of-hospital cardiac arrest have return of spontaneous circulation in the field. To date, there has been no therapy for medical cardiac arrest patients that would impact survival and was only available in the hospital. This, along with the difficulty of conducting resuscitation during transport, has strongly argued in favor of continuing resuscitation on scene for most patients. However, it may be the case that ECMO would improve survival for selected patients who would not achieve return of spontaneous circulation (ROSC) otherwise. Some systems have begun to identify potential ECMO candidates and transport them early to the hospital. Typically, these are patients with witnessed arrests, with shockable rhythms, and under 65–70 years old. Also, there have been several systems that have begun ECMO cannulation in the field, but this is highly resource intensive and requires both significant financial investment and extensively trained physician responders.

13. What is targeted temperature management and should it be performed in the out-of-hospital environment?

It is well established that unconscious survivors of out-of-hospital cardiac arrest have a high risk of death or poor neurologic function. The initiation of therapeutic hypothermia is recommended by international guidelines, although the supporting evidence is limited. Despite several options for starting hypothermia protocols in the out-of-hospital setting, it remains logistically difficult to implement and the optimal target temperature is not well established. Moreover, in several randomized controlled trials, prehospital induction of hypothermia did not reduce poor neurological outcome or mortality.

14. Where should you transport a cardiac arrest patient?

The American Heart Association model for cardiac resuscitation systems recommends transport to a level I resuscitation center because it can provide comprehensive cardiovascular care, including primary percutaneous coronary intervention (PCI), for the approximately 25% of patients who experience a cardiac arrest in the setting of an acute STEMI. For some areas where ambulance transport times from the scene to hospital are not prolonged, some protocols may encourage bypass of the closest hospital in order to bring the patient directly to a level I center.

KEY POINTS

- CPR quality and early defibrillation are the interventions with the largest improvement in the survival of cardiac arrest patients.
- Bystander CPR is important for survival, and emergency medical dispatch systems may aid in patient survival.
- No medication has been shown to improve survival in cardiac arrest.
- Field termination of resuscitation is appropriate in selected patients.

BIBLIOGRAPHY

Benjamin EJ, Virani SS, Callaway CW, et al. Heart disease and stroke statistics—2018 update: a report from the American Heart Association. *Circulation.* 2018;137:e67-e492.

Donnino MW, Andersen LW, Berg KM, et al. Temperature management after cardiac arrest: an advisory statement by the Advanced Life Support Task Force of the International Liaison Committee on Resuscitation and the American Heart Association Emergency Cardiovascular Care Committee and the Council on Cardiopulmonary, Critical Care, Perioperative and Resuscitation [published correction appears in *Circulation.* 2016;133:e13]. *Circulation.* 2015;132:2448-2456.

Hopkins CL, Burk C, Moser S, et al. Implementation of pit crew approach and cardiopulmonary resuscitation metrics for out-of-hospital cardiac arrest improves patient survival and neurological outcome. *J Am Heart Assoc.* 2016;5(1).

Jabre P, Penaloza A, Pinero D, et al. Effect of bag-mask ventilation vs endotracheal intubation during cardiopulmonary resuscitation on neurological outcome after out-of-hospital cardiorespiratory arrest: a randomized clinical trial. *JAMA.* 2018;319:779-787.

Kudenchuk PJ, Brown SP, Daya M, et al. Amiodarone, lidocaine, or placebo in out-of-hospital cardiac arrest. *N Engl J Med.* 2016;374:1711-1722.

Link MS, Berkow LC, Kudenchuk PJ, et al. Part 7: adult advanced cardiovascular life support: 2015 American Heart Association Guidelines update for cardiopulmonary resuscitation and emergency cardiovascular care. *Circulation.* 2015;132:S444-S464.

McNally B, Robb R, Mehta M, et al. Out-of-hospital cardiac arrest surveillance—Cardiac Arrest Registry to Enhance Survival (CARES), United States, October 1, 2005–December 31, 2010. *MMWR Surveill Summ.* 2011;60:1-19.

National Association of EMS Physicians. Termination of resuscitation in nontraumatic cardiopulmonary arrest. *Prehosp Emerg Care.* 2011;15:542.

Nielsen N, Wetterslev J, Cronberg T, et al. Targeted temperature management at 33 °C versus 36 °C after cardiac arrest. *N Engl J Med.* 2013;369(23):2197-2206.

Nikolaou N, Dainty KN, Couper K, et al. A systematic review and meta-analysis of the effect of dispatcher-assisted CPR on outcomes from sudden cardiac arrest in adults and children. *Resuscitation.* 2019;138:82-105.

Panchal AR, Berg KM, Hirsch KG, et al. 2019 American Heart Association focused update on advanced cardiovascular life support: use of advanced airways, vasopressors, and extracorporeal cardiopulmonary resuscitation during cardiac arrest: an update to the American Heart Association guidelines for cardiopulmonary resuscitation and emergency cardiovascular care. *Circulation.* 2019;140:e881-e894.

Perkins GD, Ji C, Deakin CD, et al. A randomized trial of epinephrine in out-of-hospital cardiac arrest. *N Engl J Med.* 2018; 379(8):711-721.

Wang HE, Schmicker RH, Daya MR, et al. Effect of a strategy of initial laryngeal tube insertion vs endotracheal intubation on 72-hour survival in adults with out-of-hospital cardiac arrest. *JAMA.* 2018;320:769-778.

Wang PL, Brooks SC. Mechanical versus manual chest compressions for cardiac arrest. *Cochrane Database Syst Rev.* 2018;8(8):CD007260.

CHAPTER 12

HYPOTENSION AND SHOCK

Duane D. Siberski

QUESTIONS AND ANSWERS

1. What is hypotension?

   Decreased blood pressure relative to a person's baseline blood pressure.

   Hypotension is a systolic blood pressure less than 90 mm Hg or a mean arterial pressure of less than 60 mm Hg for a duration of at least 30 minutes. Another definition is a decrease in a person's baseline blood pressure of 30%. The absolute point of hypotension varies between individuals. A normal adult whose systolic blood pressure is chronically 90 mm Hg may have no symptoms. Another adult with chronic hypertension, whose chronic systolic blood pressure is 185 mm Hg, may be symptomatic at 120 mm Hg. The blood pressure below which a person becomes symptomatic is hypotension.

2. What is needed for adequate blood pressure?

   A closed, functional, filled cardiovascular system with the body in homeostasis.

   Blood pressure is the result of multiple, interactive components. The vascular structures, arteries, arterioles, capillaries, venioles, and veins are intact and without significant leaks. There is an adequate and appropriate volume of blood and blood components to fill the vascular structures. Heart function must be sufficient to propel the blood forward through the body with total volume return for redistribution. Renal function balances fluids, electrolytes, and pH while removing wastes. Neurohormonal oversight and management detect and adjust the systems (e.g., vascular tone, heart rate, respiratory rate, glomerular filtration rate, gluconeogenesis) to control the variables that can affect the homeostatic state of the body.

3. What are the symptoms of hypotension?

   Evidence of organ dysfunction or compensation.

   General—fatigue, thirst, syncope, depression
   Cardiac—tachycardia, chest pain
   Cerebral—confusion, dizziness, light-headedness, blurred vision, decreased concentration
   Dermal—pallor, diaphoresis
   Gastrointestinal—nausea
   Pulmonary—tachypnea, palpitations, dyspnea

4. What is shock?

   Inadequate tissue perfusion.

   Shock is a syndrome in which hypotension is the hallmark. The absolute definition of undifferentiated shock is inadequate tissue perfusion. Unmet metabolic demands due to inadequate perfusion result from hypotension and hypoxia. The inadequate supply of fuels (e.g., oxygen, glucose or electrolytes) or the inability to distribute the fuels to cells, tissues, and organs impacts the cellular function. A cascade of events resulting from the lack of perfusion begins a process that can lead to cellular injury, cellular death, tissue injury, organ dysfunction, multiorgan failure, and death.

   Compensated shock is a response that occurs when heart rate increases, increasing cardiac output, attempting to normalize and maintain blood pressure for adequate perfusion.

   Decompensated shock occurs when blood pressure drops, resulting in hypotension, despite the tachycardic response.

   Decreased perfusion causing cellular hypoxia stimulates cells to utilize anaerobic metabolism. Production of metabolic by-products and lactic acid and inadequate production of adenosine triphosphate (ATP) occur during anaerobic metabolism compared with aerobic metabolism. Inadequate levels of ATP affect cellular function, causing the depolarization of the cell membrane. Swelling of the cell occurs and leads to cell necrosis. Reversal of shock, by treating its cause, may halt this progression. Death from shock is a result of hypoxia causing multiorgan failure.

5. Other than blood pressure, are there other methods of recognizing shock?

   Serum lactate and end-tidal carbon dioxide ($EtCO_2$) can also be measured as indicators of poor perfusion, especially in sepsis.

   Point of care testing can measure serum markers, such as lactic acid, indicating poor perfusion. An elevated lactate level of 2 mmol/L or greater is associated with higher in-hospital mortality. Such testing is invasive and may not be available for use in all areas. $EtCO_2$ can also be used as a marker for poor perfusion. Low readings of $EtCO_2$ have been shown to correlate with lactic acidosis, organ dysfunction, and mortality in sepsis and trauma patients. Readings of EtCO$_2$ of 25 mmHg or less, when used with a sepsis screening tool, showed a correlation with metabolic acidosis and in-hospital lactate levels. As a noninvasive measurement, this could be used in conjunction with vital signs in patients with shock and poor perfusion.

6. What are the different types of shock?
   There are four types of shock: cardiogenic, distributive, hypovolemic, and obstructive.
   Cardiogenic—myocardial infarction, dysrhythmia, toxins
   Distributive—decreased autonomic tone, sepsis, toxins, spinal cord injury, anaphylaxis
   Hypovolemic—blood loss, plasma loss, dehydration
   Obstructive—tension pneumothorax, cardiac tamponade, pulmonary embolism, atrial myxoma

7. What can cause the different types of shock?
   Disruption of one or more of the components of the cardiovascular system and metabolic substrates can cause shock.
       Cardiogenic shock results from pump failure, decreasing cardiac output.
       Cardiac output, typically 4.7 L/min (5 qts/min), is calculated based on stroke volume multiplied by heart rate. Myocardial tissue dysfunction caused by ischemia or toxins leads to impaired contractility. Ischemia impacting at least 45% of the left ventricle can result in significantly decreased cardiac output, hypotension, and hypoperfusion. Cardiotoxic chemicals can have chronotropic and/or ionotropic effects causing decreased cardiac output. Dysrhythmias decrease cardiac output either by decreasing the effective rate or decreasing the stroke volume from inadequate diastolic filling time.
       Distributive shock—septic, neurogenic, anaphylactic
       Chemical, hormonal, or immunologic mediators cause vascular instability due to capillary bed leakage or decreased vascular tone. This effectively increases the relative volume of the vascular system or allows the escape of plasma to the extravascular space. There may, in cases of septic shock, be additional cardiosuppressive effects. Compensatory tachycardia may result, as in cases of anaphylaxis. In neurogenic shock, damage to the spinal cord results in loss of sympathetic tone due to the disruption of the autonomic chain. Compensatory tachycardia does not occur in neurogenic shock. In fact, when parasympathetic input is unopposed, from the loss of sympathetic balance, bradycardia may occur.
       Hypovolemic shock is caused by inadequate circulation blood volume.
       Hemorrhagic hypovolemic shock results from external or internal loss of blood. Hemorrhage from vascular damage, hemothorax, and gastrointestinal hemorrhage may result in blood loss of greater than 40% of total blood volume, impacting the body's compensatory mechanisms and causing shock. Nonhemorrhagic hypovolemic shock is caused by loss of plasma volume, without cell loss. It can result from the gastrointestinal tract, such as by vomiting, diarrhea, insufficient intake resulting in dehydration, or necrotizing pancreatitis. Dermatologic plasma losses can be caused by significant burns, TENS (toxic epidermal necrolysis syndrome), or Stevens-Johnson syndrome.
       Obstructive shock is caused by disruption of blood flow, decreased cardiac output, and/or decreased venous return.
       Tension pneumothorax occurs from pulmonary parenchymal damage, allowing air to escape into the potential space in the chest cavity between the chest wall and the lung. Without the ability to exit, there is a buildup of trapped air within the chest, increasing the intrathoracic pressure in the hemithorax and collapsing the lung on the affected side. Mediastinal structures, vena cava, aorta, trachea, esophagus, and heart shift contralaterally. Venous return through the vena cava is decreased with increasing external pressure and mediastinal shift. As venous return decreases, cardiac output also decreases. Hypoxia occurs due to shunting through the pulmonary vasculature past collapsed alveoli without uptake of oxygen. Shock occurs from the combination of decreased cardiac output and hypoxia. Pericardial tamponade results from fluid accumulation in the pericardial sac. Hemorrhagic or nonhemorrhagic fluid collection in the pericardium exerts external pressure of the heart restricting adequate filling. Decreased filling of the ventricles decreases stroke volume. As stroke volume decreases, cardiac output will decrease with a resultant drop in blood pressure. Massive pulmonary embolism disrupts flow through the pulmonary vasculature. Decreased vascular return from the pulmonary beds leads to decreased cardiac output. Mismatched areas of functional alveoli and decreased pulmonary vasculature result in decreased oxygenation of blood. Decreased cardiac output leading to hypotension, combined with hypoxia, produces a shock state. Atrial myxoma, a rare tumor arising in the right atrium, can obstruct venous return flow, decreasing cardiac output. With increasing size of the tumor, flow decreases, and decreased perfusion can result in a shock state. Surgical excision can be curative.

8. How do you treat shock?
   Treat the cause.
       Dependent on the cause, treatment will vary accordingly.
       Cardiogenic shock treatment utilizes chronotropic and ionotropic agents to increase cardiac output or increase vascular tone. Antidysrhythmic agents treat cardiac rhythms causing decreased cardiac output impacted by fast, slow, irregular, or absent rhythms. Electrical stimulation of the myocardium with transcutaneous pacing, synchronized cardioversion, or unsynchronized defibrillation may also be utilized.

Distributive shock, whether by neurogenic, anaphylactic, or septic cause, occurs when cardiac function and circulating volume are adequate but there is an inappropriately low systemic vascular resistance. Loss of vascular autonomic tone leading to vasodilatation results in decreased systemic resistance, increased capillary permeability, and hypotension. Vasopressors and inotropic agents are utilized with intravenous fluid. In septic shock, antimicrobials are utilized to treat the infectious agent.

Hypovolemic shock from decreased circulating volume is treated with volume expansion utilizing isotonic intravenous fluid. Hypovolemic shock from a hemorrhagic cause is best treated with whole blood or blood products for volume expansion. Correction of ongoing losses may require surgical intervention.

Obstructive shock from causes such as tension pneumothorax, pleural effusion, pericardial effusion with tamponade, and atrial myxoma requires intervention to relieve the pressure of buildup either in the intrathoracic, pericardial, or intracardiac cavity.

9. Are there cases where shock should not be treated?

Generally, no.

In some cases of hypovolemic, hemorrhagic shock, permissive hypotensive or damage control resuscitation may allow for improved outcome of patients when appropriate surgical intervention is readily available. In hemorrhagic shock, fluid resuscitation with crystalloids or nonblood products to a normalized blood pressure may result in further worsening of condition. As blood pressure elevates, the ongoing hemorrhagic losses accelerate the loss of red blood cells and further decrease oxygen-carrying capacity. Dilution of clotting factors, with the intravenous crystalloid fluids, worsens coagulopathy. Newly formed clots may be disrupted as blood pressure rises with fluid resuscitation. Hypothermia can occur from combined decreased intrinsic metabolic heat generation and intravenous crystalloid fluid infusion. Permissive hypotension may allow for interoperative management of the injuries combined with resuscitation. Limited intravenous fluid infusion is utilized to attempt to support perfusion with a target systolic blood pressure of 90–100 mmHg. Prehospital plasma infusion of two units has been investigated in damage control resuscitation for trauma victims with unstable vital signs and resulted in decreased 30-day mortality. Higher elevation of blood pressure, with aggressive fluid resuscitation, is avoided to minimize hemodilution, decreased oxygen-carrying capacity, clotting factor dilution, and hypothermia.

KEY POINTS

- Hypotension is the hallmark symptom in shock.
- Shock syndrome results from inadequate tissue perfusion.
- Treating the causes of shock targets reversal before the progression of cell hypoxia to cell death to multisystem organ failure.

BIBLIOGRAPHY

American Heart Association. *Advanced Cardiovascular Life Support.* 19th ed. Dallas, TX, Santoni Continuum, 2020.

Bickell W, Wall M, Pepe P, et al. Immediate versus delayed fluid resuscitation for hypotensive patients with penetrating torso injuries. *N Engl J Med.* 1994;331:1105-1109.

Bonanno F. Clinical pathology of the shock syndromes. *J Emerg Trauma Shock.* 2011 Apr-Jun;4(2):233-243.

Cannon JW. Hemorrhagic shock. *N Engl J Med.* 2018;378:370-379.

Hunter CL, Silvestri S, Ralls G, et al. A prehospital screening tool utilizing end-tidal carbon dioxide predicts sepsis and severe sepsis. *Am J Emerg Med.* 2016;34:813-819.

Myburgh M, Mythen M. Resuscitation fluids. *N Engl J Med.* 2013;369:1243-1251.

National Association of Emergency Medical Technicians. *Tactical Combat Casualty Care Guidelines for Medical Personnel.* Clinton, MS: Jones & Bartlett Learning; 2019.

Selde W. Damage control resuscitation principles adapted for EMS civilian trauma. *J Emerg Med Serv.* 2017;42(4.).

Sperry JL, Guyette FX, Brown JB, et al. Prehospital plasma during air medical transport in trauma patients at risk for hemorrhagic shock. *N Engl J Med.* 2018;379:566-572.

Tobias AZ, Guyette FX, Seynour CW, et al. Pre-resuscitation lactate and hospital mortality in prehospital patients. *Prehosp Emerg Care.* 2014 Jul-Sep;18(3):321-327.

Tran A, Yates J, Lau A, Lampron J, Matar M. Permissive hypotension versus conventional resuscitation strategies in adult trauma patients with hemorrhagic shock. *J Trauma Acute Care Surg.* 2018 May;84(5):802-808.

Worthley L. Shock: a review of pathology and management, part I. *Crit Care Resusc.* 2000;2:55-65.

CHAPTER 13

ALTERED MENTAL STATUS

Elizabeth Barrall Werley

QUESTIONS AND ANSWERS

1. What does altered mental status mean?

   Altered mental status is a disorder of consciousness; disorders of consciousness are divided into issues of arousal, thought content, or some combination of both. Dementia is more progressive in nature. Coma can be acute or progressive. Delirium is typically more abrupt in onset, over hours or days.[1,2] Both coma and delirium can fall under the category of acute "altered mental status."

   With dementia, content degrades over time, but arousal remains relatively intact. Delirium is abnormal function of both arousal and content, although some variable function remains. Coma is outright failure of those functions.[1]

2. What other terms may be used to describe altered mental status?

   A wide variety of terminology may be used to describe the spectrum of illness that is "altered mental status": mental status change, delirium, confusion, acute confusional state, organic brain syndrome, stupor, obtunded, encephalopathy, among others.[1,2]

3. How frequent is altered mental status?

   Estimates show that anywhere from 3% to 10% of patients presenting to the Emergency Department are altered.[3,4] Other estimates show that up to 40% of elderly patients present to the Emergency Department with a complaint of altered mental status, and up to 10% to 25% of all elderly patients meet the definition of delirium at the time of admission.[1,4] The rate of mortality is higher in those patients presenting with delirium. Therefore, every provider should be cognizant of the frequency of altered mental status.[5]

4. What causes altered mental status?

   A simplistic approach to altered mental status is to consider structural neurologic pathology, which represents about 15% of cases, and metabolic or other systemic factors (including external factors, such as toxins), which represents the other 85% of cases.[1,3]

   Causes of altered mental status differ by age. In adolescents and young adults, traumatic injuries, recreational drug use, and other toxic ingestions are most frequent. The elderly are also subject to trauma and are particularly sensitive to prescription and nonprescription medications or medication changes. In addition, they are more prone to other causes, such as stroke and infection, and even environmental changes.[3]

   Regarding the danger associated with altered mental status, the timing of onset correlates with severity. Slowly progressive causes, such as dementia, are less likely to be acutely life-threatening. The converse is also true; the more acute in presentation and the more deranged from baseline the patient is, the increased likelihood of a life-threatening condition.[4]

   When considering all patients, the spectrum of causes is broad and not limited to[2,3]:
   - Central nervous system disease, such as seizure, stroke, mass, trauma
   - Respiratory abnormalities leading to hypoxia, hypercapnia
   - Endocrine problems including glucose disorders (hypoglycemia and hyperglycemia), thyroid disorders, and others
   - Metabolic disorders
   - Decreased cerebral perfusion states due to shock
   - Fluid, electrolyte, and acid-base disturbances
   - Infections
   - Endogenous toxins (i.e., ammonia, uremia, carbon dioxide)
   - Exogenous toxins: alcohols, medications, drugs of abuse, environmental toxins, and other chemicals
   - Drug or alcohol withdrawal
   - Temperature extremes, both environmental temperatures and temperature-regulation disorders
   - Idiopathic

5. If the patient is altered, how does an EMS provider acquire any information?

   The best approach to the altered patient is to obtain as much historical information as possible, patient status permitting. Sometimes, there will be little or no information to obtain on the scene, and the patient will be promptly transported to the hospital. Whenever possible, a provider should attempt to obtain a brief history from the patient, family or friends, other bystanders, or staff if at a residential care facility.[2,3,6] It is important to ascertain the

- Timing of events
- Associated or preceding symptoms
- Relevant past medical history
- Medications, including prescriptions, over-the-counter, and herbals/supplements. Consideration should be taken to other medications available in the house (those not prescribed to the patient) as well as to any recent medication changes.
- Physical exam, which may point to a source: signs of trauma, elevated body temperature indicating fever, signs of toxidromes, etc.
- Discernable information from the surrounding environment: blood or disruption of the scene, drug abuse paraphernalia, medication bottles or pills, suicide note, possible environmental exposures

6. What is the role of point-of-care laboratory testing?

If available, a point-of-care glucose should be obtained on all patients. There are few absolutes in medicine, but ruling out a rapidly correctable problem such as hypoglycemia is one thing that should always occur.[4] An elevated glucose may also guide prehospital management.

7. What is the role of EMS in the overdose patient?

EMS and emergency physicians and staff share similar roles in managing the acute known or presumed overdose. The initial management does not change whether it is an intentional or accidental overdose; the primary goal is airway and cardiovascular stabilization. The second step is obtaining a history. The final step includes initiating therapies if a specific overdose is suspected.[7] Therefore, it is relevant for prehospital providers to at least know some common toxidromes. It is also helpful to be aware of common drugs of abuse and slang terminology for these drugs. The National Institute on Drug Abuse provides such a reference (https://www.drugabuse.gov/drugs-abuse/commonly-abused-drugs-charts).[8]

The ABCs of resuscitation (airway, breathing, circulation) remain a priority. Due to the sometimes rapid progression of illness seen with these patients, the ABCs should be evaluated first and reevaluated frequently.[7] History should focus on past medical history, history supplemented by family or friends, as well as environmental cues, such as pill bottle, etc.[2,7] Electrocardiogram testing and interpretation are especially important in the intoxicated patient. Specific findings, such as QR and QT prolongation, are concerning for developing cardiac toxicity.[7]

8. Are there any common treatments of overdose patients?

After the ABCs have been assessed, there are certain measures that can be trialed. Known or suspected hypoglycemia should be treated with intravenous dextrose. Those patients with respiratory depression, pinpoint pupils, and coma or near coma should have a trial of the opioid antagonist naloxone.[7] If a patient responds to an initial dose of naloxone but then declines, this is an indication to give more. If the patient has minimal or no response, there may be another drug involved or a non-opioid-related cause of the altered mental status.[2] Intravenous fluids may be warranted to replete volume losses. Agitated or violent patients may require chemical sedation. Routine gastrointestinal decontamination has fallen out of favor. Gastric lavage and activated charcoal have specific indications and can be deferred to the hospital setting; both require a protected airway, which in the case of altered mental status or coma typically means intubation.[7]

9. What if there are signs of trauma in the altered patient?

In addition to the ABCs, in the secondary survey, there should be a head-to-toe assessment of the patient. Look for evidence of head and neck injury, as well as other signs of trauma. Evidence of head and neck injury may include lacerations, contusions, abrasions, soft tissue avulsions, depressed skull fractures, hemotympanum, periauricular and periorbital ecchymosis, otorrhea, and rhinorrhea.[8] If there is any penetrating trauma to the head or neck, it should remain in place until definitive management in the hospital.[9]

A Glasgow Coma Scale (GCS) score should be calculated for every patient. The patient's motor and sensory function should be grossly assessed. Brainstem function can be assessed by pupillary size, symmetry and reactivity to light, extraocular eye movements, and respiratory patterns. Deterioration in neurologic function or development of focal findings when there previously were none may be signs of developing brain herniation.[9]

10. In addition to identifying signs of trauma, are there any other precautions that need to be taken?

In the setting of significant head trauma, associated cervical spine injury is seen frequently enough to warrant proper immobilization in transport.[9]

Depending on the injuries found on scene and the patient's mental status upon EMS arrival or enroute to the hospital, criteria may be met for transport to a designated trauma center. There are criteria for the specific levels of trauma centers, and the risks and benefits of diverting to a higher level of care must be considered depending on how stable the patient is. The same can be said when deciding between air and ground medical transport.[10]

Unfortunately, there is not much prehospital providers can do for primary brain injury in the field beyond appropriate recognition, triage, initial stabilization, and transport. However, prehospital care can make a significant impact on outcomes by preventing or minimizing secondary brain injury that results from hypotension, hypoxia, hypocarbia and hypercarbia, anemia, and hyperpyrexia.[9]

11. What do you do if the altered patient is agitated or violent?

If an altered patient is agitated or violent, various efforts should be made to calm the patient. The safest strategy is to attempt verbal and environmental deescalation, although this may not work if the patient is already altered. The next strategy is to attempt anxiolysis with oral medications, safety of the patient and staff permitting and if available in the prehospital setting. If these measures are unsuccessful, the acutely agitated or violent patient may require intramuscular (IM) or intravenous (IV) sedation. Occasionally, patients may also need to be physically restrained, but this is typically preferred in conjunction with chemical restraint than as an isolated measure. It is best to use the lowest possible dose necessary to safely provide care to the patient.[4,11]

Various agents are available for sedation should an agitated or violent patient require them. Two mainstays of treatment options include benzodiazepines (often lorazepam and midazolam in this setting) and butyrophenones (such as haloperidol and droperidol). Atypical antipsychotics are also being used in increasing frequency.[4,11] Ketamine is also an alternative option.[4] All drugs used for chemical sedation should be guided by regional and state protocols.

12. Can an altered patient refuse care?

It is unlikely that the altered patient is capable of refusing care. Medical personnel may be protected by implied consent laws if a patient is altered.[2] Competency is a more complex and time-intensive medical evaluation. In the prehospital setting, the relevant question is that of patient capacity. In determining capacity, the patient must comprehend their medical problem, as well as the potential alternative treatments, if any, and the risks and benefits of refusing care. They should also be making the decision freely of their own accord, not under duress or influence of anyone else.[2,5] If they cannot do so, they are unlikely to have capacity to make such decisions. Prehospital personnel may require assistance of family or police to encourage the patient to cooperate with care or require chemical and/or physical restraint to safely transport the patient. All supporting documentation should acknowledge the lack of capacity and the contributing factors in play.[2]

KEY POINTS

- The likelihood of a life-threatening emergency is directly related to the rapidity in which symptoms develop and how far from baseline the patient's mental status varies.
- All patients with altered mental status should be assessed for rapidly correctable etiologies, such as hypoglycemia, and treated accordingly.
- If the patient can provide little or no history, it is important to get as much historical information from the persons with the patient and environmental cues.

REFERENCES

1. Huff SJ. Altered mental status and coma. In: Tintinalli JE, Stapczynski JS, Ma O, Yealy DM, Meckler GD, Cline DM, eds. *Tintinalli's Emergency Medicine: A Comprehensive Study Guide*. New York, NY: McGraw-Hill; 2016.
2. Stackpool M. Altered mental status. In: Pons PT, Markovchick VJ, eds. *Prehospital Care: Pearls and Pitfalls*. Shelton, CT: People's Medical Pub. House; 2012:257-266.
3. Bassin BS, Cooke JL, Barsan WG. Altered mental status and coma. In: Adams JG, Barton ED, Collings J, DeBlieux PMC, Gisondi MA, Nadel E, eds. *Emergency Medicine Clinical Essentials*. Philadelphia, PA: Saunders; 2013:811-817e1.
4. Smith AT, Han JH. Altered mental status in the emergency department. *Semin Neurol.* 2019;39(01):5-19.
5. Wilber ST, Ondrejka JE. Altered mental status and delirium. *Emerg Med Clin N Am.* 2016;34(3):649-665.
6. Lei C, Smith C. Depressed consciousness and coma. In: Walls RM, Hockberger RS, Gausche-Hill M, eds. *Rosen's Emergency Medicine: Concepts and Clinical Practice*. Philadelphia, PA: Elsevier; 2018:123-131e1.
7. Chatterjee P, Perrone J. Drug overdoses and toxic ingestions. In: Lanken PN, Manaker S, Kohl BA, Hanson CW, eds. *Intensive Care Unit Manual*. Philadelphia, PA: Elsevier; 2014:557-567e1.
8. National Institute on Drug Abuse. Commonly abused drugs charts. Modified July 2019. https://www.drugabuse.gov/drugs-abuse/commonly-abused-drugs-charts.
9. Papa L, Goldberg SA. Head trauma. In: Walls RM, Hockberger RS, Gausche-Hill M, eds. *Rosen's Emergency Medicine: Concepts and Clinical Practice*. Philadelphia, PA: Elsevier; 2018:301-329e5.
10. Reid T, Spain DA. Prehospital management of the trauma patient. In: Cameron JL, Cameron AM, eds. *Current Surgical Therapy*. Philadelphia, PA: Elsevier; 2017:1121-1125.
11. Isaacs E. The violent patient. In: Adams JG, Barton ED, Collings J, DeBlieux PMC, Gisondi MA, Nadel E, eds. *Emergency Medicine Clinical Essentials*. Philadelphia, PA: Saunders; 2013:1630-1638e1.

CHAPTER 14

ARRHYTHMIAS AND ELECTROCARDIOGRAM INTERPRETATION

Christopher Tems

QUESTIONS AND ANSWERS

1. What is an EKG?
   An electrocardiogram (EKG/ECG) is a graphic recording of electrical potentials produced by the cardiac tissue and measured by electrodes placed at different sites on the body.

2. How does electrical activity travel through the heart?
   Cardiac conduction typically starts at the sinoatrial (SA) node near the top of the right atrium (Fig. 14.1). This impulse carries across the atria until it reaches the atrioventricular (AV) node, which is located near the junction of the atria and ventricles. The impulse is slightly delayed here as the atria contract. Conduction then continues down the bundle of His to the left and right bundle branches, which then break into Purkinje fibers in the ventricles. Heart rate is usually controlled by the fastest firing pacemaker. This should be the SA node at 60–100 beats per minute (bpm), but the controlling pacemaker activity may drop to lower sites in the setting of conduction system problems.

3. How do you interpret an EKG?
   The key is to be systematic! Read every EKG the same way every time. For prehospital purposes, the most critical points of EKG interpretation are identifying rate, rhythm, and evidence of myocardial ischemia.

4. What is a normal heart rate?
   The rate should normally be between 60 and 100. A heart rate <60 is considered bradycardia. A heart rate >100 is considered tachycardia.

5. How do you identify the rhythm?
   We will examine specific rhythms later. To understand rhythm, it is essential to ask four questions:
   - Is the rate fast or slow?
   - Are the QRS complexes narrow or wide?
   - Are the QRS complexes spaced regularly or irregularly?
   - Are there P waves present and what is their relation to the QRS complex?

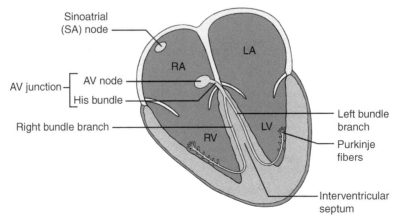

Fig. 14.1. Cardiac conduction system of the heart. *AV,* Atrioventricular; *RA,* right atrium; *LA,* left atrium; *RV,* right ventricle; *LV,* left ventricle. *(From Goldberger A, Goldberger Z, Shvilkin A. Goldberger's Clinical Electrocardiography. Philadelphia: Elsevier; 2018.)*

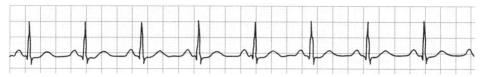

Fig. 14.2. Normal sinus rhythm. *(Courtesy of Christopher Tems, MD, FACEP.)*

6. What is a normal rhythm?
   Normal sinus rhythm (NSR) has a rate of 60–100, narrow and regular QRS complexes, P waves present, and every P wave associated with a QRS complex with a regular PR interval (Fig. 14.2).

7. What are the important bradycardias to know?
   You should be able to identify sinus bradycardia, AV blocks, and junctional and idioventricular rhythms (Fig. 14.3).

8. What is sinus bradycardia?
   Sinus bradycardia has a rate less than 60, narrow and regular QRS complexes, P waves present, and every P wave associated with QRS complex (Fig. 14.4). This is just NSR with a slower rate.

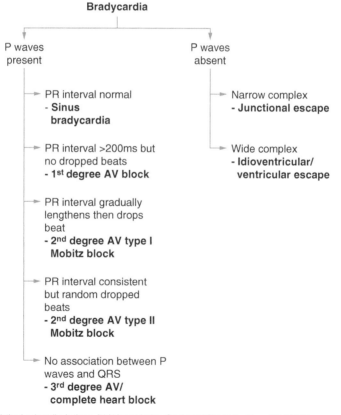

Bradycardia

P waves present

- PR interval normal
  - **Sinus bradycardia**

- PR interval >200ms but no dropped beats
  - **1st degree AV block**

- PR interval gradually lengthens then drops beat
  - **2nd degree AV type I Mobitz block**

- PR interval consistent but random dropped beats
  - **2nd degree AV type II Mobitz block**

- No association between P waves and QRS
  - **3rd degree AV/ complete heart block**

P waves absent

- Narrow complex
  - **Junctional escape**

- Wide complex
  - **Idioventricular/ ventricular escape**

Fig. 14.3. Differentiating bradycardic rhythms. *AV,* Atrioventricular. *(Courtesy of Christopher Tems, MD, FACEP.)*

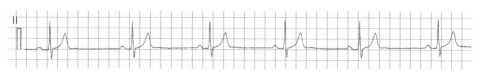

Fig. 14.4. Sinus bradycardia. *(From Goldberger A, Goldberger Z, Shvilkin A.* Goldberger's Clinical Electrocardiography. *Philadelphia: Elsevier; 2018.)*

This can be a normal variant seen during sleep or in young healthy adults or athletes. It may also be seen in the setting of pathologic processes such as myocardial infarction, beta-blockers or calcium channel blockers, hypothermia, hypoxia, or Cushing's reflex with high intracranial pressure. Arrhythmia treatment is usually not required. Address underlying causes if needed.

9. What are AV blocks?

There are four types of AV blocks.

- 1st degree AV block can have a rate that is slow, normal, or even fast! It will have a regular rhythm with narrow QRS complexes, P waves present, and every P wave associated with QRS complex (Fig. 14.5A). It is defined by a consistently long PR interval (>200 ms). It is caused by delayed conduction through the AV node with similar causes to sinus bradycardia earlier. Treatment is typically not required.
- 2nd degree AV block type I Mobitz is also known as Wenckebach. It can have a rate that is slow, normal, or fast. There are narrow QRS complexes but an irregular rhythm (look for "clumps" of beats) (Fig. 14.5B). P waves are present but sometimes are *not* associated with QRS complexes. It is defined by a PR interval that gradually lengthens until there is a nonconducting P wave and dropped beat. This is usually caused by a reversible conduction block at the AV node. Treatment is typically not required.
- 2nd degree AV block type II Mobitz can have a rate that is slow, normal, or fast. There are narrow QRS complexes but an irregular rhythm (Fig. 14.5C). P waves are present but sometimes are *not* associated with QRS complexes. It is defined by a constant PR interval but an intermittently nonconducting P wave and dropped beat. This is caused by conduction block below the AV node (His/Purkinje fibers). This is more frequently due to structural damage to the conducting system but may also be seen with hyperkalemia or medications. Treatment is more frequently needed and this rhythm may progress to 3rd degree heart block. Many of these patients will require a permanent pacemaker.
- 3rd degree AV block typically is also known as complete heart block. It has a slow rate, usually a regular rhythm, and there may be a narrow or wide complex QRS depending on the underlying escape rhythm (Fig. 14.5D). It is defined by complete absence of AV conduction. P waves are present, but the PR interval is

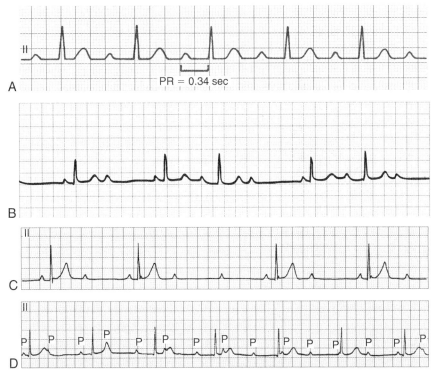

Fig. 14.5. Atrioventricular (AV) blocks. (A) First-degree AV Block. (B) Second-degree AV type I Mobitz. (C) Second-degree AV type II Mobitz. (D) Third-degree AV block. *(A, C, D, From Goldberger A, Goldberger Z, Shvilkin A.* Goldberger's Clinical Electrocardiography. *Philadelphia: Elsevier; 2018. B, From Yealy DM, Kosowsky JM. Dysrhythmias. In: Walls RM, Hockberger RS, Gausche-Hill M, eds.* Rosen's Emergency Medicine: Concepts and Clinical Practice. *Philadelphia: Elsevier; 2018.)*

random and there is *no association* between P waves and QRS complexes. This is most commonly due to fatigue of AV nodal cells or sudden loss of conduction through the His/Purkinje system. Treatment is usually required as these patients are often hemodynamically unstable or at least symptomatic from their arrhythmia. These patients will often require emergent transcutaneous pacing. These patients will usually require a permanent pacemaker.

10. What are junctional rhythms?

These rhythms are narrow complex and regular, but normal P waves are *not* present. You may just see the QRS complex without a preceding P wave or retrograde P waves (after the QRS) may be present (Fig. 14.6). These are usually slow junctional escape rhythms at 40–60 but may be accelerated junctional rhythms with a normal rate or isolated junctional beats. It is caused by enhanced automaticity near the AV node and decreased automaticity of the SA node. Treatment is aimed at the underlying cause. If symptomatic or unstable, you can use medications or pacing as discussed later.

11. What are idioventricular rhythms?

These are slow ventricular escape rhythms at 20–40. These rhythms are wide complex and usually regular. P waves may or may not be present but will not be associated with the QRS (Fig. 14.7). This is caused by a decreased automaticity of higher pacemakers resulting in cardiac contractions that originate in the ventricles. Treatment is usually required, and these patients are frequently critically ill. This may not be a perfusing rhythm, so be sure to check for a pulse! Medications may be ineffective, and these patients often require transcutaneous pacing.

12. Is there a general treatment algorithm that can be used for bradycardia?

Yes! First, make sure you are addressing underlying causes such as hypothermia, hyperkalemia, hypoxia, or increased intracranial pressure. If the patient is symptomatic and you suspect this is due to the slow heart rate, you should start with atropine 0.5 mg IV. This can be repeated every 3–5 minutes to a total dose of 3 mg. If atropine does not seem to be effective, consider starting an intravenous (IV) infusion of epinephrine (2–10 mcg/min) or dopamine (2–20 mcg/kg/min). If the patient is unstable and not responding rapidly to medications, start transcutaneous pacing.

Atropine will not work in patients who have had a heart transplant. In these cases, move directly to epinephrine, dopamine, or pacing.

13. What are bundle branch blocks?

Bundle branch blocks result from a conduction delay in one of the two bundle branches (Fig. 14.8). Both right (RBBB) and left (LBBB) bundle branch blocks are common. An LBBB is defined by a long QRS (>120 ms), a broad prominent S wave in V1, and a broad notched/slurred upright QRS complex in V6. LBBB often has discordant (in an opposite direction to the QRS complex) ST elevation of <5 mm. An RBBB is defined by a long QRS (>120 ms), an rSR' pattern in V1, and wide deep S waves in V6. With an RBBB, any ST elevation is abnormal.

14. What are the important narrow complex tachycardias to know?

You should be able to identify sinus tachycardia, supraventricular tachycardia (SVT), atrial fibrillation (AF), and atrial flutter (Fig. 14.9).

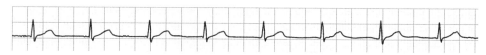

Fig. 14.6. Junctional rhythm. *(Courtesy of Christopher Tems, MD, FACEP.)*

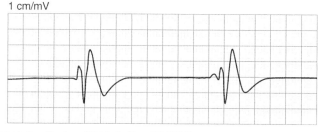

1 cm/mV

Fig. 14.7. Idioventricular rhythm. *(Courtesy of Christopher Tems, MD, FACEP.)*

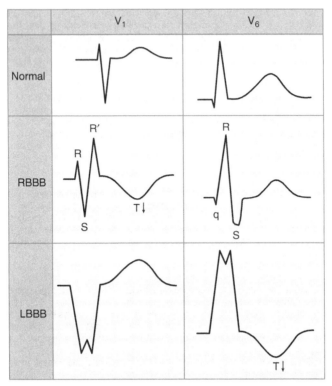

Fig. 14.8. Bundle branch blocks. *LBBB*, Left bundle branch block; *RBBB*, right bundle branch block. *(From Goldberger AL, Goldberger ZD, Shvilkin A. Goldberger's Clinical Electrocardiography: A Simplified Approach. 9th ed. Philadelphia: Elsevier; 2017.)*

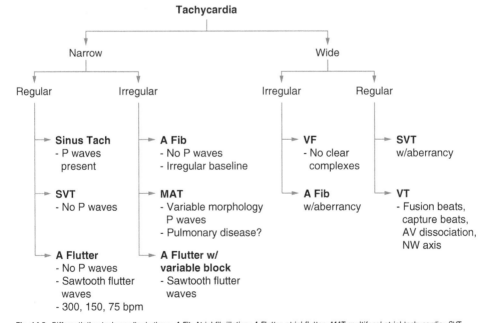

Fig. 14.9. Differentiating tachycardic rhythms. *A Fib*, Atrial fibrillation; *A Flutter*, atrial flutter; *MAT*, multifocal atrial tachycardia; *SVT*, supraventricular tachycardia; *VF*, ventricular fibrillation; *VT*, ventricular tachycardia. *(Courtesy of Christopher Tems, MD, FACEP.)*

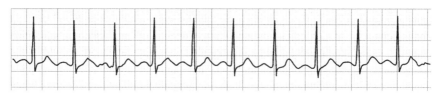

Fig. 14.10. Sinus tachycardia. *(Courtesy of Christopher Tems, MD, FACEP.)*

15. What is sinus tachycardia?

Sinus tachycardia has a rate >100, narrow and regular QRS complexes, P waves present, and every P wave associated with QRS complex (Fig. 14.10). This is just NSR with a faster rate. It is always secondary to another process. It may be due to exercise, dehydration, pain, fever, sepsis, hypoxia, pulmonary embolism, shock, or medications or drugs such as sympathomimetics or caffeine. Treatment is directed at the underlying cause.

16. What is SVT?

SVT has a rate >100 and narrow, regular QRS complexes (Fig. 14.11). It is often much faster than 100 bpm, and the rate typically does not vary by more than 5 bpm. P waves are usually not seen, but if P waves are present, they will be retrograde. SVT is caused by reentry circuits arising above the bundle of His.

Treatment should start with vagal maneuvers. Progress to adenosine 6 mg IV if vagal maneuvers fail. If this is unsuccessful, use adenosine 12 mg IV. If adenosine is not successful, you can consider a calcium channel blocker such as diltiazem (0.25 mg/kg IV) or a beta-blocker such as metoprolol (5 mg IV) if the blood pressure is stable. If the patient is unstable, treatment should be synchronized cardioversion (50–100 J).

17. What are AF and atrial flutter?

Atrial fibrillation (AF) can have a fast, normal, or slow rate. It is an irregularly irregular rhythm usually with narrow QRS complexes (Fig. 14.12). There are random atrial depolarizations so P waves are not seen and the EKG baseline will have rough fibrillatory waves. When the pulse is palpated, an irregularly irregular rhythm with different pulse amplitudes will be felt. When the heart rate is >100, it is termed AF with rapid ventricular response (RVR).

Atrial flutter is similar to AF both in etiology and in treatment. Atrial flutter can be fast, normal, or slow. It is typically a regular, narrow complex rhythm with "sawtooth" flutter waves. P waves are not seen (Fig. 14.13). There is often a variable AV block, most typically 2:1 block with two flutter waves for each QRS complex, but you may also see 3:1, 4:1, or variable block. If there is a variable block, the rhythm will be irregular.

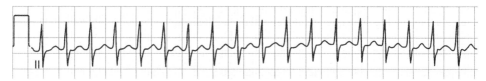

Fig. 14.11. Supraventricular tachycardia. *(Courtesy of Christopher Tems, MD, FACEP.)*

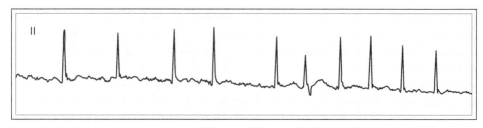

Fig. 14.12. Atrial fibrillation. *(From Adams J, Barton E, Collings J, et al.* Emergency Medicine: Clinical Essentials. *2nd ed. Philadelphia: Elsevier; 2013.)*

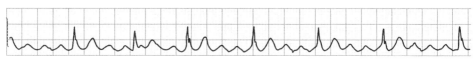

Fig. 14.13. Atrial flutter. *(Courtesy of Christopher Tems, MD, FACEP.)*

Atrial flutter and fibrillation are the most common sustained arrhythmias. Treatment depends on the heart rate and symptoms. It will most frequently be an episode of AF with RVR that brings the patient to seek emergency care. In this situation, if the patient is stable but symptomatic from their tachycardia, generally start with diltiazem (0.25 mg/kg IV) or metoprolol (5 mg IV) for rate control. If the patient is unstable, proceed with synchronized cardioversion (120–200 J).

18. What are the important wide complex tachycardias to know?
You should be able to identify ventricular tachycardia (VT) and differentiate this from one of the previous rhythms with aberrant conduction.

19. What is aberrant conduction?
Aberrant conduction results from an abnormal conduction system. This may be seen when the earlier arrhythmias occur in a patient with an underlying RBBB or LBBB or with accessory pathways such as in Wolff-Parkinson-White syndrome. This can make a typically "narrow complex tachycardia" appear to be wide complex. The most important arrhythmia with aberrant conduction to be able to identify is wide complex AF. This appears to be an irregularly irregular wide complex rhythm. Especially in a young patient, this is most commonly due to an accessory pathway. In this subset of AF, calcium channel and beta-blockers should be avoided as they can lead to ventricular fibrillation (VF). These patients should be treated with synchronized cardioversion if unstable and discussed with medical control if stable.

20. What is VT?
VT has a rate >100, usually 150–200. It has a regular rhythm with wide QRS complexes. This can be difficult to differentiate from SVT with aberrancy. Monomorphic VT originates from a single ventricular focus with identical QRS complexes (Fig. 14.14A). Polymorphic VT originates from multiple ventricular foci with variable morphology QRS complexes. Torsades de Pointes (TdP) is a subset of polymorphic VT that is due to QT prolongation (Fig. 14.14B). QRS complexes are seen to rotate around an isoelectric line.

21. How are wide complex tachycardias treated?
If debating whether a wide complex is VT or SVT with aberrancy, it is safer to assume the rhythm is VT as 80% of the time this is correct. In patients with a history of heart disease or advanced age, it is even more likely that the underlying rhythm is VT. If the patient is stable, start management with amiodarone (150 mg IV) or lidocaine (1.5 mg/kg IV). If the patient has TdP, treat with magnesium sulfate (2 g IV bolus). If the patient is unstable but has a pulse, perform synchronized cardioversion (100–200 J). If the patient is pulseless, proceed with cardiopulmonary resuscitation (CPR) and immediate defibrillation at 200 J.

22. What agonal (cardiac arrest) rhythms are important to know?
In addition to VT, you should be able to identify VF, pulseless electrical activity (PEA), and asystole.

23. What is VF?
VF has disorganized ventricular depolarizations that appear as a coarse baseline without clear QRS complexes (Fig. 14.15). The amplitude of VF tends to decrease with time with coarse VF degenerating to fine VF to asystole. These patients will always be pulseless. If you see what looks like VF in a patient who is talking to you, it is not VF! Consider shivering, tremor, or lead placement issues.
Treatment is aimed at restoration of circulation. Immediately start CPR. Defibrillate at 200 J. Follow standard advanced cardiac life support (ACLS) algorithms.

24. What is PEA?
PEA can be any organized rhythm on the EKG but without a pulse. Treatment is aimed at addressing underlying potentially reversible processes. Consider the "H's and T's"—hypovolemia, hypoxia, hypoglycemia, hypothermia,

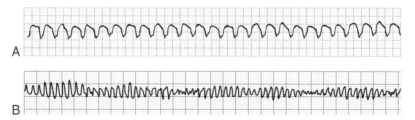

Fig. 14.14. Ventricular tachycardia. (A) Monomorphic ventricular tachycardia. (B) Torsades de Pointes. *(A, From Yealy DM, Kosowsky JM. Dysrhythmias. In: Walls RM, Hockberger RS, Gausche-Hill M, eds. Rosen's Emergency Medicine: Concepts and Clinical Practice. Philadelphia: Elsevier; 2018.)*

1 cm/mV

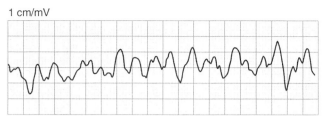

Fig. 14.15. Ventricular fibrillation. *(Courtesy of Christopher Tems, MD, FACEP.)*

hyperkalemia, hydrogen ion (acidosis), trauma, toxins, tension pneumothorax, tamponade (cardiac), and thrombosis (myocardial infarction or pulmonary embolism).

Address potentially reversible causes as earlier. Follow standard ACLS algorithms. There is no role for atropine, transcutaneous pacing, or cardioversion/defibrillation.

25. What is asystole?

Asystole is a "flatlined" EKG, but there may be occasional irregular electrical complexes (Fig. 14.16). The patient will always be pulseless. Treatment is aimed at addressing reversible causes of the arrest and restoring circulation. Start immediate CPR and initiate ACLS algorithms. There is no indication for atropine, pacing, or cardioversion/defibrillation.

26. What does ischemia look like on an EKG?

Myocardial ischemia most frequently manifests as changes to the ST segment or T wave of the EKG. This can manifest as ST depression, T wave inversions, or ST elevation (Fig. 14.17A and B). The most crucial manifestation of ischemia to identify is ST elevation myocardial infarction (STEMI). This is diagnosed with ST elevation of at least 1 mm (1 small box) in two contiguous leads, and there is often reciprocal ST depression in other leads. STEMI is important to identify as these patients are candidates for rapid reperfusion therapy with either cardiac catheterization or thrombolysis. All prehospital systems should incorporate prehospital STEMI notification into catheterization lab activation protocols.

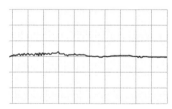

Fig. 14.16. Asystole. *(Courtesy of Christopher Tems, MD, FACEP.)*

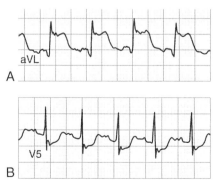

Fig. 14.17. Ischemic manifestations. (A) ST elevation. (B) ST depression. *(Courtesy of Christopher Tems, MD, FACEP.)*

27. Can the EKG show you which part of the heart is affected or which vessel may be occluded in a STEMI?
Inferior STEMI is identified with ST elevation in leads II, III, and aVF. Reciprocal changes (ST depression) are frequently seen in I and aVL. This is typically caused by an occlusion of the right coronary artery (RCA). Inferior STEMI also frequently involves infarction of the right ventricle so nitroglycerin should be avoided in these patients. Anteroseptal STEMI is identified with ST elevation in leads V1–V4. This is typically caused by an occlusion of the left anterior descending artery (LAD). Lateral STEMI is identified with ST elevation in leads V5–V6, I, and aVL and is usually due to an occlusion of the left circumflex artery. Posterior STEMI can be difficult to diagnose but is identified with ST depression in V1–V2 with tall R waves and upright T waves. It may be easier to identify with posterior placement of EKG leads. It is typically caused by an occlusion of the posterior descending artery.

KEY POINTS

- Systematically approach every EKG the same way every time to become expert at interpretation.
- Look at the rate, whether the rhythm is regular or irregular, if QRS complexes are wide or narrow, and for the presence of P waves to discern the cardiac rhythm.
- Treatment of arrhythmias in the prehospital setting should be based on whether the patient is symptomatic or unstable.

BIBLIOGRAPHY

Adams J, Barton E, Collings J, et al. *Emergency Medicine Clinical Essentials*. Philadelphia: Elsevier; 2013.
Dubin D. *Rapid Interpretation of EKGs*. 6th ed. Tampa: Cover Publishing; 2000.
Goldberger A, Goldberger Z, Shvilkin A. *Goldberger's Clinical Electrocardiography*. Philadelphia: Elsevier; 2018.
Link MS, Berkow LC, Kudenchuk PJ, et al. Part 7: adult advanced cardiovascular life support: 2015 American Heart Association guidelines update for cardiopulmonary resuscitation and emergency cardiovascular care. *Circulation*. 2015;132(suppl 2):S444-S464.
Mirvis DM, Goldberger AL. *Braunwald's Heart Disease: A Textbook of Cardiovascular Medicine*. Philadelphia: Elsevier; 2019.
Morris F, Edhouse J, Brady WJ, Camm J. *ABCs of Clinical Electrocardiography*. London: BMJ Books; 2003.
Yealy DM, Kosowsky JM. Dysrhythmias. In: Walls RM, Hockberger RS, Gausche-Hill M, eds. *Rosen's Emergency Medicine, Concepts and Clinical Practice*. Philadelphia: Elsevier; 2018.

CHAPTER 15

CARDIAC EMERGENCIES—CHEST PAIN, STEMI, ACS, CHF

Michael J. Burla

CHEST PAIN

1. Name some life-threatening causes of chest pain.
   Chest pain can be due to a variety of causes. In the prehospital setting, it is always important to consider some of the more life-threatening etiologies to chest pain. Listed here are the "serious 6" concerning etiologies for chest pain:
   - Tension pneumothorax
   - Pulmonary embolism (PE)
   - Ruptured esophagus
   - Cardiac tamponade
   - Aortic dissection
   - Acute coronary syndrome (ACS)

2. What are some initial questions to assessing the type of chest pain a patient is experiencing?
   Having a good description of the chest pain can help identify the etiology of the symptoms. Asking about duration of symptoms, quality, intensity, frequency, location, and if it radiates to other parts of the body is a good start. In addition, identifying the precipitating factors or associated symptoms can provide important clues.

3. What are some initial steps in your physical exam to assessing chest pain in the prehospital setting?
   It is important to always start by assessing the patient's heart rate and breathing. If the patient is tachycardiac (fast heart rate) or tachypneic (fast breathing), it could be signs of heart or lung pathology. **In general, a heart rate above 100 beats per minute and respirations over 20 respirations per minute are abnormal.** Checking a pulse and observing respirations can be very helpful to determine how sick a patient is. Next, auscultating the heart and lungs can help guide management.

4. What are some findings that can be suggested with an electrocardiogram (EKG)?
   An EKG can detect and suggest many things clinically. One of the main reasons to obtain an EKG is to assess for ST-segment elevation myocardial infarction (STEMI) and ACS; however, there are EKG findings that can suggest pericardial effusion, pericarditis, PE, heart failure, left ventricular aneurysm, hypothermia, and electrolyte abnormalities (i.e., hyperkalemia, hypercalcemia, etc.). For this reason, an EKG should be performed on all patients with the complaint of chest pain or shortness of breath.

KEY POINTS: INITIAL ASSESSMENT OF CHEST PAIN

- Obtain vital signs (heart rate, respiratory rate, blood pressure, O_2 saturation).
- Auscultate the heart and lungs.
- Obtain an EKG.
- Develop a differential diagnosis.

STEMI AND ACS

1. What is a STEMI?
   STEMI stands for ST-segment elevation myocardial infarction. A STEMI is an episode of transmural infarction involving the entire thickness of the myocardium, demonstrated on EKG.

2. What are the EKG findings for a STEMI?
   - 1 mm of ST-segment elevation in two or more anatomically continuous leads (see Fig. 15.2) with reciprocal depression over areas opposite to the ST-segment elevation, or of injury.
   - Isolated ST-segment depression in V1–V4 is an indication of posterior STEMI and should be evaluated with a posterior lead EKG.

3. What parts of the heart correlate to EKG findings where a STEMI can be located?
Different areas on the EKG correlate with different regions of the heart.
- Septal: V1 and V2
- Anterior: V3 and V4
- Lateral: V5 and V6
- Anteroseptal: V1–V4
- Anterolateral: V3–V6
- Extensive anterior: V1–V6
- Inferior: II, III, aVF
- High lateral: I, aVL
- Posterior: tall R wave and ST depression in V1–V2

4. What are some STEMI mimics that could cause ST-segment elevation?
It is important to consider other causes of ST-segment elevation on an EKG other than a STEMI, especially when the patient's complaints do not correlate with typical ACS symptoms.
- Left ventricular hypertrophy
- Early repolarization
- Acute pericarditis
- Cor pulmonale
- Hyperkalemia
- Hypercalcemia
- Hypothermia
- Left ventricular aneurysm

5. What medications should be given to a patient with a STEMI or ACS?
In patients with possible STEMI or ACS, aspirin should be given. A dose of 160–325 mg PO or PR is acceptable. Aspirin alone can lead to a **23% reduction in mortality.**
Other medications that can help in the prehospital setting are as follows:
- Nitroglycerin for persistent chest pain (typically 0.4 mg sublingual, every 5 minutes for three doses as needed)
- Morphine for persistent chest pain (typically 0.1 mg/kg, or a 4-mg dose)
- Supplemental oxygen if the patient is hypoxic
Other medications such as heparin, clopidogrel, and abcixmab are best utilized in a hospital setting in collaboration with the emergency medicine physician and a cardiologist.

6. What is percutaneous coronary intervention (PCI)?
PCI is a procedure that uses a catheter inserted into a patient's femoral or radial artery to gain direct visualization of the patient's coronary arteries with dye injection. Primary PCI is utilized to treat STEMIs and other forms of myocardial infarctions. This is accomplished by placing a stent or angioplasty to open the narrowing of the coronary artery.

7. In patients with a STEMI, what are the recommendations for PCI?
The American Heart Association recommends PCI as the preferred treatment for STEMI or ACS. **Expected first medical contact to first balloon inflation time is ≤90 minutes**. From a prehospital standpoint, it is important to know which facilities have PCI capabilities.

8. What if PCI cannot be performed in under 90 minutes?
Immediate transfer to a PCI-capable facility is recommended if first medical contact to device is ≤120 minutes. If anticipated transfer time is >120 minutes, thrombolytics should be administered. This means possibly transferring a patient to a closer facility to receive thrombolytics and stabilization as opposed to attempting to get to the nearest PCI-capable facility.

9. Name some of the medications that should *not* be given to a patient with a STEMI or ACS in the acute, prehospital setting.
- Avoid beta-blockers in the presence of STEMI or ACS.
- Avoid supplemental oxygen if the patient is **not** hypoxic.

10. Are there any EKG findings that are considered STEMI equivalents?
Yes. There are a few EKG findings that would be considered STEMI equivalents in the presence of someone experiencing symptoms of ACS. Illustrated in the following are relevant STEMI equivalents.
- Proximal left anterior descending artery (LAD) or left main coronary artery occlusion (Fig. 15.1)
- Widespread ST-segment depression with ST elevation in aVR.
de Winter's T waves (Fig. 15.2)

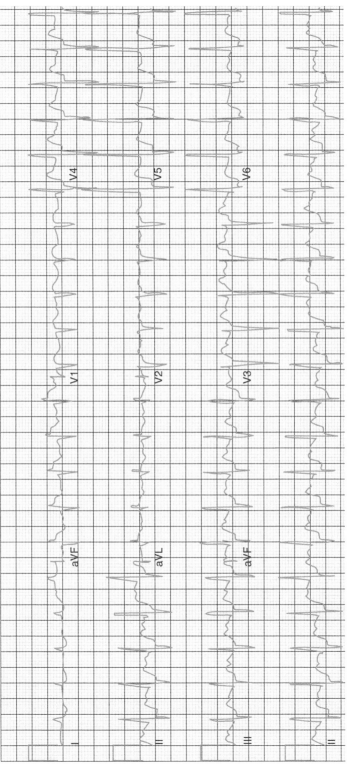

Fig. 15.1. This electrocardiogram demonstrates a proximal left anterior descending artery (LAD) or left main coronary artery (LMCA) occlusion. This is illustrated by the ST elevation in lead aVF, and the diffuse ST depression in all of the other leads. Proximal left anterior descending artery (LAD) or left main coronary artery (LMCA) occlusion. *Knotts RJ, Wilson JM, Kim E, Huang HD, Birnbaum Y. Diffuse ST depression with ST elevation in aVR: Is this pattern specific for global ischemia due to left main coronary artery disease? J Electrocard. 2013;46(3):240–248.*

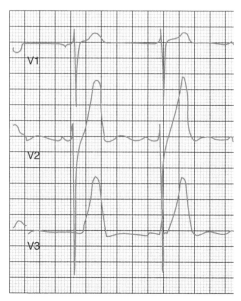

Fig. 15.2. de Winter's T waves. *Lawner BJ, Nable JV, Mattu, A, Novel patterns of ischemia and STEMI equivalents.* Cardiol Clin. *2012;30(4):591-599.*

- Tall peaked T waves in the precordial leads with precordial ST-segment depression at the J-point. Lead aVR might show slight ST elevation. This finding suggests proximal LAD lesion.
  Wellens' syndrome (Fig. 15.3)
- There are two types of morphology for Wellens' syndrome. Type A EKG findings are described as a biphasic T-wave pattern in V2 and V3. Type B EKG findings are described as deeply inverted and symmetric T waves. Both can have isoelectric or minimally elevated ST segments (<1 mm) and the absence of precordial Q waves with preserved R waves. These findings typically represent stenosis of the LAD and require PCI in the next 24 to 48 hours.

11. What about patients with a possible new left bundle branch block?
    While a new left bundle branch block in the setting of ACS symptoms is concerning, it is not considered a true STEMI equivalent anymore. For this reason, patients in this clinical scenario should not necessarily have immediate PCI with catheter lab activation but rather be treated as a high-risk ACS patient.

12. Describe EKG findings that can suggest a STEMI in the presence of a left bundle branch block.
    It can be difficult to interpret EKG changes when a patient has a left bundle branch block. Sgarbossa's criteria are a set of criteria to help identify a STEMI in the presence of a left bundle branch block or pacemaker.
    Sgarbossa's criteria:
- ≥3 points = 98% probability of STEMI
- ST-segment elevation ≥1 mm in a lead with upward (concordant) QRS complex—5 points
- ST-segment depression ≥1 mm in lead V1, V2, or V3—3 points
- ST-segment elevation ≥5 mm in a lead with downward (discordant) QRS complex—2 points

13. What about chest pain that is ACS but not a STEMI?
    ACS is defined as damage to the heart from decreased blood flow into the coronary arteries. There are different classifications to ACS, including angina, unstable angina, non-STEMI, and STEMI. It is important to note that even if the patient's EKG is normal, if they are having concerning symptoms of ACS, they should be treated as if they have ACS.

14. Describe the classic signs of ACS.
    One the most common presenting symptoms is **central chest pain or discomfort**. This chest discomfort is usually described as a pressure or squeezing sensation, worse with exertion, often associated with diaphoresis and/or nausea. The discomfort can radiate to the left arm, right arm, both, or the patient's jaw.

15. Do the signs of ACS change for the elderly?
    Yes. Patients above the age of 75 tend to have more atypical symptoms. These symptoms can include nausea, vomiting, light-headedness, upper back pain, fatigue, and dyspnea. In fact, dyspnea is the most common complaint for ACS in the elderly.

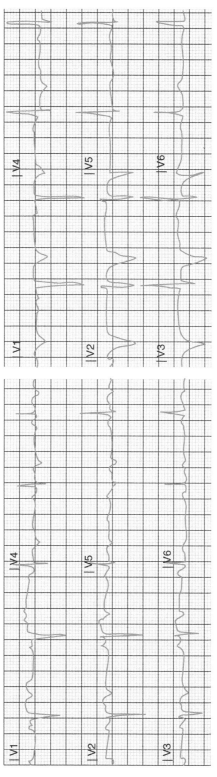

Fig. 15.3. Wellens' syndrome. *Lawner BJ, Nable JV, Mattu, A, Novel patterns of ischemia and STEMI equivalents. Cardiol Clin. 2012;30(4):591-599.*

16. Are there other populations that are also more prone to present with atypical symptoms?
   Yes. Women and diabetic patients are also well known to present with more atypical symptoms for ACS. However, it is important consider other populations that could present with atypical symptoms, which include patients with chronic kidney disease (CKD), chronic steroid use, psychiatric patients, altered mental status patients, human immunodeficiency virus (HIV) patients, and patients with lupus or other autoimmune conditions. It is also important to note that conditions such as CKD, HIV, autoimmune diseases, and vasculitis put patients at higher risk of ACS.

17. Describe the classic risk factors for ACS.
   The most common classic risk factors for ACS are smoking, hyperlipidemia, hypertension, family history of heart disease, obesity, and diabetes mellitus.

18. What are some EKG findings that can suggest ACS?
   - T-wave inversions or bimodal T waves.
   - Pathologic Q waves, ≥1 square wide, ≥1/3 height of R waves.
   - As stated earlier, a new left bundle branch block is still concerning for ACS.

19. Why is it important to obtain an EKG in the prehospital setting to assess for STEMI and ACS?
   Early recognition of STEMI in the prehospital setting has been shown to decrease time to PCI and achieve definitive care through prenotification. It is important to obtain an EKG in a patient who exhibits signs and symptoms of ACS to assess for ischemic EKG changes and STEMI. Early intervention leads to less ischemic time and better outcomes for the patient.

KEY POINTS: STEMI AND ACS

- Always give aspirin for STEMI and ACS.
- Obtain a prehospital EKG to assess for STEMI.
- Always consider the closest facility with PCI capabilities for STEMI.
- Consider morphine and/or nitroglycerin for symptom control.

CONGESTIVE HEART FAILURE

1. What is congestive heart failure (CHF)?
   CHF is cardiac dysfunction that leads to an inability of the heart to work as a pump to meet the circulatory demands of the patient. As a result, pulmonary congestion occurs, and when the problem is severe enough, pulmonary edema (lungs filled with fluids) results. This phenomenon occurs due to the increased pulmonary vascular volume, leading to an increase in hydrostatic pressure that pushes fluid out of the vascular and into the lung tissue.

2. What causes CHF?
   CHF can result for many reasons. There are typically four different causes for CHF, and in the prehospital setting, it can be important to try to identify them to help determine what other comorbidities a patient might have.
   - Ischemic (myocardial infarction)
   - Congestive (volume overload of the ventricle from valvular insufficiencies)
   - Hypertrophic (long-standing hypertension or valvular stenoses)
   - Restrictive (hemochromatosis, pericardial disease)

3. What types of symptoms are typical for CHF?
   CHF can have a variety of symptoms. The most common symptom that patients will describe is being short of breath, or dyspnea. This dyspnea is usually exacerbated with exertion; however, as CHF progresses, patients can experience symptoms even at rest. Patients may also complain of dyspnea while laying supine (orthopnea) or sudden onset of dyspnea at night (paroxysmal nocturnal dyspnea). These symptoms become worse with an exacerbation of CHF, which lead to an increase in preload.

4. Describe the vital signs that would be expected with a CHF exacerbation.
   Patients typically present with an elevated blood pressure, typically with a systolic blood pressure >180. Patients will also likely be tachycardic and tachypneic. If the patient is sick enough with pulmonary edema, they may be hypoxic as well.

5. Describe some physical exam findings of a CHF exacerbation.
   As stated earlier, the main symptom of CHF is dyspnea, so patients may present with labored breathing or tachypnea. This can be assessed by counting the patient's respirations per minute and observing if the patient is

using accessory muscles to help with breathing (i.e., subcostal retractions, use of neck muscles, etc.). The patient may also appear sweaty (diaphoretic) or exhibit jugular venous distension (JVD), which is an observation of jugular venous engorgement and pulsatile presentation due to right-sided heart strain from heart failure. The patient may also be coughing up frothy sputum and have rales on auscultation.

6. What is an initial intervention that can help in the prehospital setting?
It is important to check pulse oximetry to see if the patient is hypoxic. If a patient is hypoxic, placing them on a nasal cannula or continuous positive airway pressure (CPAP) for oxygen supplementation can be helpful. It can also be helpful to place the patient in a 30°–90° upright position, as laying the patient supine can worsen their respiratory status.

7. What medication can be given if the patient is in acute respiratory distress?
If a patient is in respiratory distress due to CHF, nitroglycerin is a first-line therapy that can quickly decrease a patient's preload. Typically, a 0.4-mg sublingual tablet can be given every 5 minutes up to three doses, which can also help reduce the patient's blood pressure. If possible, it can be administered intravenously at 0.1 mcg/kg/min—5 mcg/kg/min, and titrate up to blood pressure tolerance. Nitro paste is also an option, which can be spread across the patient's chest, although the onset time for this medication is much longer than the oral or IV routes.

8. Are there other interventions that can be done to help a patient in acute respiratory distress from CHF?
Noninvasive positive pressure ventilation (NPPV) has been shown to decrease the need for intubation in patients with acute respiratory distress.

9. What is NPPV and how does it work?
NPPV reduces preload by increasing intrathoracic pressure. This is accomplished by creating an airtight seal with the mask and the device pushing air into the patient's airway during inspiratory and expiratory phases. There are two types of NPPV, CPAP and bilevel positive airway pressure (BiPAP). Both methods can help increase positive end-expiratory pressure (PEEP), by recruiting compressed alveoli, which can allow for better oxygenation and gas exchange. Continuous positive airway pressure achieves this with constant pressure, while BiPAP utilizes a different inspiratory and expiratory pressure. Typically starting with an inspiratory pressure of 10–12 cm/H_2O and expiratory pressure of 5-6 cm/H_2O is reasonable.

10. Are there contraindications to NPPV?
Most contraindications to NPPV involve the patient's inability to participate in the treatment. This is due to the fact that the device will either not work or create a potential aspiration risk.
- Uncooperative patients
- Vomiting or aspiration risk
- Obtunded or unresponsive patients
- Facial trauma or burns to where the mask would be placed
- Poor mask fitting, inability to get good seal
    One other scenario to be cautious when using NPPV is when the patient is hypotensive. This is because the increased intrathoracic pressure caused by NPPV that leads to decreased preload is due to a decrease in venous return to the heart and thus lowers the patient's blood pressure.

11. What about diuretics? Do diuretics help in the prehospital setting?
In the prehospital setting, medications such as furosemide and other diuretics have not been shown to provide a benefit acutely. In addition, early administration of furosemide has the potential to be harmful, as patients with symptoms of CHF could also have other underlying pathologies of infection, dehydration, and other disease processes, in which a diuretic would be counterproductive.

12. Are there other medications to avoid?
In patients with CHF, typically, it is important to avoid antiarrhythmic medications other than digoxin and amiodarone. Although digoxin and amiodarone can have some indication for CHF in the acute setting, more often, these interventions are initiated in the hospital setting as opposed to the prehospital setting. In addition, medications like calcium-channel blockers can worsen heart failure. **One other medication to avoid is morphine**; although it was potentially used for CHF in the past, it has actually been shown to increase morbidity.

13. What is the most important part of CHF management in the prehospital setting?
Respiratory stabilization in the acute CHF patient is the most important aspect of treating these patients in the prehospital setting. This includes supplemental oxygen, NPPV, and nitroglycerin or alternatives to nitroglycerin. Since in the prehospital setting, it is hard to know the exact etiology for a CHF exacerbation, it is important to avoid additional medications such as diuretics, arrhythmics, and other interventions until the patient is in the hospital setting.

KEY POINTS: CHF

- Sublingual nitroglycerin can help acutely.
- Early NPPV in an acutely ill CHF patient can help prevent intubation.
- Avoid morphine and early diuretics.

BIBLIOGRAPHY

Alexander KP, Newby LK, Cannon CP, et al. Acute coronary care in the elderly, part I: non-ST-segment-elevation acute coronary syndromes: a scientific statement for healthcare professionals from the American Heart Association Council on Clinical Cardiology: in collaboration with the Society of Geriatric Cardiology. *Circulation.* 2007;115:2549-2569.

de Winter RJ, Verouden NJ, Wellens HJ, Wilde AA. Interventional Cardiology Group of the Academic Medical Center. A new ECG sign of proximal LAD occlusion. *N Engl J Med.* 2008;359:2071-2073.

ECC Committee, Subcommittees and Task Forces of the AHA 2005 American Heart Association guidelines for cardiopulmonary resuscitation and emergency cardiovascular care. *Circulation.* 2005;112:IV1-IV203.

Knotts RJ, Wilson JM, Kim E, Huang HD, Birnbaum Y. Diffuse ST. depression with ST elevation in aVR: is this pattern specific for global ischemia due to left main coronary artery disease? *J Electrocard.* 2013;46(3):240-248.

Lawner BJ, Nable JV, Mattu A. Novel patterns of ischemia and STEMI equivalents. *Cardiol Clin.* 2012;30(4):591-599.

Mattu A, Lawner B. Prehospital management of congestive heart failure. *Heart Fail Clin.* 2009;5:19-24.

Mosesso VN, Dunford J, Blackwell T, Griswell JK. Prehospital therapy for acute congestive heart failure: state of the art. *Prehosp Emerg Care.* 2003;7:13-23.

O'Gara PT, Kushner FG, Ascheim DD, et al. 2013 ACCF/AHA guideline for the management of ST-elevation myocardial infarction: executive summary: a report of the American College of Cardiology Foundation/American Heart Association Task Force on Practice Guidelines. *Circulation.* 2013;127:529-555.

Rhinehardt J, Brady WJ, Perron AD, Mattu A. Electrocardiographic manifestations of Wellens' syndrome. *Am J Emerg Med.* 2002;20: 638-643.

Zègre-Hemsey JK, Patel MD, Fernandez AR, Pelter M, Brice J, Rosamond W. A statewide assessment of prehospital electrocardiography approaches of acquisition and interpretation for ST-elevation myocardial infarction based on emergency medical services characteristics. *Prehosp Emerg Care.* 2020;24:550-556.

CARDIAC DEVICE EMERGENCIES

Jordan B. Schooler and Joshua J. Davis

CHAPTER 16

QUESTIONS AND ANSWERS

Case: *You arrive on scene to find a 69-year-old female with a past medical history of atrial fibrillation, hypertension, and heart failure and an implantable defibrillator with a pacemaker. She called because her defibrillator shocked her.*

1. What are the types of implantable devices and their purposes?

   An implantable pacemaker is used to ensure that the heart rate is adequate when the native conduction system is not working properly. Indications for pacemakers are provided in Table 16.1. An implantable cardiac defibrillator (ICD) is an implantable device designed to provide electrical cardioversion to the heart when it goes into a dysrhythmia. Indications for an ICD are also provided in Table 16.1. All modern ICDs are also capable of acting as pacemakers, but not the reverse.

2. Your patient says she has a DDD pacemaker mode. What are the different settings for pacemakers?

   Pacemakers have a three- (or four-) letter abbreviation. The first letter indicates paced chamber, the second letter indicates the sensed chamber, and the third chamber indicates the response to sensing. Table 16.2 shows the different modes of pacemakers. A DDD pacemaker is what is nearly universally implanted in recent years. These pacemakers sense both chambers, pace both chambers, and have inhibitory and trigger modes for each chamber.

3. What are the major types of pacemaker malfunctions?

   Oversensing occurs when the pacemaker recognizes native beats that are not present. Output failure occurs when the pacer fails to generate a beat. Failure to capture occurs when the pacer fires, but the heart does not contract. Undersensing is when the pacemaker does not detect native beats and results in asynchronous pacing. Pacemaker associated tachycardia is a re-entrant tachycardia caused by sensing of retrograde p waves. Finally, leads can become dislodged or fractured, causing intermittent or complete failure to capture.

4. What are the treatments for pacemaker malfunction?

   This depends on the patient's heart rate and rhythm. In cases of bradycardia or ventricular tachycardia or fibrillation, the patient should be treated as though the pacemaker were not present. If there is bradycardia, medications may include atropine, epinephrine, dopamine, or isoproterenol. Transcutaneous pacing may also be performed. Patients in ventricular tachycardia or ventricular fibrillation can be defibrillated, but it is ideal to avoid placing the pads directly over the pacemaker. On the other hand, patients experiencing pacemaker-mediated tachycardia may require temporary suspension of pacemaker sensing using a magnet.

5. What does a magnet do when placed over a pacemaker?

   The most common response is for the device to go into asynchronous mode, often around 60 bpm (this would correspond to DOO, AOO, or VOO, depending on the paced chambers). Usually, normal function will resume when the magnet is removed. However, this response can vary depending on the pacemaker and its programming.

Table 16.1. Indications for an Implantable Cardiac Defibrillator or Pacemaker

CARDIAC DEFIBRILLATOR	PACEMAKER
Left ventricular function <30%–35%	Third-degree heart block, or high risk or symptomatic second-degree and occasionally first-degree heart block
Syncope of presumed cardiac cause (e.g., Brugada, long QT syndrome)	Irreversible symptomatic bradycardia
Inducible ventricular tachycardia or ventricular fibrillation	Intermittent asystole or prolonged sinus pause
Sustained ventricular tachycardia	Symptomatic sinus node dysfunction
Survivors of cardiac arrest from ventricular tachycardia or ventricular fibrillation	Symptomatic carotid dysfunction with prolonged asystole

Table 16.2. Types of Pacemaker Settings

PACING		SENSING		RESPONSE		RATE CONTROL	
0	None	0	None	0	None	0	None
A	Atrial	A	Atrial	I	Inhibit	P	Single programmable
V	Ventricular	V	Ventricular	T	Trigger	M	Multiprogrammable
D	Dual chamber	D	Dual chamber	D	Dual	R	Rate modulated

Note that most pacemakers are reported as only their three-letter abbreviation.

6. What is Twiddler's syndrome?

Twiddler's syndrome is a rare cause of lead fracture or dislodgement, resulting from repetitive movement of the pacemaker, either due to the patient playing with it or excessive mobility in adipose tissue.

7. What are the most common ways an ICD can malfunction?

The most common defibrillator complication is inappropriate shock. Most ICDs cannot interpret the patient's rhythm, so any tachycardia including atrial or sinus may trigger a shock if the rate is above the programmed threshold. Patients will often feel shocks but only an interrogation can tell whether they are appropriate or not. Frequent shocks may indicate an underlying problem with the heart or the device that needs further investigation. Just as with pacemakers, ICD leads may fracture or become dislodged, preventing shocks from being delivered.

8. What is the treatment for a patient who has been shocked by their ICD?

The key is to determine whether the shock is appropriate, and treat underlying causes of dysrhythmia. A patient who is receiving appropriate shocks should have external defibrillator pads placed, but they can continue to receive shocks from their defibrillator. Antiarrhythmic medications and analgesia should be considered. A patient with an ICD who experiences cardiac arrest should receive standard care according to basic life support (BLS) and advanced cardiac life support (ACLS) guidelines, including defibrillation with an external defibrillator. A patient receiving inappropriate shocks should have a magnet placed over the ICD to temporarily turn off the defibrillation function.

9. The patient says she got her pacemaker just 1 month ago. Are there any specific procedural risks after placement of a pacemaker or ICD?

Placement of either type of device may cause complications, including pneumothorax, lead infection, hematoma, pocket infection, or deep vein thrombosis (DVT).

10. What is the hospital going to do for this patient?

Any ICD that delivers a shock to a patient should be interrogated to determine the cause. The patient should be evaluated for dysrhythmia, lead fracture, infection, and causes of dysrhythmia such as cardiac ischemia or electrolyte abnormalities. This will frequently require an electrocardiogram, blood count, electrolyte panel, cardiac troponin, and a chest x-ray. Some patients may require additional testing including echocardiography or coronary angiography.

Case: You are called to the scene of an unresponsive patient. His wife notes that he has an LVAD. You cannot feel pulses.

11. What is an LVAD?

An LVAD is a left ventricular assist device. It is an implanted mechanical pump that supplements or replaces the function of the left side of the heart. It is often used for refractory or end-stage heart failure. It can be implanted as a bridge to a heart transplant or a "destination" therapy in patients who are not candidates for heart transplant. There are, very rarely, right ventricular assist devices placed (called RVADs), which have a similar mechanism but support the right ventricle instead.

12. What does it mean that you cannot feel a pulse in this patient?

Patients with most LVADs do not have a palpable pulse, as the machine pumps blood in a continuous fashion, and the patient's own cardiac contractility is often minimal or absent. Pulselessness alone is not an indication of cardiac arrest.

13. How do I know if an LVAD patient is in cardiac arrest?

If the LVAD is working, a hum should be heard on auscultation of the precordium. Tissue perfusion should be assessed, particularly mental status, spontaneous respiration, and capillary refill. End-tidal capnography can be very helpful, if available. Blood pressure may not be able to be measured without a Doppler ultrasound even if the LVAD is functional. Pulse oximetry may be falsely low or unreadable due to the low pulse pressure, although a normal value would be reassuring.

14. What are the most important aspects of prehospital care for a patient with an LVAD?

If the patient is in cardiac arrest, he or she should receive standard ACLS care including medication and defibrillation. Although there is some controversy regarding chest compressions due to the risk of disrupting the grafts, the consensus is that compressions should be performed if the patient truly appears to have no cardiac output (unresponsive, $EtCO_2$ <20 mm Hg). It is important to remember that if an LVAD is not functioning, the patient likely has very little native cardiac output and may need inotropic support to maintain perfusion.

The LVAD controller and at least one functioning battery must be transported with the patient. Backup batteries should be brought if possible. Any LVAD alarms, the flow and rotations per minute (RPMs), and the type of device should be noted and ideally transmitted in advance to the receiving hospital.

15. What are some common complications of LVADs?

LVADs have a driveline that passes through the skin and is connected to a battery-operated external controller. This is often a nidus for infection. If the driveline is disconnected, the LVAD will stop. Patients with LVADs are at risk of thrombosis due to the extensive artificial surface in contact with blood. This can lead to pump failure or stroke. For this reason, patients with LVADs must be anticoagulated, generally with aspirin and coumadin. This in turn often leads to bleeding, commonly in the gastrointestinal (GI) tract, nose, and brain. Anemia may also be caused by hemolysis of red blood cells as they travel through the LVAD pump. Patients with LVADs have underlying heart failure and are usually on diuretics. This predisposes them to electrolyte abnormalities and hypovolemia. While hypovolemic, patients can be at risk for "suction events" on the LVAD itself. This can also predispose them to dysrhythmias as the mechanical portion of the LVAD comes into contact with a large portion of the ventricular myocardium.

KEY POINTS

- In patients with an ICD or pacemaker, consider that the device may be malfunctioning and firing more than it should or not firing when it should be.
- Obtain a 12-lead EKG for any patient with an ICD or pacemaker who has chest pain, shortness of breath, palpitations, or receives a shock.
- Patients with nonfunctioning cardiac devices should be treated per ACLS algorithms. They can receive defibrillation and chest compressions.
- Patients with an LVAD routinely do not have a pulse. Evaluate for LVAD hum, mental status, and $EtCO_2$.

BIBLIOGRAPHY

Allison MG, Mallemat HA. Emergency care of patients with pacemakers and defibrillators. *Emerg Med Clin North Am.* 2015;33:653-667.
Greenwood J, Herr D. Mechanical circulatory support. *Emerg Med Clin North Am.* 2014;32:851-869.
McMullan J, Valento M, Attari M, Venkat A, Care of the pacemaker/implantable cardioverter defibrillator in the ED. *Am J Emerg Med.* 2007;25:812-822.
Partyka C, Taylor B. Review article: ventricular assist devices in the emergency department. *Emerg Med Australas.* 2014;26:104-112.
Peberdy MA, Gluck JA, Ornato JP, et al. Cardiopulmonary resuscitation in adults and children with mechanical circulatory support: a scientific statement from the American Heart Association. *Circulation.* 2017;135:e1115-e1134.

CHAPTER 17

GASTROINTESTINAL EMERGENCIES

Erica Bates

QUESTIONS AND ANSWERS

1. What elements of history are helpful to elicit from a patient with abdominal pain?

   Establish the location, severity, duration, and a description of the pain. Any associated symptoms, such as fevers, vomiting, diarrhea, dysuria, hematuria, or passing out, should be noted. Identify factors that improve or worsen the pain, such as movement or eating. Ask about any recent trauma. Women of childbearing age should be asked about pregnancy status. Obtain a complete past medical and surgical history, with special attention to any previous abdominal surgeries. A history of multiple abdominal surgeries increases the risk of bowel obstruction, and absence of the gallbladder, appendix, or ovary can help rapidly eliminate possibilities. Alcohol use should be assessed. Ask if the patient has experienced similar symptoms in the past and, if so, what diagnosis they received at that time.

2. Describe the key elements of the abdominal examination.

   Patients with abdominal pain should have a full set of vital signs including temperature. Assess the patient's general appearance and level of distress. The abdominal examination begins with inspection for distention, bruising, rash (such as shingles), previous surgical scars, or obvious hernia. Palpate all four quadrants of the abdomen, starting away from the area of greatest pain. Note any masses, enlargement of the liver, or focal tenderness. A pulsatile abdominal mass is a sign of abdominal aortic aneurysm. Guarding occurs when the patient tenses his or her muscles to protect against pain with palpation. It is called "voluntary guarding" when the patient can intentionally relax the muscles or stops guarding with distraction. "Involuntary guarding" occurs when the patient is unable to relax the abdomen and is worrisome. To assess for rebound tenderness, slowly push in on the abdomen, then release the pressure. Increased pain with removal of your hand is positive rebound tenderness and can be a sign of peritonitis from infection or organ perforation. Patients with peritonitis are often exquisitely sensitive to any movement of their stretcher or the ambulance.

3. What non-gastrointestinal (GI) conditions can present with abdominal pain or vomiting?

   Abdominal pain is not specific to the GI system. Abdominal aortic aneurysm or abdominal aortic dissection can present with abdominal pain. Diabetic ketoacidosis frequently causes vomiting and abdominal pain. Pneumonia in the lower lobes can also be felt as abdominal pain due to irritation of the diaphragm. A wide variety of toxic ingestions, including alcohol intoxication, can present with abdominal pain or vomiting. Myocardial infarction can present atypically with upper abdominal pain, nausea, or vomiting, especially in diabetic patients, women, and the elderly. Increased intracranial pressure from intracranial hemorrhage, stroke, a brain mass, or meningitis can cause vomiting. Genitourinary conditions such as testicular or ovarian torsion, renal stone, pyelonephritis, urinary retention, or pregnancy-related complications can also present with abdominal pain and vomiting. Have a low threshold to obtain a 12-lead electrocardiogram (EKG) or fingerstick glucose level in patients with abdominal pain or vomiting, especially if there is not a specific area of tenderness on palpation to suggest an intra-abdominal cause.

4. What is "bilious" vomiting and why does it matter?

   Bilious vomit is greenish vomit that receives its color from bile backing up into the stomach from the intestine. Even one episode of bilious vomiting in an infant is considered a surgical emergency until proven otherwise because it can be the first sign of bowel obstruction.

5. Describe the common serious causes of abdominal pain and vomiting in pediatric patients.

   Although many children who complain of abdominal pain and vomiting have viral illnesses, a number of potentially life-threatening conditions can present similarly. The differential diagnosis depends on the age of the patient. Young, especially premature, infants are at risk for a severe intestinal infection called necrotizing enterocolitis or congenital problems that cause obstruction. Pyloric stenosis usually occurs in infants less than 2 months old and is associated with projectile vomiting after feeds due to blockage of food from entering the small intestine. Infants and toddlers can have testicular torsion, intussusception, urine infections, volvulus, and incarcerated hernias. Appendicitis, diabetic ketoacidosis, ectopic pregnancy, ovarian torsion, pneumonia, sexually transmitted infections, and inflammatory bowel disease all affect pediatric patients. Even children with vomiting from a viral gastroenteritis can become profoundly dehydrated and require fluid resuscitation.

6. Does administering pain medication inhibit diagnosis of a patient with abdominal pain after they arrive at the hospital?

   No. Studies have shown that administering narcotic pain medication to patients with abdominal pain does not decrease the accuracy of physician examination and diagnosis. Appropriate pain control should be provided as indicated on a case-by-case basis.

7. **Does a patient with abdominal pain who has normal vital signs and a normal, nontender abdomen on examination still need to be transported to the hospital?**
    Yes. As discussed earlier, a wide range of serious medical conditions can cause abdominal pain in any age group. Most patients require some kind of diagnostic testing. Elderly patients with abdominal pain are at particularly high risk for having a life-threatening or surgical condition, even if their pain is not severe. The abdominal examination is also less reliable in elderly patients because they often do not experience pain the same way as younger people. Geriatric patients are less likely to show classic signs of peritonitis and are less likely to mount a fever during a serious infection.

8. **Name several potential complications of cirrhosis.**
    Patients with cirrhosis are at risk for serious bleeding because their liver does not produce clotting factors normally. Advanced liver disease also causes low platelets, which further worsens the ability to clot. The scarred liver causes high pressures in the venous system of the body, which produces varices (extremely dilated veins) in the esophagus, stomach, and rectum. These varices can rupture at any time and bleed profusely. Reduced filtration of waste products by the damaged liver can lead to a buildup of ammonia in the bloodstream, causing mental status changes ranging from mild confusion to coma (hepatic encephalopathy). Scarring of the liver also causes fluid retention, leading to shortness of breath from pulmonary edema or from tense buildup of abdominal fluid inhibiting expansion of the diaphragm. Finally, patients with cirrhosis are at risk for infections, including an infection of the fluid in the abdomen called spontaneous bacterial peritonitis. Cirrhosis also can affect the patients' ability to metabolize certain medications. For this reason, certain pain medications and sedatives like morphine or benzodiazepines should be avoided or be given at lower doses when possible. Cirrhotic patients also often have baseline blood pressures that are on the lower than normal range—ask the patient or family what their normal blood pressure usually runs at to gauge how far they are from their baseline.

9. **What are the most important steps to take in a patient with known or suspected GI bleed?**
    Hemodynamic status can deteriorate rapidly in a patient with GI bleeding. Obtain intravenous (IV) access early; two large-bore IVs should be established. Start fluid resuscitation as needed. Assess patients with hematemesis or altered mental status from shock to determine whether they are able to protect their airway. Vomiting alone without evidence of aspiration, respiratory distress, or poor mental status does not usually require intubation. If a patient has nausea or vomiting, elevate the head of the stretcher and position them with their head to the side to minimize the risk of aspiration. Antiemetics should be administered to vomiting patients. Cardiac monitoring and frequent blood pressure assessments should be performed. If the patient is not able to provide reliable history, it is very helpful to ask family whether the patient has a bleeding disorder or takes blood thinners so that the emergency department can rapidly initiate appropriate reversal medications if necessary. The patient should be made NPO in case they require an emergent endoscopy procedure.

10. **What are the common causes of upper and lower GI bleeding in adults?**
    Upper GI bleeding is bleeding that occurs above the ligament of Treitz, a structure located in the distal duodenum. Upper GI bleeding classically presents with either hematemesis or melena. Melena appears very dark or black because the blood is partially digested during transit through the GI tract. Patients with rapid upper GI bleeding can still have red blood in their stool, and it is not always possible to determine the source of the bleeding without endoscopy.
    Gastric or duodenal ulcers are a common cause of upper GI bleeding. Forceful vomiting can cause a rip in the lining of the esophagus, called a Mallory-Weiss tear. A Mallory-Weiss tear should be suspected when a patient reports bouts of nonbloody vomiting that later became streaked with red blood. Patients with a history of cirrhosis are also at risk for bleeding from esophageal or gastric varices.
    Lower GI bleeding comes from below the ligament of Treitz and typically presents with maroon or bright red blood mixed with the stool. Hemorrhoids are a very common cause of hematochezia. Diverticulosis is the development of outpouchings of bowel as we age. These diverticula sometimes bleed spontaneously, which is usually painless. Small blood vessel malformations, certain bacterial infections, and colon cancer can also cause lower GI bleeding.

11. **What causes of GI bleeding are seen in children, and how does treatment differ?**
    Ulcers, hemorrhoids, anal fissures, infections, intussusception, inflammatory bowel disease, Meckel's diverticulum, and bleeding disorders can cause gastrointestinal bleeding in children. Just like adults, the first steps are to assess the patient for hemodynamic stability, evaluate their airway if vomiting, start fluids when necessary, obtain the relevant history, and monitor vitals closely during transport. If you are transporting a pediatric patient with GI bleeding and hemophilia, notify the receiving facility early so they can have the correct medications available.

12. **What is biliary colic, and what are common infections involving the biliary system (cholecystitis, cholangitis)?**
    "Biliary colic" refers to abdominal pain in the right upper quadrant caused by gallstones. The pain often comes and goes as gallstones shift, may be associated with nausea and vomiting, and is classically worse after eating fatty foods. Unless a gallstone is blocking a duct in the biliary system, patients with recurrent gallstone pain

are often scheduled for gallbladder removal nonemergently. Gallstones alone do not cause fever. Cholecystitis, an infection of the gallbladder, causes right upper quadrant pain with or without fever. Cholecystitis requires antibiotics and surgical management. Cholangitis, an infection in the bile ducts themselves, can also present with fever and right upper quadrant pain. Cholangitis is a medical emergency that can progress rapidly to septic shock without treatment. Cholangitis is treated with antibiotics and drainage by a gastroenterologist.

KEY POINTS

- Patients with GI bleeding should have two large-bore IVs, cardiac monitoring, and frequent blood pressure measurements.
- Non-GI conditions, such as myocardial infarction and diabetic ketoacidosis, can present with abdominal pain and vomiting.
- Providing analgesia for severe abdominal pain does not prevent adequate diagnosis at the hospital.
- Patients with cirrhosis are at increased risk for serious bleeding, altered mental status, and infection.

BIBLIOGRAPHY

Kim BS, Li BT, Engel A, et al. Diagnosis of gastrointestinal bleeding: a practical guide for clinicians. *World J Gastrointest Pathophysiol.* 2014;5(4):467.

Magidson PD, Martinez JP. Abdominal pain in the geriatric patient. *Emerg Med Clin.* 2016;34(3):559-574.

Neidich GA, Cole SR. Gastrointestinal bleeding. *Pediatr Rev.* 2014;35(6):243-254.

Ranji SR, Goldman LE, Simel DL, Shojania KG. Do opiates affect the clinical evaluation of patients with acute abdominal pain? *JAMA.* 2006;296(14):1764-1774.

Smith J, Fox SM. Pediatric abdominal pain: an emergency medicine perspective. *Emerg Med Clin.* 2016;34(2):341-361.

Tsochatzis EA, Bosch J, Burroughs AK. Liver cirrhosis. *Lancet.* 2014;383(9930):1749-1761.

DIABETIC EMERGENCIES

Sarah K. Lewis and Susan B. Promes

CHAPTER 18

QUESTIONS AND ANSWERS

Case: *A neighbor calls 911 for someone continuously pounding trying to enter the apartment next door. They are worried that the person knocking is high on drugs. Police arrive to a confused male in his 20s and recognize a medical emergency. EMS is called. Meanwhile, the pale, diaphoretic male passes out across the doorway. With the noise of the sirens, the patient's girlfriend wakes up and comes to the door and finds her boyfriend's limp body is blocking the threshold and the officer right outside the door. She shouts, "He's diabetic!" She then proceeds to deliver a rescue glucagon injection to the patient. He wakes up slowly, is still weak, and vomits. The EMS crew arrives, notes a glucose level of 34, establishes an IV, gives a bolus of D10, and hangs 500 mL of normal saline. The patient arrives at the emergency department nauseated, with a glucose level of 60. When asked about the events leading up to the emergency, he remembers suddenly having a feeling of "being low" and knew he needed help. He could not unlock the door to their apartment in his hypoglycemic state, which is why he was pounding.*

1. What is diabetes and what do type 1 and type 2 diabetes have in common?

   Both types of diabetes involve abnormal glucose regulation. Although the pancreas is especially involved in insulin production and release into the blood, other organs, including the liver, kidneys, and intestines, also affect glucose regulation in the body.

2. How are type 1 and type 2 diabetes different from each other?

   Type 1 diabetes is caused by an autoimmune attack of the pancreatic cells that make insulin. Imagine insulin is a key that unlocks doors for glucose to get into cells. Without insulin, there are no keys to unlock the cell's doors so glucose cannot get in. Without insulin therapy, type 1 diabetic patients can build up high glucose levels in their blood, because the cells cannot get glucose into cells. Cells without glucose start to break down fats, spill ketones, and develop systemic acidosis. Your type 1 diabetes patients will need multiple daily insulin injections or continuous insulin via an insulin pump to avoid going into diabetic ketoacidosis, also known as DKA.

   Type 2 diabetes differs from type 1 in that the pancreatic cells make insulin, but the cells are resistant to this insulin. Using the key analogy again, the insulin keys are being made in response to elevated glucose levels, but the insulin keys can only fit a few locks. Again, the inability to autoregulate intravascular glucose results in hyperglycemia but is less likely to cause DKA as some insulin is functioning and allowing some glucose to enter cells. Additionally, when oral or injectable type 2 diabetes therapies are no longer regulating glucose levels well, type 2 diabetics can also require insulin injections. The insulin therapy increases the likelihood of insulin keys finding a matching lock, shifts glucose intracellularly, and allows the pancreas to not work so hard making insulin.

3. How prevalent is diabetes?

   About 9% of the US population has type 2 diabetes, and 0.5% have type 1.

4. At what level is a patient considered hypoglycemic?

   The American Diabetes Association defines hypoglycemia at or below 70 mg/dL.

5. What is the most important treatment needed in the care of a diabetic coma patient?

   Medications used to treat patients with diabetes, especially insulin, can cause dangerously low glucose levels of hypoglycemia and even coma. For this reason, an infusion of dextrose, most commonly as D10 or D50, remains an essential treatment. D50 use is becoming less common because of concerns for rebound hypoglycemia after administration, overshooting of glycemic targets after treatment, and its hypertonic toxicity.

   If a known diabetic is found unresponsive and establishing an IV is not possible, another therapeutic option is to give glucagon IM, which causes a sudden surge of glucose into the bloodstream from the liver. Many patients on insulin carry a glucagon rescue kit in a long red case. The rescue kit contains glucagon in powder form within a vial and a syringe prefilled with saline. Rapidly plunge the syringe's saline into the vial, and quickly mix the saline with the powder into solution. Draw the glucagon solution back up into the syringe to then give the unresponsive diabetic patient an IM injection. And get a glucose reading. Glucagon side effects include a headache, and nausea with vomiting, so also be prepared to place the patient on their side.

6. How do you treat an alert diabetic patient who is hypoglycemic?

   An alert hypoglycemic (glucose ≤70 mg/dL) patient can be given about 15 g of carbohydrates orally, preferably rapidly absorbing (low fat, low fiber) carbohydrates such as a couple of inches of juice in a cup, sugary candy, or simply four dextrose tablets. Icing certainly could raise the glucose, but the fat content may slow the absorption. Since it takes time to absorb the 15 g, the next step is to wait 15 minutes to recheck the glucose reading. If the patient is experienced in their hypoglycemic management and wants to take extra carbohydrates for the low glucose level, that is ok too. They just are more likely to have a rebound hyperglycemia if given too many carbohydrates too fast. While waiting, continue your other assessments, and establish an IV in case they become less responsive and need a dextrose bolus. If after 15 minutes, the patient still has a low glucose level, administer another 15 g and wait an additional 15 minutes. Repeat 15 g every 15 minutes until their glucose level is over 100 or you have transitioned their care to the emergency department team.

7. Do all patients with hypoglycemia who are treated at home need to be transported to the hospital?
No, not all patients with a history of hypoglycemia will need to be transported. Local protocols may vary, but per national EMS guidelines, a patient needs to meet ALL of these criteria to be released without transport:
1. Repeat glucose measurement over 80 mg/dL
2. Patient takes insulin or metformin to control diabetes
3. Patient returns to normal mental status, with no focal neurologic signs or symptoms after receiving glucose/dextrose
4. Patient can promptly obtain and will eat a carbohydrate meal
5. Patient or legal guardian refuses transport and EMS providers agree transport not indicated
6. A reliable adult will be staying with patient
7. No major comorbid symptoms occur, such as chest pain, shortness of breath, seizures, intoxication
8. A clear cause of the hypoglycemia is identified (e.g., skipped meal)
   Please note that if a patient takes other oral diabetes medications other than metformin, the medication could cause hypoglycemia for a long time. Sulfonylureas are especially notorious for prolonged hypoglycemia risks.

8. At what level is a patient considered hyperglycemic?
The American Diabetes Association defines hyperglycemia at or above 180 mg/dL.

9. How do you support a hyperglycemic diabetic patient who is clinically stable but unable to lower their glucose level after repeated insulin doses at home?
On the way to your local emergency department, get a glucose reading. A finger prick can be accidentally elevated by food left on the skin, so be sure to clean the digit with alcohol. The patient may have just checked their glucose level, but after stacked insulin doses at home, or with ongoing food metabolism, their glucose level could shift and you want to be prepared with an updated glucose reading. With hyperglycemia intravascularly, water is drawn from the cells into the blood vessels, to balance out the electrolyte shift. The kidneys spill both glucose and water into the urine, to lower the glucose level, but this also worsens the cellular dehydration. As long as the patient is not in active heart failure (edema, shortness of breath, or known heart failure history), giving a normal saline bolus is helpful, as is drawing a blood for labs. Clinicians in the emergency department will need to check the patient's potassium level before giving insulin, as insulin shifts potassium intracellularly, and critical hypokalemia can cause a critical heart conduction abnormality.

10. What is diabetic ketoacidosis or DKA?
DKA occurs when cells are starving for glucose, especially in type 1 diabetics who have not had enough insulin. The cells without glucose instead break down fatty acids, which causes ketones to build up in the blood and urine. The buildup of ketones depletes the bicarbonate buffer in the blood and eventually makes the blood acidic. Patients in DKA can feel sick, weak, short of breath, and confused and it can even cause coma or death. On examination, you may note Kussmaul breathing—a rapid breathing pattern used by the body to breathe off some acid, which might smell fruity. A diabetic patient can test their urine for ketones at home, and the presence of ketones may trigger a call to EMS for help. Initiating IV access, rechecking glucose level, and beginning fluid resuscitation are all helpful. DKA can shift potassium out of cells, which is concerning because elevated or low potassium levels can cause cardiac arrhythmias. If you have time, obtaining an electrocardiogram (EKG) could show peak T waves with hyperkalemia (high potassium) and flat T waves plus U waves in hypokalemia (low potassium). In the emergency department, DKA patients will have their potassium corrected, IV fluids given, and an insulin drip started. Pediatric patients are especially at risk for cerebral edema if fluid resuscitation is too rapid.

11. How is DKA different from nonketotic hyperosmolar coma (NKHC)?
When there is not enough insulin, or if the cells are resistant to insulin, hyperglycemia can occur. Hyperglycemia causes a shift of water and electrolytes into the blood. The kidneys begin to then spill the excessive glucose into the urine at levels of 160–180 mg/dL. Excessive urine production can be a clue that a diabetic patient has hyperglycemia, and although the excessive urination of glucose will help to lower the blood glucose level, it also can lead to severe dehydration. In extreme hyperglycemia with dehydration, but no ketones, patients can present with an altered mental status, lethargy, seizures, or even coma. The treatment of NKHC is similar to DKA, with electrolyte correction, fluid resuscitation, and an IV infusion of insulin.

12. Aside from hypoglycemia and hyperglycemia symptoms, how does diabetes affect the body?
Chronic hyperglycemia can cause damage to many organs, especially of an organ's vasculature. For example, diabetic damage to coronary arteries of the heart increases the risk of occlusion and heart attack. Diabetes can also damage the kidneys, leading to poor autoregulation of fluid retention and blood pressure control and diminished protein retention, and alter electrolyte levels such as potassium. Microvascular damage to the skin of the feet, combined with diabetic nerve damage and collapse of bony foot anatomy, can also cause patients with diabetes to develop life-threatening foot ulcers. Another site of diabetic disease can be the eyes and lead to diabetic retinopathy and blindness. Unfortunately, hypoglycemia can also be damaging to critical organs such as the brain and peripheral nerves.

13. Your diabetic patient is wearing a continuous glucose monitor and refuses a finger stick. What will you do about this when your protocol advises a finger stick to obtain a glucose reading?
Continuous glucose monitors, also known as CGMs, are Food and Drug Administration–approved subcutaneous glucose measuring devices that reduce finger sticks in diabetic patients. They can be as accurate, or more accurate, than a glucometer in reading the glucose level in interstitial fluid around cells. CGMs show trends in glucose, with readings every 5 minutes. Since these devices are new, they may not be included in EMS protocols. EMS providers should discuss CGM use with their medical directors, ideally before encountering one on a call. If the patient with diabetes has a glucose level ≤70 mg/dL on their CGM, start treating them for the low sugar with oral carbohydrates as discussed earlier. Then confirm the hypoglycemia by finger stick if necessary, but again, these devices are an accurate alternative to finger sticks.

14. If a diabetic patient with an insulin pump is hypoglycemic, should you remove the pump?
The most important first step is treating the hypoglycemia. If the hypoglycemic patient is awake, treat their hypoglycemia first with rapid-acting oral carbohydrates. If they are awake, you can ask them to pause their insulin delivery, but this reduction does not impact their glucose level for nearly an hour.
If they are not responsive, focus on getting IV access, delivering a dextrose infusion, and consider glucagon IM if IV access is not available. The rapid-acting insulin they are receiving through their pump will not affect their current glucose level for at least 30–60 minutes and is not your immediate priority.
If their family or you can pause the pump, that is preferred. If the pump is too complicated to stop, remove a patient's insulin cannula and gently lift the cannula from their skin.
Insulin pumps deliver a continuous stream of insulin, to allow glucose to enter cells. Without a functioning insulin pump, a type 1 diabetic patient can go into DKA in only 4 hours! Be certain to relay to the medical team that the patient had a pump that was disconnected.

15. Are there any special conditions or presentations where a glucose check is especially important?
Glucose levels need to be closely managed in patients with a stroke or with seizures. The brain is very sensitive to low or high glucoses.

KEY POINTS

- Whenever possible, check the glucose level of patients with diabetes.
- Hypoglycemia can be treated with oral carbohydrates in an awake patient, or when the patient is unconscious, treat with D10 and/or glucagon.
- Hyperglycemia is initially supported with fluid resuscitation in the prehospital setting.
- Patients with diabetes may be wearing glucose monitors or insulin pumps.
- Assessing a glucose level is appropriate in any patient who has an altered level of consciousness.

BIBLIOGRAPHY

Agiostratidou G, Anhalt H, Ball D, et al. Standardizing clinically meaningful outcome measures beyond HbA$_{1c}$ for type 1 diabetes: a consensus report of the American Association of Clinical Endocrinologists, the American Association of Diabetes Educators, the American Diabetes Association, the Endocrine Society, JDRF International, The Leona M. and Harry B. Helmsley Charitable Trust, the Pediatric Endocrine Society, and the T1D Exchange. *Diabetes Care.* 2017;40(12):1622-1630.

American Diabetes Association. Statistics about diabetes. https://www.diabetes.org/resources/statistics/statistics-about-diabetes.

Calderón DIA. Can you leave them be? A review of the recommendations of hypoglycemia treat and release protocols. http://www.naemsp-blog.com/emsmed/2018/6/30/can-you-leave-them-be-a-review-of-the-recommendations-of-hypoglycemia-treat-and-release-protocols.

Moore C, Woollard M. Dextrose 10% or 50% in the treatment of hypoglycaemia out of hospital? A randomised controlled trial. *Emerg Med J.* 2005;22(7):512-515.

Seaquist ER, Anderson J, Childs B, et al. Hypoglycemia and diabetes: a report of a workgroup of the American Diabetes Association and the Endocrine Society. *Diabetes Care.* 2013;36(5):1384-1395.

CHAPTER 19

SEPSIS

Marina Boushra

QUESTIONS AND ANSWERS

1. What is sepsis and why is it important?

    Describing sepsis, Sir William Osler wrote: "Except on few occasions, the patient appears to die from the body's response to infection rather than from (the infection itself)." Simply put, sepsis is a dysregulated exaggeration of the normal immune mechanisms set in place to fight infection. Sepsis may be caused by any infection, including bacterial, viral, and fungal etiologies, and can occur in patients of any age, demographic background, or state of health. The treatment of sepsis accounts for over $20 billion in annual healthcare expenditure in the United States. Sepsis has approximately 10% mortality, with mortality as high as 40% in septic shock, and sepsis-spectrum disorders are the most common cause for admission and death in the intensive care unit (ICU) in the United States.[1]

2. What is the role of EMS professionals in the care of septic patients and how can they help improve patient outcomes?

    Early EMS recognition and intervention for time-sensitive conditions have resulted in outcome benefits in the case of stroke, ST-elevation myocardial infarction (STEMI), and penetrating trauma. Like those conditions, sepsis is a time-critical illness requiring early recognition and intervention. Approximately one- to two-thirds of septic patients enter the healthcare system through the emergency department (ED), and over half of those patients arrive through EMS.[2] This places EMS professionals in a unique position to initiate early intervention that translates into outcome improvements for septic patients. In fact, one study showed an odds ratio of 3.19 in favor of survival for patients with severe sepsis identified by EMS personnel rather than those identified later by ED staff.[3] Additionally, as EMS professionals become responsible for increasingly longer transport times, recognition of sepsis and knowledge of its management have become vital to patient outcomes.

3. What is our understanding of the pathophysiology of sepsis?

    Despite decades of research, the pathophysiology of sepsis is still poorly understood. It has been theorized that sepsis may be due to a pathologic imbalance of the proinflammatory and anti-inflammatory mediators of the immune response, leading to cellular injury and multiorgan dysfunction. Genetic susceptibility and direct effects of the etiologic microorganism or its toxic by-products are also thought to play a role in the development of sepsis.

4. How are the spectrum of sepsis disorders defined?

    Unfortunately, there is no gold standard laboratory test, imaging study, or universally accepted clinical criteria to define sepsis. The definition of sepsis has been an evolving one, and the history of defining sepsis mirrors the increasing recognition of its pathophysiology as a *multisystemic process* resulting in *end-organ dysfunction*. The first consensus definition defined the spectrum of sepsis to septic shock by the presence of two or more elements of the patient's systemic inflammatory response syndrome (SIRS) (Table 19.1).

    Most recently, in 2016, the Sepsis-3 consensus statement defined sepsis as the presence of a suspected or documented infection in addition to two or more of the quick Sequential Organ Failure Assessment (Table 19.2).[4] Septic shock was defined clinically as sepsis requiring vasoactive agents to maintain mean arterial pressure

Table 19.1. Systemic Inflammatory Response Syndrome (SIRS) and the Definition of Sepsis

SIRS	Two or more of the following: Temperature $>38°C$ or $<36°C$ Heart rate >90 beats per minute (bpm) Respiratory rate >20 breaths/minute or $PaCO_2$ <32 mmHg White blood cell count $>12,000$ cu/mm, <4000 cu/mm, $>10\%$ bands
Sepsis	The presence of two SIRS criteria in the setting of known or suspected infection
Severe sepsis	Sepsis associated with end-organ dysfunction
Septic shock	Sepsis with a systolic blood pressure <90 mmHg or >40 mmHg decrease in baseline systolic blood pressure

Adapted from the 1991 American College of Physicians/ Society of Critical Care Medicine consensus statement.

Table 19.2. Quick Sequential Organ Failure Assessment Criteria (qSOFA)	
qSOFA	Altered mental status Systolic blood pressure <90 mmHg Respiratory rate ≥22 breaths/minute

(MAP) ≥65 mmHg despite adequate fluid resuscitation and a lactic acid >2 mmol/L. Importantly, this paper eliminated the category of severe sepsis entirely, reflected in the most recent Surviving Sepsis Campaign (SSC) guidelines released in early 2017. The most important thing to remember in the diagnosis of sepsis is that it requires an assessment of the whole clinical picture: not every patient with fever has sepsis and afebrile patients may be septic.

5. What are the most common sources of sepsis? What signs and symptoms should raise concern for the diagnosis of sepsis in a patient?
   Infections of the respiratory and urinary tracts account for the majority of sepsis diagnoses. Other potential sources of infection include musculoskeletal (cellulitis, septic joints, discitis, osteomyelitis, abscesses), cardiac (endocarditis, myocarditis), abdominal (enteritis, diverticulitis, appendicitis, abscesses), neurologic (meningitis, encephalitis, cerebral and epidural abscess), and infected indwelling devices (Foley catheters, central lines, and ports). Recognition of sepsis is hampered by the remarkable variability in its presentation, and almost any chief complaint could be a warning sign of sepsis. Table 19.3 outlines the signs and symptoms that should raise concern for the diagnosis of a sepsis-spectrum disorder in the appropriate clinical setting.

6. What are the Surviving Sepsis Guidelines and what are their recommendations for the treatment of septic patients?
   The SSC is a program that aims to decrease sepsis mortality through protocolized and bundled care. The following is a summary of the most current recommendations from the SSC.
   - Continuous administration of crystalloid fluids as long as hemodynamic factors continue to improve up to a total volume of 30 mL/kg.
   - If the administration of fluids fails to achieve a MAP ≥65 mmHg, the use of vasoactive agents is recommended, with norepinephrine being the vasopressor of choice.
   - Prompt and aggressive source control is of utmost importance. This can be achieved through the administration of broad-spectrum antimicrobials and, in some cases, through surgical intervention.
   - Cultures should be collected prior to the initiation of antimicrobials if doing so does not significantly delay the administration of antimicrobials.

7. What tools are available to help EMS professionals identify septic patients?
   The development of early detection tools for EMS providers is hampered by the broad definition of sepsis as well as the lack of availability of laboratory testing to EMS providers. Several screening tools exist to aid EMS professionals in recognizing sepsis. These include the Rapid Acute Physiology Score (RAPS), the Robson screening tool, the BAS tool, the Prehospital Sepsis Score (PRESS), and the Prehospital Early Sepsis Detection Score (PRESEP). The best screening tool for a particular EMS service depends on its available resources: some scores require measurement of temperature and/or a point-of-care lactic acid, which may not be feasible in all systems. Two

Table 19.3. Signs and Symptoms Concerning for Sepsis	
SYSTEM	**SIGNS AND SYMPTOMS**
Pulmonary	Cough, shortness of breath, hypoxia
Urinary	Pain with urination, foul-smelling or cloudy urine
Musculoskeletal	Skin redness, drainage or ulcers Joint swelling or redness Bony tenderness Purulent drainage
Cardiac	New murmur, chest pain, shortness of breath
Gastrointestinal	Abdominal pain, poor appetite, nausea, vomiting, diarrhea
Neurologic	Altered mental status, seizure, neck pain or stiffness, weakness in an extremity, speech difficulty
Indwelling devices	Redness, drainage, or pain around the insertion site

Table 19.4. Prehospital Sepsis Score (PRESS)

PARAMETER	POINTS
Chief concern: sick person	3
Nursing home transport	4
Age (years)	
18–39	0
40–59	4
≥60	2
Hot tactile temperature	3
SBP (mmHg)	
100–109	0
90–99	1
80–89	2
70–79	5
60–69	4
< 60	5
Oxygen saturation (%)	
≥90	0
80–89	1
70–79	3
60–69	4
< 60	5

This score can only be used in patients ≥18 years old with an SBP <110 mmHg, heart rate >90 bpm, and a respiratory rate >20 who do not have a traumatic injury, cardiac arrest, pregnancy, a psychiatric emergency, or a known toxic ingestion. A score of ≥2 is associated with an increased risk of sepsis.
SBP, systolic blood pressure.

Table 19.5. Prehospital Early Sepsis Detection Score (PRESEP Score)

VITAL SIGN	POINTS
Temperature >38°C	4
Temperature <36°C	1
Heart rate >90 bpm	2
Respiratory rate >22 breaths/minute	1
Oxygen saturation <92%	2
Systolic blood pressure <90 mmHg	2

A score ≥4 is suggestive of sepsis.

examples of scoring systems that do not rely on laboratory data, PRESS and PRESEP, are outlined in Tables 19.4 and 19.5, respectively. More recently, end-tidal CO_2 ($EtCO_2$) has emerged as a useful prehospital inverse indicator of increased lactic acid and a marker of sepsis and severe sepsis.[5,6] In patients with suspected infection, an $EtCO_2$ of ≤25 mmHg when found in conjunction with two or more SIRS criteria has been demonstrated to have a 90% sensitivity, 58% specificity, and 93% negative predictive value for the presence of severe sepsis.[10]

8. What are possible EMS interventions in septic patients and how do they affect outcomes?
   A variety of trials have investigated the role of early EMS interventions in sepsis, including the administration of antibiotics and intravenous fluids.[7,8] A study investigating the role of EMS fluid administration did demonstrate a mortality benefit in the subset of patients with initial systolic hypotension. Unfortunately, EMS administration of antibiotics has not been shown to improve outcomes.[9] Another study found that EMS recognition of a patient as "sick," measured by whether or not a prehospital IV was started, was enough to lead to a mortality benefit, even when no medications or fluids were infused through that IV in the prehospital setting.[8] Until more data are available on how EMS providers can intervene in sepsis, one thing is clear: the most important thing EMS providers can do in sepsis is recognize that it is there.

KEY POINTS

- Sepsis-spectrum disorders are multisystemic, difficult to recognize, and result in significant patient morbidity and mortality.
- Sepsis is a time-critical illness requiring early recognition and intervention. EMS recognition of sepsis in the prehospital setting results in significant patient mortality benefit.
- The presentation of sepsis is variable and vital sign abnormalities are not universally present. Several scoring systems exist to help EMS professionals identify and risk-stratify patients with sepsis-spectrum disorders.

REFERENCES

1. Torio CM, Andrews RM. *National Inpatient Hospital Costs: The Most Expensive Conditions by Payer, 2011: Statistical Brief #160. Healthcare Cost and Utilization Project (HCUP) Statistical Briefs*. Rockville (MD): Agency for Healthcare Research and Quality (US); 2006.
2. Smyth MA, Brace-McDonnell SJ, Perkins GD. Identification of adults with sepsis in the prehospital environment: a systematic review. *BMJ Open*. 2016;6(8):e011218.
3. Hunter CL, Silvestri S, Stone A, et al. Prehospital sepsis alert notification decreases time to initiation of CMS sepsis core measures. *Am J Emerg Med*. 2019;37(1):114-117.
4. Napolitano LM. Sepsis 2018: definitions and guideline changes. *Surg Infect (Larchmt)*. 2018;19(2):117-125.
5. Hunter CL, Silvestri S, Ralls G, Stone A, Walker A, Papa L. A prehospital screening tool utilizing end-tidal carbon dioxide predicts sepsis and severe sepsis. *Am J Emerg Med*. 2016;34(5):813-819.
6. Weiss SJ, Guerrero A, Root-Bowman C, et al. Sepsis alerts in EMS and the results of pre-hospital $ETCO_2$. *Am J Emerg Med*. 2019; 37(8):1505-1509.
7. Smyth M, Brace-McDonnell S, Perkins G. Impact of prehospital care on outcomes in sepsis: a systematic review. *West J Emerg Med*. 2016;17(4):427-437.
8. Lane DJ, Wunsch H, Saskin R, et al. Association between early intravenous fluids provided by paramedics and subsequent in-hospital mortality among patients with sepsis. *JAMA Netw Open*. 2018;1(8):e185845.
9. Alam N, Oskam E, Stassen PM, et al. Prehospital antibiotics in the ambulance for sepsis: a multicentre, open label, randomised trial. *Lancet Respir Med*. 2018;6(1):40-50.

CHAPTER 20

OBSTETRIC AND GYNECOLOGIC EMERGENCIES

Matthew J. Streitz

QUESTIONS AND ANSWERS

OBSTETRICAL AND GYNECOLOGIC EMERGENCIES

1. What are the typical expected physiologic/anatomic changes in pregnancy?

   A number of changes occur. Average weight gain is 25–35 lbs (11.5–16 kg).[1] Most weight gain is from the enlarged uterus/fetus, blood volume, breast tissue, and extracellular fluid. Physiologic changes include 1500 mL increase in blood volume,[2] heart rate increases of 15 to 20 bpm, increased cardiac output (30%–50% above baseline), and a trend toward lower mean arterial pressure.[3] Functional residual capacity (FRC) also decreases in pregnancy, up to 10% to 25% depending on gestational age, due to uterine enlargement resulting in an upward movement toward the diaphragm and elevating.[3] Minute ventilation with a subsequent respiratory alkalosis and increased oxygen consumption are the leading reasons for increased hypoxemia in a pregnant patient with decreased or absent respirations.

Case: A 23-year-old female calls EMS for sudden-onset lower abdominal pain. She was running and felt a sudden "pain." She is nauseated and reports vaginal bleeding that started today. Her friend reports a possible syncopal episode. She denies trauma and reports her period is 3 weeks late. She denies sexual activity. Vital signs (VS): blood pressure (BP), 83/45; heart rate (HR), 123; respiratory rate (RR), 16; temperature (T), 100.4 (oral); and 100% room air (RA).

2. What diagnoses are included in her differential and what actions need to be taken?

   The differential for this patient is wide, including ovarian torsion, ectopic pregnancy, appendicitis, tuboovarian abscess (TOA), pelvic inflammatory disease (PID), and threatened miscarriage. Maintaining a high index of suspicion is key for not missing these diagnoses in female patients. The patient is hypotensive, tachycardic, febrile, and in pain. Given the sudden onset of pain, ovarian torsion and ruptured ectopic are higher on the differential. The delay in her normal menstrual period also leads toward an ectopic. The patient should receive intravenous (IV) fluids and pain medication and be transported to a facility where an obstetrician/gynecologist or general surgeon with surgical capabilities can evaluate her. Prompt transport and further evaluation can decrease morbidity as well as mortality in these cases.

3. What is an ectopic pregnancy?

   Any pregnancy implanted outside the endometrial cavity, occurring in 1.5% to 2.6% of pregnancies, with an increased risk if there is a history of PID.[4–7]

Case: A 35-year-old female 35 weeks pregnant with twins calls EMS for sudden-onset central abdominal pain. She was sitting at home and her 3-year-old child jumped on her stomach. She is nauseated and reports vaginal bleeding that started after he jumped on her. She reports chronic hypertension, and her first delivery was by cesarean section. VS: BP, 142/82; HR, 123; RR, 22; T, afebrile; 100% RA. The patient smokes socially.

4. What are risk factors for placental abruption?

   Placental abruption is premature separation of the placenta from the uterine wall and accounts for upward of 30% of second trimester bleeding.[8] Abdominal pain and vaginal bleeding should lead you to concerns for abruption, but vaginal bleeding can be absent with a concealed hemorrhage. Risk factors include chronic hypertension with or without preeclampsia, smoking, multiple gestation pregnancies, trauma, and cocaine/drug use.[9]

5. What if the patient in the case had a more severe trauma mechanism? Does this change your concerns?

   Uterine rupture can occur in late-term pregnancies or those with multiple gestations due to a thinning uterine wall and increased intrauterine volume. Loss of fundal height or a fetal presenting part that is easily palpable through the abdominal can occur. Vaginal bleeding, VS instability, and fetal heart rate abnormalities (bradycardia) are common.[10]

6. What if the patient has painless vaginal bleeding and no trauma? Does this change your concerns?
   Yes, painless vaginal bleeding can be seen in the setting of a vasa/placenta previa occurring in the second half of pregnancy. In previa, the placenta or umbilical cord (vasa) overlies the internal cervical os.[11] Digital cervical examinations are contraindicated; any further examination should be deferred to the treating facility. Large-bore IV above the diaphragm access should be obtained.

Case: A 43-year-old female who is 39 weeks pregnant with twins calls EMS for sudden-onset blurred vision and headache. She is nauseated, reports good fetal movement, and denies vaginal bleeding or loss of fluid. She has 2+ pitting edema in her lower extremities. Past medical history (PMH): chronic hypertension. Past surgical history (PSH): cesarean section. VS: BP, 172/112; HR, 98; RR, 18; T, afebrile; 100% RA. Repeat BP 5 minutes later is 175/110.

7. What defines preeclampsia?
   Preeclampsia is the presence of hypertension (>140/90 on two occasions over 4 hours apart) and proteinuria after 20 weeks' gestation in the absence of chronic hypertension.

8. What defines preeclampsia with severe features?
   A blood pressure of >160/110 mmHg meets the definition or a blood pressure ≥140/90 mmHg (with or without proteinuria) coupled with signs and symptoms of significant end-organ dysfunction meet diagnostic criteria. Altered mental status, flashes of light (photopia), or dark areas or gaps in the visual field (scotomata) are signs of end-organ dysfunction. In addition, severe headache ("the worst headache I've ever had") or a headache that persists despite treatment also meets the definition. Epigastric or right upper quadrant pain is also a feature and can indicate liver involvement.

9. How does her diagnosis change if she has a seizure?
   If the patient has a seizure, she is now diagnosed with eclampsia.

10. How do you treat eclampsia?
    A 4–6 g loading dose of magnesium sulfate intravenously over the course of 15–20 minutes followed by a 2 g/hour continuous infusion is the treatment for eclampsia.[12,13] Give antihypertensives during transport.[14]

11. What can be done when an umbilical cord prolapse is found?
    If a cord prolapse is found, placing the patient in Trendelenburg and lifting the presenting part (typically the head) off of the cord can help prevent cord compression.[15,16]

12. What defines a shoulder dystocia?
    Shoulder dystocia is the delayed delivery of the shoulders (>60 seconds) after the head has been delivered and occurs in 0.2% to 3% of deliveries.[17–19] The "turtle sign" is a retrograde (toward the perineum) movement of the head once it has been delivered after the cessation of pushing. The McRoberts maneuver—hyperflexion of the maternal hips—is the first step in conjunction with suprapubic pressure. Importantly, suprapubic pressure is accomplished by placing pressure just above the symphysis pubis on the anterior shoulder of the fetus. Pressure should be in the same direction as that of the baby's face in order to help collapse the anterior shoulder, thus decreasing the AP diameter. Fundal pressure should be avoided. Emergency transport should be undertaken as soon as possible in the event these are not successful. Placing the patient on "all fours" (Gaskin maneuver) should follow unsuccessful attempts to reduce the dystocia.[20]

13. How do you support a patient through childbirth?
    Women typically contract every 2–4 minutes during active labor. Place the patient in the dorsal lithotomy position (lying prone, hips flexed with someone supporting her feet/legs). Encourage her to take a deep breath just prior to the peak of the contraction, holding her breath and bearing down for 10 seconds. As you begin to see the baby's scalp, gently support the perineum and head to aid in a controlled delivery, decreasing the chance of a large perineal tear. Once the head is delivered, sweep around the neck for a nuchal cord. If one is felt, attempt to reduce the cord to help with delivery. After delivery of the head, apply downward traction with both hands flatly on either side of the head to help reduce the anterior shoulder. Once the anterior shoulder is reduced, apply upward traction to deliver the posterior shoulder. The rest of the delivery should happen easily and quickly.

14. What is an APGAR score?
    The APGAR score, which stands for activity (muscle tone/activity), pulse, grimace, appearance, and respiration, is used as a standard method to evaluate a newborn at 1 and 5 minutes of life. See Table 20.1.

15. What are common causes of postpartum hemorrhage (PPH)?
    PPH is the leading cause of maternal mortality and can occur weeks after delivery. Uterine atony (most common), perineal and cervical lacerations, placenta accreta, uterine inversions, and retained products of conception can cause profound bleeding.[21]

Table 20.1. APGAR Score for Neonates

	0	1	2
A (activity/muscle tone)	Absent	Flexed arms and legs	
P (pulse)	Absent	Below 100	Above 100
G (grimace/reflex irritability)	Floppy	Minimal response to stimulation	Prompt response to stimulation; active motion
A (appearance)	Blue/pale	Pink body, blue extremities	Pink
R (respiration)	Absent	Slow and irregular	Vigorous cry

16. How do EMS crews treat PPH?

    Large-bore IV access, administering fluid boluses, as well as vigorous uterine massage can help with PPH. While massaging the uterus, place one hand above the pubic bone to prevent uterine inversion while the other massages the fundus. Medications such as oxytocin, misoprostol (cytotec), methylergonovine (Methergine), and prostaglandins such as hemabate and dinoprostone are medication adjuncts. Tranexamic acid (TXA) is also often indicated in these patients. The use of methergine in patients with hypertension and the use of hemabate in patients with asthma are not advised.[21] If all else fails, vaginal packing can be a temporizing measure until arrival at a facility.

17. What are common neonatal complications encountered by EMS crews?

    Apnea, prematurity, neonates requiring resuscitation (bagging/intubation), hypothermia, and hypoglycemia are commonly seen.[22]

18. What are common causes of cardiac arrest in the pregnant patient?

    Cardiovascular, trauma, sepsis, hypovolemia, thromboembolic disease, hypoxia, intracranial hemorrhage, eclampsia, and amniotic fluid embolus are the leading causes.

19. Is treating a pregnant patient in cardiac arrest different from a nonpregnant patient?

    Yes and no.
    - Administer oxygen via facemask at 100% and obtain IV/IO access above the diaphragm.
    - Chest compressions (supine position) should be performed at the standard rate of 100–120/minute at a depth of 2 inches with complete recoil.
    - Defibrillation should be done promptly if indicated after the anterolateral placement of pads; the lateral pad should be placed under the lateral breast tissue against the chest wall.
    - Medications used during cardiac arrest are unchanged (i.e., epinephrine, amiodarone).
    - After 20 weeks, aortocaval compression can occur in the supine position. Leftward manual uterine displacement (pulling the uterus) can assist in blood return.
    - If after 4 minutes, there is no return of spontaneous circulation (ROSC), a resuscitative cesarean delivery (RCD) should be considered.[3]

20. Should PMCD be performed in the field?

    If trained personnel are present at a witnessed arrest of an over 20 weeks' gestational pregnancy, ROSC has not been obtained by 4 minutes, and there are appropriate resources for both potential patients, the procedure should be considered.[3,23] If the gestational age is <20 weeks, if ROSC has already been achieved, and if there has been a prolonged downtime of >15 minutes, no PMCD should be performed.[23]

KEY POINTS

- Emergency medical technicians and paramedics are likely to be the first health professionals to attend a patient in the prehospital setting.
- Planning, training, and preparing for obstetrical and gynecologic emergencies are paramount.
- Interventions for the mother are interventions for the unborn fetus.
- Understanding maternal anatomic and physiologic changes during pregnancy allows for improved treatment of patients and provides an improved understanding of the potential complications as well as disease processes that affect pregnant patients.
- Prehospital treatment of patients has the potential to have drastic positive effects on pregnant patients and their unborn fetus.

REFERENCES

1. Rasmussen KM, Yaktine AL. *Committee to reexamine IOM pregnancy weight guidelines. Food and Nutrition Board, Board on Children, Youth and Families, Institute of Medicine, National Research Council. Weight Gain During Pregnancy: Reexamining the Guidelines.* Washington, DC: National Academies Press; 2009.
2. Pritchard JA. Changes in the blood volume during pregnancy and delivery. *Anesthesiology: The Journal of the American Society of Anesthesiologists.* 1965;26(4):393-399.
3. Jeejeebhoy FM, Zelop CM, Lipman S, et al. Cardiac arrest in pregnancy: a scientific statement from the American Heart Association. *Circulation.* 2015;132(18):1747-1773.
4. Berg, CJ, Chang, J, Elam-Evans, L, et al. (2003). Pregnancy-related mortality surveillance—United States, 1991-1999.
5. Hoover KW, Tao G, Kent CK. Trends in the diagnosis and treatment of ectopic pregnancy in the United States. *Obstetrics & Gynecology.* 2010;115(3):495-502.
6. Trabert B, Holt VL, Yu O, Van Den Eeden SK, Scholes D. Population-based ectopic pregnancy trends, 1993-2007. *American Journal of Preventive Medicine.* 2011;40(5):556-560.
7. Kamwendo F, Forslin L, Bodin L, Danielsson D. Epidemiology of ectopic pregnancy during a 28 year period and the role of pelvic inflammatory disease. *Sexually Transmitted Infections.* 2000;76(1):28-32.
8. Ananth CV, Berkowitz GS, Savitz DA, Lapinski RH. Placental abruption and adverse perinatal outcomes. *JAMA.* 1999;282(17):1646-1651.
9. Oyelese Y, Ananth CV. Placental abruption. *Obstetrics & Gynecology.* 2006;108(4):1005-1016.
10. Ridgeway JJ, Weyrich DL, Benedetti TJ. Fetal heart rate changes associated with uterine rupture. *Obstetrics & Gynecology.* 2004;103(3):506-512.
11. Oyelese Y, Smulian JC. Placenta previa, placenta accreta, and vasa previa. *Obstetrics & Gynecology.* 2006;107(4):927-941.
12. ACOG Committee on Obstetric Practice/ACOG practice bulletin. Diagnosis and management of preeclampsia and eclampsia. Number 33, January 2002. American College of Obstetricians and Gynecologists. *International Journal of Gynaecology and Obstetrics: The Official Organ of the International Federation of Gynaecology and Obstetrics.* 2002;77(1):67.
13. Sibai BM. Magnesium sulfate prophylaxis in preeclampsia: evidence from randomized trials. *Clinical Obstetrics and Gynecology.* 2005;48(2):478-488.
14. Beaird DT, Kahwaji CI. EMS, prehospital deliveries. StatPearls [Internet]. StatPearls Publishing; 2018.
15. Mercado J, Brea I, Mendez B, Quinones H, Rodriguez D. Critical obstetric and gynecologic procedures in the emergency department. *Emergency Medicine Clinics of North America.* 2013;31(1):207-236.
16. Kahana B, Sheiner E, Levy A, Lazer S, Mazor M. Umbilical cord prolapse and perinatal outcomes. *International Journal of Gynecology & Obstetrics.* 2004;84(2):127-132.
17. Wolfson AB, Hendey GW, Ling LJ, Rosen CL, Schaider JJ, Sharieff GQ. *Harwood-Nuss' Clinical Practice of Emergency Medicine.* Philadelphia: Lippincott Williams & Wilkins; 2012.
18. Benrubi GI. *Obstetric and Gynecologic Emergencies.* Philadelphia: Lippincott Williams & Wilkins; 1994.
19. Gabbe SG, Niebyl JR, Simpson JL, et al. *Obstetrics: Normal and Problem Pregnancies E-Book.* Philadelphia: Elsevier Health Sciences; 2016.
20. Sokol RJ, Blackwell SC. ACOG practice bulletin: Shoulder dystocia. Number 40, November 2002. (Replaces practice pattern number 7, October 1997). *International Journal of Gynaecology and Obstetrics: The Official Organ of the International Federation of Gynaecology and Obstetrics.* 2003;80(1):87.
21. American College of Obstetricians and Gynecologists/ACOG practice bulletin: clinical management guidelines for obstetrician-gynecologists number 76, October 2006: postpartum hemorrhage. *Obstetrics and Gynecology.* 2006;108(4):1039.
22. McLelland GE, Morgans AE, McKenna LG. Involvement of emergency medical services at unplanned births before arrival to hospital: a structured review. *Emerg Med J.* 2014;31(4):345-350.
23. Parry R, Asmussen T, Smith JE. Perimortem caesarean section. *Emerg Med J.* 2016;33(3):224-229.

CHAPTER 21

DYSPNEA

Sarah K. Lewis and Susan B. Promes

QUESTIONS AND ANSWERS

1. What is dyspnea?

   The word stem dys- means difficult and -pnea means breath. Combined, the word dyspnea means difficult breath. The symptom of dyspnea or shortness of breath is very subjective and is included in the patient's history.

2. How is respiratory distress described and documented?

   General inspection: While collecting the history, you will already have begun a general examination of the patient. If the patient is talking and oriented, you can be reassured that respiration is occurring, the heart is pumping, and at least some oxygen is being supplied to the brain. Do you note any color change to the extremities, such as cyanosis or pallor? If they are perfusing their brain and skin, that is reassuring.

   Airway: If the patient is talking normally the airway is clear or patent. If they need to pause midsentence, that is more concerning for respiratory distress. If they need to pause to breathe after every word or two, they are in severe respiratory distress and could collapse quickly, requiring an advanced airway.

   Breathing: Moving on to B for Breathing, note the presence of nasal flaring, use of accessory muscles for chest wall retractions, and patient's chosen position, such as tripoding. Note respiratory rate and end-tidal CO_2 ($EtCO_2$) with associated waveform and obtain a pulse ox. Hearing audible sounds of breathing without your stethoscope is an ominous sign.

   Examples include:

   - Stridor in a narrowed airway from croup
   - Wheezing from asthma
   - Snoring breath sounds in patient with chronic obstructive pulmonary disease (COPD).

     Localizing lung sounds can help to further identify the cause, as described further later.

Case: A 76-year-old male calls 911 for worsening shortness of breath today. He complains of a cough, chest discomfort, and leg swelling. His house smells like tobacco smoke, and he confirms he does indeed smoke as well. He has a long list of medical conditions and a countertop lined with pill bottles.

3. As you consider the long list of possible causes for the patient's shortness of breath, where will you begin?

   One simple line of discussion to consider would be asking the patient whether he has felt this way before, and if so, what caused it. This may show history to repeat itself, but certainly, there could be multiple reasons working to cause shortness of breath in this patient. What past medical history does he have?

   Shortness of breath could be caused by many systems, including respiratory, cardiac, hematologic, endocrine, toxic exposures, or others.

   - His cough might be from pneumonia, a PE, lung damage from smoking such as COPD, or cancer.
   - His chest discomfort could be a heart attack, tamponade, chest wall injury, or even reflux from the stomach.
   - His leg swelling may be from heart failure, peripheral vascular disease, renal failure, or liver failure.

     After hearing him speak (checks the airway, too), the vital signs may be a helpful clue.

   - Pulse oximeter saturation on room air is helpful to document, before and after putting the patient on oxygen.
   - Respiratory rate before and after oxygen should be noted as well.
   - Place the patient on $EtCO_2$ when possible—the associated number and waveform can indicate possible causes to his respiratory distress.
   - Fever most likely is from an infectious source, such as pneumonia.
   - Hypotension is a serious red flag, associated with shock, septic shock, heart failure, heart attack, tamponade, PE, and others.
   - Tachycardia could be from many sources.

4. What three areas of the body would you check first in the patient described earlier?

   When time is of the essence and the examination needs to be focused, high-yield quick examinations will be key. Certainly Airway, Breathing, and Circulation examinations will be the first systems to check.

   Airway: He is speaking in half sentences, with pauses to breathe in between sentences.

   Breathing:

   - Accessory muscle use or nasal flaring seen?
   - Lung auscultation:
     - Rales in the lower lungs could indicate fluid overload from cardiac (heart), renal (kidney), or hepatic (liver) failure.

- A focal area of rhonchi could point to pneumonia.
- Course breath sounds or diffuse rhonchi could be from bronchitis or COPD.
- Circulation:
  - Cardiac auscultation:
    - An irregular rhythm may be a cause of both shortness of breath and edema.
    - A loud murmur could contribute to heart failure or be from a heart attack.
  - Examining the extremities:
    - Poor perfusion can be associated with shock, causing pale and cold extremities.
    - Edema can have multiple causes:
      - Sudden new edema most likely is from a heart failure source.
      - Renal failure can build up fluid over days as the kidney filters less urine.
      - Liver failure is from decreased protein in the blood and also occurs more gradually. Look for jaundice (yellow skin) and icteric sclera (whites of the eyes are now yellow) as a clue for liver disease.
    - Skin for pallor in anemia or hemorrhage.
    - Diaphoresis (sweating) with severe pain, heart attack, infection, or hypoxia.

Simply put, is oxygen exchange occurring in the lungs, is there enough blood to circulate the oxygen, and a functioning pump to distribute it? In a rapid focused assessment, these are the essential questions.

Case: On examination, this patient is found to be tripoding, speaking in half sentences, followed by a gasp. He has a respiratory rate of 40, blood pressure (BP) of 160/90, and pulse of 110. His pulse ox was 88% on room air and improved to 94% on 6 liters per minute of oxygen via nasal cannula. He has rales in the lower lungs bilaterally, and rhonchi diffusely too. Heart murmur is heard loudest over the aorta. He has pitting edema in both ankles. An IV was started and blood was drawn. His electrocardiogram (EKG) shows left ventricle hypertrophy, without ST segment changes. In the emergency department, he was found to have severe aortic stenosis with associated congestive heart failure (CHF), as well as COPD flare. He was given Lasix to remove fluid hopefully from his lungs and placed on bilevel positive airway pressure (BiPAP) for both COPD and heart failure. His medications for heart failure and COPD were optimized. And a cardiothoracic surgeon will replace his aortic valve.

5. How do you differentiate COPD vs. CHF?

The presentation of COPD flare causes acute inflammation and spasm of the already chronically thickened bronchioles and alveoli. COPD symptoms include progressive shortness of breath and a cough that tries to open the airway. COPD can have diffuse rhonchi. IV steroids reduce the inflammation. Albuterol can help with spasm, or positive pressure ventilation such as with continuous positive airway pressure (CPAP) can help support the work of expiration and inhalation. The most important early intervention for a patient in severe respiratory distress from COPD, asthma, or CHF is early noninvasive positive pressure.

Heart failure can occur from too much preload, heart valve disease, heart wall diseases (cardiomyopathy, hypertrophy, myocardial infarct), and increased afterload. Heart failure causes fluid to accumulate in the legs, and the lungs, so it can also cause shortness of breath. The lung exam for heart failure starts with rales in the lower lungs, but abnormal lung sounds can be heard across the lungs as the fluid spreads. However, noninvasive positive pressure (CPAP) again can support the work of breathing.

The similarities of COPD and CHF can make it difficult to differentiate the two in the field. Capnography may be helpful. Lower levels of $EtCO_2$ may be associated with CHF and may serve as an objective diagnostic adjunct. Capnography waveforms may also help (see later). Oxygen and CPAP will generally help both causes. An EKG would be appropriate, as a heart attack could present with shortness of breath. Getting IV access will help to expedite the patient's care in the emergency department. Once at the hospital, lab work and a chest x-ray will help to determine COPD, CHF, or both.

6. Should oxygen be restricted for a COPD patient with shortness of breath?

In a patient with new or worsening shortness of breath, there is no reason to restrict oxygen. It is important to target oxygen saturations in the 90s; you do not need to get to 100%.

7. What are signs of worsening respiratory distress?

- Rigorous accessory muscle use becomes labored, or the patient looks more tired.
- Needs to pause more often when speaking, to take a breath.
- Altered mental status including combativeness.
- An increase in the respiratory rate.
- A drop in the pulse oximeter saturation.

8. What respiratory conditions are most urgent to detect prehospital?

- Airway obstructions need to be removed or a surgical airway will be needed.
- Severe asthma flares benefit from early administration of epinephrine, noninvasive positive pressure, and albuterol.
- Tension pneumothorax needs a needle decompression.

9. What cardiac causes of dyspnea need to be considered emergently in the prehospital setting?
   - Heart attack (myocardial infarction [MI]): need an EKG, aspirin, IVs, and consider nitroglycerin.
   - Aortic dissection (chest pain that radiates to the back, with absent pulses in a limb): two large IVs, EKG, notify the emergency department of your concern, and rapid transport.
   - Cardiac tamponade: Fluid between the heart and pericardium causes pump failure; presents with Becks triad of muffled heart sounds, jugular venous distention, and low BP; treatment is pericardiocentesis.

10. How does anemia or hemorrhage cause shortness of breath?
    If there are not enough red blood cells to transport oxygen, then tissues will become hypoxic. The heart will compensate by pumping more quickly, and the lungs will breathe more rapidly. Examples of hematologic causes of shortness of breath include internal hemorrhage from a dissection, a severe gastrointestinal (GI) bleed, or a chemotherapy patient, all of whom have fewer red blood cells to transport oxygen.

11. What is pleuritic chest pain?
    Pleuritic chest pain is pain with inspiration. The lung is coated in a visceral (organ) pleura, and with every breath, the visceral pleura slides against the parietal pleura of the inner surface of the chest wall. The space between the pleural membranes is the pleural space. We breathe all day and normally do not feel pain from friction in the pleural space. However, if there is inflammation or an irregular surface on either surface, breathing will cause painful friction. Examples of causes include pneumonia, a pneumothorax, PE, or a general diagnosis of "pleurisy." Most often, pleurisy is from a viral infection.

12. What is the classic presentation of pneumonia?
    Pneumonia is an infection of one or multiple regions of the lungs' alveoli. Most often, pneumonia is caused by a viral infection but can also be bacterial. In both viral and bacterial pneumonia, patients will feel sick and have a fever and cough. Viral pneumonias tend to present with or just after other viral infection symptoms such as nasal congestion, sore throat, aches and pains, and even GI complaints. Bacterial pneumonias tend to have a thicker sputum produced by cough, without upper respiratory involvement. Another type of pneumonia is caused from aspiration of food, drink, or gastric contents. This can cause severe inflammation to the lungs, with cough and shortness of breath. For example, someone who has had a stroke can easily aspirate. On examination of the lungs, patients with pneumonia may have rhonchi over a focal area of infection. Viral pneumonias can affect all of both lungs. Aspiration can affect any or all of the lungs, depending on where the aspirate settled.

    Any type of pneumonia patient with shortness of breath and hypoxia should receive oxygen, noting vitals and pulse ox before and after treatment. If they look really sick, or have low BP, starting an IV and starting IV fluids will be helpful, too, following your sepsis protocols.

    Pneumonias can also trigger an asthma or COPD flare, so also consider a bronchodilator albuterol if the patient has a history of these conditions or if you hear wheeze.

13. What causes PEs?
    Most often, a deep venous thrombosis, or DVT, forms in a leg, a piece breaks off and lodges in the lung, causing a PE. Virchow's triad summarizes the common causes of venous thrombotic events, or VTEs (such as PEs and DVTs). The more components of Virchow's triad that patients have, the more likely they will have a VTE:
    - Intimal trauma (damage to the inner surface of the blood vessels)
      - Examples: crush injury to a limb with vessel damage, or vascular surgery
    - Venous stasis (blood staying still)
      - Examples: recent surgery, casted limb, bed-bound or immobile patients, recent long travel, recent hospitalization
    - Hypercoagulable (prone to forming clots) state
      - Clotting-prone blood disorders, including Factor V Leiden
      - Cancer, pregnancy, smoking, estrogen use
        PE can cause shortness of breath, pleuritic chest pain, tachycardia, anxiety, and occasionally blood in the sputum. A small percentage of PE patients will have sudden heart failure and hypotension and can die in the first 1–2 hours. If PE is in your differential, vigilant BP monitoring is important, with IV access, and ability to support hypotension. An EKG and drawing labs would help expedite the patient's emergency department care as well. Again, support shortness of breath with oxygen.

14. How can capnography be useful in the prehospital environment?
    Capnography is the measurement of the pressure of carbon dioxide in exhaled air as measured through a device placed at the lips, combining a numerical readout of $EtCO_2$ with a waveform. Three physiological processes are critical for capnography use and interpretation: metabolism, circulation, and ventilation. In addition to verifying endotracheal tube placement, there are numerous roles for capnography in the prehospital environment. These include evaluating for return of spontaneous circulation in cardiac arrest and evaluating shock states. In addition, the shape of the waveform can give information about the underlying disease process. For example, the classic

"shark fin" shape is indicative of obstructive diseases like asthma. In patients with a pneumothorax, the shape will start high and then trail off as air leaks from the lung, producing a high on the left, lower on the right shape.

KEY POINTS

- Documentation of pulse oximetry and respiratory rate on room air before and after treatment is helpful to show objective improvement.
- Use of $EtCO_2$ can help predict the cause of dyspnea and monitor the efficacy of treatment.
- A trial of noninvasive positive pressure ventilation can help support the work of breathing.
- In new or worsening shortness of breath, there is no reason to restrict oxygen, with the target pulse oximetry of saturations in the 90s.

BIBLIOGRAPHY

Goodacre S, Stevens JW, Pandor A, et al. Prehospital noninvasive ventilation for acute respiratory failure: systematic review, network meta-analysis, and individual patient data meta-analysis. *Acad Emerg Med.* 2014 Sep;21(9):960-970.

Hunter CL, Silvestri S, Ralls G, Papa L. Prehospital end-tidal carbon dioxide differentiates between cardiac and obstructive causes of dyspnoea. *Emerg Med J.* 2015;32(6):453-456.

Markovchick VJ, Pons PT, Bakes KM, Buchanan JA. *Emergency Medicine Secrets.* 6th ed. Philadelphia: Elsevier; 2016.

Prekker ME, Feemster LC, Hough CL, et al. The epidemiology and outcome of prehospital respiratory distress. *Acad Emerg Med.* 2014;21(5):543-550.

Thompson JE, Jaffe MB. Capnographic waveforms in the mechanically ventilated patient. *Respir Care.* 2005;50(1):100-109.

Tintinalli JE, Stapczynski JS, Ma OJ, Cline D, Meckler GD, Yealy DM. *Tintinalli's Emergency Medicine: A Comprehensive Study Guide.* 8th ed. New York: McGraw-Hill Education; 2016.

CHAPTER 22

SEIZURES

Ethan J. Young

QUESTIONS AND ANSWERS

1. What is a seizure?
   A seizure occurs when there is an abnormal surge of coordinated electrical impulses in the brain. It can have many different objective appearances such as shaking of the whole body, part of the body, or staring off. Seizures themselves are not a disease, but rather they are a symptom of several different disorders.

2. What types of seizures are there?
   There are several general types of seizures. These include focal seizures, generalized seizures, and absence seizures. See Table 22.1 for seizure types and basic characteristics.

3. What is a generalized seizure?
   Generalized seizures (formerly known as grand mal seizures) are when a patient loses consciousness and experiences abnormal muscle movements. They are caused by abnormal electrical activity within the entire brain. There are different phases within a generalized seizure. The tonic phase is when the muscles in the body stiffen. The clonic phase is when there is rhythmic jerking of the muscles. A seizure can also be primarily tonic or primarily clonic. There is a postictal period after a generalized seizure where a patient should slowly return to their mental baseline. A typical generalized seizure should not last longer than 5 minutes.

4. What is a focal seizure?
   Focal seizures (formerly known as petit mal seizures) occur when the abnormal electricity of the brain occurs only within one area of the brain. The clinical appearance of the seizure depends on the area of the brain that is affected. For example, if the seizure is in the part of the brain that controls motor movement of the left arm, there will be abnormal movement of that arm. A patient can either be conscious or unconscious during a focal seizure. Focal seizures can evolve into a generalized seizure.

5. What is an absence seizure?
   An absence seizure is a mild type of seizure during which there is no full-body generalized seizure activity. Instead, the patient will have a loss of consciousness and may appear to have a blank stare. These usually last for a matter of a few seconds. You may also witness some other physical examination clues such as rapid breathing, rhythmic blinking, or a chewing motion. These usually occur in children.

6. What is a febrile seizure?
   These are seizures related to a febrile illness. They are related to a rapid rise in the patient's core temperature. Febrile seizures occur between the ages of 3 months and 6 years of age. They will generally last less than 15 minutes and usually only require supportive care.

7. What is status epilepticus?
   Status epilepticus is a life-threatening seizure presentation. It is generally considered to be present when a seizure lasts longer than 5 minutes or when a patient has multiple seizures without recovering between the seizures. It requires immediate recognition and intervention from the prehospital provider.

Table 22.1. Basic Seizure Characteristics

TYPE	LEVEL OF CONSCIOUSNESS	MOTOR INVOLVEMENT
Generalized	Impaired	Full
Focal onset aware	Normal	Focal
Focal onset impaired awareness	Impaired	Focal
Absence	Impaired	Minimal
Febrile	Impaired	Full

Table 22.2. Common Benzodiazepine Dosages for Seizures

MEDICATION	DOSAGE
Midazolam (Versed)	5–10 mg IV or IM, 0.2 mg/kg IN
Lorazepam (Ativan)	2–4 mg IV
Diazepam (Valium)	5–10 mg IV

8. What do I do if a patient is actively seizing?

The first step in caring for a seizure is always managing the ABCs. Patients experiencing seizures will often have saliva or blood in the airway that requires suctioning. These patients will also frequently have insufficient or absent respirations requiring supplemental oxygen or even ventilation. A patient's seizure can be managed with benzodiazepine medication such as midazolam (Versed), lorazepam (Ativan), or diazepam (Valium). These medications can be given through the intravenous (IV), intraosseous (IO), intranasal (IN), or intramuscular (IM) route. See Table 22.2 for common dosages.

9. What is the RAMPART trial and what does it mean for prehospital seizure management?

This was a clinical trial comparing the effectiveness of IM midazolam (Versed) versus IV lorazepam (Ativan) in controlling seizures in a patient with status epilepticus. The results of the trial suggested that IM midazolam was superior to IV lorazepam in the termination of seizures in prehospital status epilepticus.

10. What do I do for a febrile seizure?

A febrile seizure does not typically require any medication administration to stop the seizure activity. Instead, focus should be on supportive care. This includes ensuring that the airway remains clear of blood or saliva and that the respirations and oxygen status are sufficient.

11. What are some things that mimic seizures?

There are several clinical conditions that may mimic seizure activity. The most common of these would include psychogenic nonepileptic seizures (pseudoseizures), syncopal episodes, and cardiac dysrhythmias.

12. Who can have a seizure?

Anyone can have a seizure. Seizure disorders cannot be ruled out in any patient based on previous history, age, or any other factors.

13. What etiologies of seizures should I consider for a seizure activity in a patient?

There are many etiologies of seizures. The most common form is epileptic seizures. Seizures can also be induced by a number of other medical circumstances. These can include hypoxia, hypoglycemia, trauma, or medication overdose/toxicological exposure. Seizure-like activity can also be caused by psychological stress (pseudoseizures). Finally, for any female patient of childbearing age who presents with seizure, eclampsia should be in your differential.

14. What is eclampsia and how is it managed?

Eclampsia is a seizure condition related to pregnancy. It can occur any time after 20 weeks' gestation and up to 4 weeks postpartum (after the baby is delivered). Preeclampsia is a condition where a pregnant woman, after 20 weeks' gestation, has elevated systolic blood pressures >140 mm Hg or diastolic blood pressures >90 mm Hg. Preeclampsia can lead to eclampsia.

The management of eclampsia involves rapid recognition and treatment with IV magnesium, usually at a dose of 4–6 g. The definitive treatment for eclampsia is delivery of the baby.

It is important to remember that females with a preexisting seizure condition can get pregnant and not every seizure in a pregnant patient is eclampsia. The priority is always ABC management and termination of the seizure. Caring for the mother is caring for the fetus.

15. What is epilepsy?

Epilepsy is a relatively common neurological disorder that can affect people of all ages. It is characterized by recurrent unprovoked seizures throughout the patient's life. It can have a variety of causes ranging from genetics, to traumatic brain injury, to unknown.

16. What are some prescription medications that patients with a history of seizures may take?

You will see several different prescription medications used for treating patients with a seizure disorder. These can include lamotrigine, lacosamide, levetiracetam, carbamazepine, oxcarbazepine, phenobarbital, phenytoin, and valproic acid. See Table 22.3 for most the common antiepileptic drug names.

Table 22.3. Common Prescription Antiseizure Medications

GENERIC NAME	BRAND NAME
Carbamazepine	Tegretol
Lacosamide	Vimpat
Lamotrigine	Lamictal
Levetiracetam	Keppra
Oxcarbazepine	Trileptal
Phenytoin	Dilantin
Topiramate	Topamax
Valproic acid	Depakote

17. What is a postictal period?

This is the recovery phase after a seizure. Some people may be quick to return to their mental baseline, but most will take several minutes. Common symptoms include slow mental response, sleepiness, or feeling confused. There can also be changes in the patient's feelings such as fear or anxiety.

18. What are important questions to ask while taking the history of a patient who has had a seizure?

These are some of the most important questions to ask the patient or a witness to the seizure:
Was there a loss of consciousness?
Was there a fall or any other sort of trauma associated with the seizure?
Is there a history of seizures?
Have there been any recent fevers or illness?
How many seizures were there?
How long did the seizure(s) last?
What medication(s) does the patient take for seizures and have they missed any doses?

19. What are important things to include in your physical examination of a patient who has had a seizure?

Every evaluation of a seizure patient should include a prompt evaluation of the patient's airway and breathing. A close examination of the mouth and tongue can often show a tongue injury from where the patient bit their own tongue during the seizure. Every patient should also have their blood glucose checked. A thorough head-to-toe examination to evaluate for evidence of trauma and injuries should be included in your physical examination as well. If the patient is able to participate, a mental status examination and a neurologic examination should also be performed. Is there any chance this patient could be pregnant, as eclampsia should be in the differential for women of childbearing age who have a seizure? Often, a patient will experience urinary incontinence during a seizure and this can be a clue to help you with the diagnosis. If there is no history of seizures, a 12-lead electrocardiogram (EKG) should be strongly considered to rule out other etiologies of the patient's presentation.

20. What is a pseudoseizure?

These are also known as psychogenic nonepileptic seizures (PNESs). They can look like epileptic seizures but instead of being caused by abnormal electrical activity in the brain, they are caused by psychological factors. The same evaluation used for other types of seizures should be applied to these patients.

KEY POINTS

- The priority for any seizure patient is the ABCs.
- Status epilepticus is a life-threatening subset of seizure presentations that require immediate recognition and intervention.
- Benzodiazepine medication is the treatment for seizures.
- Evaluation of a seizure patient should include evaluation for trauma, hypoxia, and hypoglycemia.

BIBLIOGRAPHY

Epilepsy Foundation. What is a seizure? Available at: https://www.epilepsy.com/learn/about-epilepsy-basics/what-seizure. Accessed October 20, 2019.
Huff JS. Seizures. *Emergency Medical Services Clinical Practice and System Oversight*, Vol 1. Grover J, Lubin J (Eds.). UK: Wiley; 2009:163-170.
Silbergleit R, et al. Intramuscular versus intravenous therapy for prehospital status epilepticus. *N Engl J Med*. 2012;366(7):591-600.
Smith D, Chadwick D. The management of epilepsy. *J Neurol Neurosurg Psychiatr*. 2001;70:ii15-ii21.
Zaccara G, Giannasi G, Oggioni R, et al. Challenges in the treatment of convulsive status epilepticus. *Eur J Epilepsy*. 2017;47:17-24.

CHAPTER 23

STROKE AND TRANSIENT ISCHEMIC ATTACK

Rohit B. Sangal

QUESTIONS AND ANSWERS

1. What is a stroke?

   A stroke, more formally termed a cerebrovascular accident (CVA), is any event that disrupts blood supply to the brain and causes neurologic compromise. It is important to diagnose and treat early as lack of blood supply to the brain equates to lack of oxygen and nutrients thus leading to irreversible cell death.[1]

2. What is a transient ischemic attack (TIA)?

   A TIA is as it sounds—a transient disruption in blood supply that causes neurologic injury. Classically, it had been defined as symptoms lasting less than 24 hours; however, evidence suggests that TIAs can lead to permanent brain injury.[1]

3. Name some patient risk factors for CVAs.

   CVA risk factors are very similar to those for coronary artery disease. These include advanced age, African American race, male gender, hypertension, diabetes mellitus, and hyperlipidemia.[2] Patient lifestyle adds to risk if the patient is physically inactive and smokes. Atrial fibrillation and carotid artery stenosis also confer an added risk of stroke.

4. What is the critical first test to do before calling a stroke alert?

   Hypoglycemia is one of the great stroke mimics where patients can be confused, altered, or have odd neurologic symptoms that can easily be mistaken for a CVA. A rapid point-of-care fingerstick blood glucose test at the scene can elucidate if this is the cause and be treated. If symptoms are related to hypoglycemia, then they should rapidly improve with normalization of the blood glucose.

5. What if you do not have capabilities to perform this critical first test?

   If you cannot perform a fingerstick blood glucose (out of supplies, basic life support unit, etc.), you can try and ask the family who may be able to assist in this testing. However, given the potential devastating pathology a stroke can cause, rapid transport should not be delayed and the receiving facility should be made aware that this test was not yet performed to help in their management.

6. How are strokes classified?

   All CVAs are related to blood supply in the brain and are classified as ischemic (90%) or hemorrhagic (10%)[1,3] (Table 23.1).

7. What are common stroke symptoms?

   CVAs can present in a variety of different manners, from unilateral facial droop and hemiparesis to dizziness or gait disturbance.[2] It is important to keep a keen eye out for symptoms that seem out of the ordinary. Larger strokes may affect speech (aphasia), cause visual disturbances or gaze preference, and even unilateral neglect, where a patient has complete lack of awareness of an entire side of their body.

Table 23.1. Cerebrovascular Accident Classification

ISCHEMIC (90%)	HEMORRHAGIC (10%)
Cardioembolic: thrombi originating from the heart as a result of atrial fibrillation or valvular heart disease	Most often from hypertension or cerebral amyloid angiopathy (in the elderly) leading to bleeding of small penetrating arteries.
Large vessel disease: occlusions often from hyperlipidemia	Aneurysm rupture leading to subarachnoid hemorrhage
Small vessel disease: occlusions often from hypertension or diabetes	
Other: ischemia from arterial dissections or hypercoagulable state	

Table 23.2. Stroke Signs and Symptoms

VESSEL AFFECTED	SIGNS AND SYMPTOMS
Anterior cerebral artery	Motor and sensory deficits of the contralateral lower extremity. Usually spares the hands and face.
Middle cerebral artery	Most common lesion location and presents with complete contralateral hand and face hemiparesis and sensory loss. Often with aphasia or neglect.
Posterior cerebral artery (and basilar artery)	Subtle symptoms including ataxia and vertigo. Severe cases include locked-in syndrome consisting of complete paralysis except blinking and upward gaze.
Cerebellar artery	Coordination (ataxia, vertigo) problems among other nonspecific symptoms.
Small penetrating arteries	Causing lacunar infarcts presenting as pure motor or sensory deficits.

8. Describe the main blood supply to the brain.
   The two carotid arteries and the two vertebral arteries become the anterior and posterior circulation of the brain, respectively. Generally, the internal carotid arteries form the anterior cerebral artery and the middle cerebral artery. The vertebral arteries anastomose to form the basilar artery which supplies the brainstem, cerebellum, and becomes the posterior cerebral artery. The anastomosis of the anterior and posterior circulation forms the circle of Willis.

9. Describe the signs of different cerebral artery and cerebellar artery occlusions and lacunar infarcts.
   The symptoms vary depending on the location of the lesion (Table 23.2).[1,4]

10. What are some stroke mimics?
    Metabolic abnormalities (electrolytes), structural brain lesions (brain tumors, metastases), migraines, sepsis, and drug intoxication (alcohol) are just some of the many other conditions that can manifest with stroke symptoms.[1]

11. How can you differentiate Bell's palsy from a stroke?
    Bell's palsy is a paralysis of the facial nerve that causes unilateral facial droop and ptosis without other symptoms. A classic test is to look at the patient's forehead to see if there are wrinkles when they raise their eyebrows. Bell's palsy is a peripheral neuropathy and will NOT spare the forehead (no wrinkles) because the peripheral nerve is affected. If the forehead shows wrinkles, then it suggests a stroke because the contralateral nerve is intact. However, when in doubt, assume a stroke until further information is available.

12. What codiagnoses can occur with strokes?
    Patients can be medically complex, and CVAs sometimes are symptoms of other pathologies. Patients with an aortic dissection extending into the carotid or vertebral arteries can suffer strokes. Myocardial infarction or new-onset atrial fibrillation can lead to embolic strokes. Hemorrhagic strokes can present as seizures. It is important to keep a wide differential.

13. What tests should I perform?
    You should perform the regular airway, breathing, and circulation assessment as well as obtain a fingerstick blood glucose and an electrocardiogram.

14. What medication is contraindicated in acute stroke?
    EMS providers should not give aspirin in the field until hemorrhagic stroke has been ruled out. This can be done at the hospital.

15. Whom should I call and what information should I give over the phone?
    Call ahead to the receiving hospital because time is of the essence. The hospital can have an opportunity to notify the stroke team, prepare the computed tomography (CT) scanner and mobilize other resources to be ready on your arrival. The critical information should be age, symptoms, last known normal, and estimated time of arrival. If contact information can be provided of whoever saw the patient last, this would greatly assist the stroke team.

16. What information should I obtain?
    A focused history is important to help prepare the receiving hospital and give handoff on arrival. Specifically, age, relevant past medical history, presenting symptoms, last known normal, and vitals (specifically blood pressure) are important. If possible, determining if the patient is on blood thinners or has had a recent stroke or brain surgery will also help. Later is a list of absolute contraindications to tissue plasminogen activator (tPA) that physicians are looking for to determine the plan of action. And of course, bringing medications and family for collateral history can also help the medical team make rapid decisions. If family is not present, the contact information of whoever saw the patient last will greatly assist the stroke team.

Cincinnati Prehospital Stroke Scale
Facial Droop Normal: Both sides of face move equally Abnormal: One side of face does not move at all
Arm Drift Normal: Both arms move equally or not at all Abnormal: One arm drifts compared to the other
Speech Normal: Patient uses correct words with no slurring Abnormal: Slurred or inappropriate words or mute

Fig. 23.1. The Cincinnati Prehospital Stroke Scale. *(From Kothari RU, Pancioli A, Liu T, Brott T, Broderick J. Cincinnati Prehospital Stroke Scale: reproducibility and validity.* Ann Emerg Med. *1999;33(4):373-378.)*

Absolute contraindications[2,5,6]
(1) History or evidence of intracranial hemorrhage
(2) Clinical presentation suggestive of subarachnoid hemorrhage
(3) Known intracranial arteriovenous malformation, neoplasm, or aneurysm
(4) Systolic blood pressure exceeding 185 mm Hg or diastolic blood pressure exceeding 110 mm Hg
(5) Platelet count below 100,000/μL
(6) Prothrombin time (PT) above 15 or international normalized ratio (INR) above 1.7 or current use of direct oral anticoagulant (DOAC)
(7) Active internal bleeding or acute trauma (fracture)
(8) Neurosurgery, head trauma, or stroke in the previous 3 months
(9) Abnormal blood glucose (<50 or >400)

17. What prehospital stroke scales exist?
The **Cincinnati Stroke Scale** and **Los Angeles Prehospital Stroke Screen** are two abbreviated scales based on the National Institutes of Health Stroke Scale (NIHSS) for rapid recognition of possible CVA (Figs. 23.1 and 23.2).

18. What prehospital stroke severity scales can be used to help differentiate a small stroke from a large vessel occlusion?
Three of the stroke scales that exist in the prehospital setting for this differentiation include the Los Angeles Motor Scale (LAMS), Rapid Arterial Occlusion Evaluation (RACE), and the Vision Aphasia Neglect (VAN) screens. Both LAMS and RACE have been validated in the prehospital setting, while VAN has been validated in the inpatient setting. A summary of their criteria is in Table 23.3.

19. What is the difference between a primary and comprehensive stroke center?
Primary stroke centers have resources available to deliver and monitor patients who receive tPA, while comprehensive stroke centers have around-the-clock stroke specialists able to perform all the functions of a primary stroke center as well as endovascular therapies.[10]

20. When should a stroke patient be taken directly to a comprehensive stroke center and bypass a primary stroke center?
Based on stroke severity scales, if a patient is suspected of having a large vessel occlusion, they should be taken to a comprehensive stroke center even if it means bypassing a primary stroke center as long as the additional travel time is under 15 additional minutes.[5]

21. What is a large vessel occlusion and why should EMS be concerned about this type of stroke?
Large vessel occlusions are blockages of proximal vessels such as the basilar artery, intracranial carotid, or proximal middle cerebral artery and may be amenable to neurointerventional radiology treatment.[2] Endovascular therapies such as intra-arterial thrombolysis and mechanical thrombectomy were studied in a variety of randomized controlled trials in 2015, with comparable results. Patients in the treatment arms had improved 90-day outcomes compared to those in the control group, without difference in mortality.[1,2] Given the additional treatments available and the data supporting their use, these patients need to be transported to a comprehensive stroke center where they can receive advanced care.

Los Angeles Prehospital Stroke Scale (LAPSS)	Patient name: _____ Rater name: _____ Date: _____

Screening criteria	Yes	No
4. Age over 45 years	____	____
5. No prior history of seizure disorder	____	____
6. New onset of neurologic symptoms in last 24 hours	____	____
7. Patient was ambulatory at baseline (prior to event)	____	____
8. Blood glucose betwen 60 and 400	____	____

9. Exam: *Look for obvious asymmetry*

	Normal	Right	Left
Facial smile / grimace:	☐	☐ Droop	☐ Droop
Grip:	☐	☐ Weak grip ☐ No grip	☐ Weak grip ☐ No grip
Arm weakness:	☐	☐ Drifts down ☐ Falls rapidly	☐ Drifts down ☐ Falls rapidly

Based on exam, patient has only unilateral (and not bilateral) weakness: Yes ☐ No ☐

10. If yes (or unknown) to all items above LAPSS screening criteria met: Yes ☐ No ☐

11. If LAPSS criteria for stroke met, call receiving hospital with "CODE STROKE," if not then return to the appropriate treatment protocol. (Note: The patient may still be experiencing a stroke if even if LAPSS criteria are not met.)

Fig. 23.2. Los Angeles Prehospital Stroke Screen. *(From Kidwell CS, Saver JL, Schubert GB, Eckstein M, Starkman S. Design and retrospective analysis of the Los Angeles Prehospital Stroke Screen (LAPSS).* Prehosp Emerg Care. *1998;2(4):267-273.)*

22. What are the time constraints with regard to treatment of stroke and large vessel occlusions?
Initial data supported the use of tPA within 3 hours of symptom onset; however, advances in the field of neurocritical care are expanding this window. In 2008, data supported the use of tPA between 3 and 4.5 hours of symptom onset if the patient met the usual tPA criteria as well as was under 80 years old; had no anticoagulant use, no history of stroke, or no diabetes; and had an NIHSS score under 26.[2,11] For endovascular therapies, the aforementioned trials examined under 6 hours and found benefit. However, in 2017, the DAWN trial examined endovascular therapies for patients between 6 and 24 hours and found benefit.[12] While protocols may vary between EMS systems, there is a trend toward stroke activation and early hospital notification for any patient suspected of having a stroke within 24 hours of symptom onset.

KEY POINTS

- Early recognition of CVAs is paramount to ensure appropriate treatment.
- Obtain a fingerstick blood glucose, obtain the patient's last known time of normal neurologic status, and notify the receiving hospital to ensure appropriate resources are available for your arrival.
- Do not forget the ABCs!

Table 23.3. Prehospital Stroke Scales for Large Vessel Occlusions (LVOs)

LAMS[7]		RACE[8]		VAN[9]	
CRITERIA	**POINTS**	**CRITERIA**	**POINTS**	**CRITERIA**	**POINTS**
Facial droop	0 Absent 1 Present	Facial palsy	0 Absent 1 Mild 2 Moderate–severe	Arm weakness	Mild Moderate Severe None
Arm drift	0 Absent 1 Drifts down 2 Falls rapidly	Arm MOTOR	0 Normal–mild 1 Moderate 2 Severe	Visual disturbance	Visual field cut Diplopia New blindness None
Grip strength	0 Normal 1 Weak grip 2 No grip	Leg motor	0 Normal–mild 1 Moderate 2 Severe	Aphasia	Expressive Receptive Mixed None
		Gaze Deviation	0 Absent 1 Present	Neglect	Forced gaze Sensation deficit Ignoring side None
		Agnosia (L)/ aphasia (R)	0 Normal 1 Mild–mod 2 Severe		
	Score ≥4 high concern for LVO		Score ≥5 high concern for LVO		VAN positive if arm weakness is present with any of the other scoring components

LAMS, Los Angeles Motor Scale; *RACE*, Rapid Arterial Occlusion Evaluation; *VAN*, Vision Aphasia Neglect.

REFERENCES

1. Go S, Worman DJ. Stroke syndromes. In: Tintinalli JE, Stapczynski JS, Ma OJ, Yealy DM, Meckler GD, Cline DM, eds. *Tintinalli's Emergency Medicine: A Comprehensive Study Guide*. New York, NY: McGraw-Hill Education; 2016:1128-1129.
2. Gross H, Grose N. Emergency neurological life support: acute ischemic stroke. *Neurocrit Care*. 2017;27:102-115.
3. Hemphill 3rd JC, Lam A. Emergency neurological life support: intracerebral hemorrhage. *Neurocrit Care*. 2017;27:89-101.
4. Crocco TJ, Meurer WJ. Stroke. In: *Rosen's Emergency Medicine: Concepts and Clinical Practice*. 3rd ed. 2018:1241–1255.
5. Powers WJ, Rabinstein AA, Ackerson T, et al. Guidelines for the early management of patients with acute ischemic stroke: 2019 update to the 2018 guidelines for the early management of acute ischemic stroke: a guideline for healthcare professionals from the American Heart Association/American Stroke Association. *Stroke*. 2019: Str0000000000000211.
6. Demaerschalk BM, Kleindorfer DO, Adeoye OM, et al. Scientific rationale for the inclusion and exclusion criteria for intravenous alteplase in acute ischemic stroke: a statement for healthcare professionals from the American Heart Association/American Stroke Association. *Stroke*. 2016;47:581-641.
7. Kim JT, Chung PW, Starkman S, et al. Field validation of the Los Angeles Motor Scale as a tool for paramedic assessment of stroke severity. *Stroke*. 2017;48:298-306.
8. Perez de la Ossa N, Carrera D, Gorchs M, et al. Design and validation of a prehospital stroke scale to predict large arterial occlusion: the Rapid Arterial Occlusion Evaluation scale. *Stroke*. 2014;45:87-91.
9. Teleb MS, Ver Hage A, Carter J, Jayaraman MV, McTaggart RA. Stroke vision, aphasia, neglect (VAN) assessment—a novel emergent large vessel occlusion screening tool: pilot study and comparison with current clinical severity indices. *J Neurointerv Surg*. 2017;9:122-126.
10. Caplan LR. Primary stroke centers vs comprehensive stroke centers with interventional capabilities: which is better for a patient with suspected stroke? *JAMA Neurol*. 2017;74:504-506.
11. Hacke W, Kaste M, Bluhmki E, et al. Thrombolysis with alteplase 3 to 4.5 hours after acute ischemic stroke. *N Engl J Med*. 2008;359:1317-1329.
12. Nogueira RG, Jadhav AP, Haussen DC, et al. Thrombectomy 6 to 24 hours after stroke with a mismatch between deficit and infarct. *N Engl J Med*. 2018;378:11-21.

CHAPTER 24

SYNCOPE

Jason Jones

QUESTIONS AND ANSWERS

1. What is syncope?
   Syncope, commonly known as fainting, is a sudden and self-limited loss of consciousness with loss of postural tone. It is a symptom, not a diagnosis. Following an episode of syncope, patients should also experience a rapid and complete return to baseline.

2. What mechanism causes syncope?
   Syncope is due to a temporary episode of insufficient blood flow to the brain.

3. Which conditions can result in syncope?
   The potential etiologies of syncope are varied. Broad categories include cardiovascular diseases, arrhythmias, neurologic reflexes, orthostatic hypotension, and volume depletion. See Table 24.1 for an overview of causes.

4. When is transient loss of consciousness NOT syncope?
   Not all brief unconscious episodes are due to impaired cerebral blood flow (i.e., syncope). Nonsyncope causes include seizures, hypoglycemia, hypoxia, hyperventilation, brain injury from head trauma, intoxication, metabolic disorders, and psychogenic episodes.

5. What is presyncope?
   Presyncope, or near-syncope, encompasses the symptoms that often occur before syncope. These include light-headedness, visual sensations like "tunnel vision" or "graying out," nausea, and diminished awareness. Presyncope may or may not lead to loss of consciousness. The evaluation of presyncope and syncope is essentially the same.

6. How can the cause of syncope be determined?
   It is often impossible to determine the exact cause of a syncopal episode. However, when the cause can be identified, it is most often found in the patient's history, physical examination, or electrocardiogram (EKG) interpretation.

7. What are important questions to ask after syncope?
   Questioning should attempt to elicit the likely cause of the episode. Inquire about symptoms preceding and following the episode. You should also address whether the patient has had any history of prior syncopal events. Ask witnesses for a description of events. See Table 24.2 for common associations.

Table 24.1. Select Causes of Syncope

Cardiac arrhythmias	Brady- or tachyarrhythmias
	Inherited syndromes (long QT syndrome, Brugada syndrome)
	Pacemaker malfunction
Neurally mediated (reflex)	Vasovagal syncope
	Situational (postmicturition, defecation, cough, sneeze, etc.)
Orthostatic hypotension	Autonomic failure
	Hypovolemia (dehydration, hemorrhage)
Cardiovascular diseases	Acute myocardial infarction
	Aortic dissection
	Cardiac outflow obstruction
	Cardiac tamponade
	Heart failure or valve disease
	Pulmonary embolism

Table 24.2. Possible Syncope Associations by History	
After change in position	Orthostatic or vasovagal
After exertion, or with known heart disease or concerning family history	Cardiac cause
Palpitations or chest pain	Possible arrhythmia
After sudden neck movement	Carotid sinus disease
During or after urination, defecation, harsh coughing, or an emotional event	Situational syncope
Vomiting, diarrhea, poor oral intake, diuretic use, or heat exposure	Hypovolemia from dehydration
Recent bleeding, bloody or tarry stools	Hypovolemia from bleeding

8. Which findings in the history are concerning for nonsyncope causes?
   Prolonged unconsciousness or confusion, seizure-like activity, preceding head trauma, persistent chest pain or shortness of breath, or neurologic deficits suggest dangerous nonsyncope causes.

9. What are important physical examination findings?
   Assess mental status and determine whether the patient has returned to their baseline. Carefully auscultate heart sounds for irregular rhythms or murmurs. Evaluate the patient's speech, strength, sensation, ability to effectively touch their nose and your index finger, and pupillary response to screen for neurologic deficits. Assess for signs of dehydration or hemorrhage such as dry mucous membranes, weak pulse, prolonged capillary refill, poor skin turgor, or pallor.

10. What interventions are critical in the evaluation of syncope?
    Prehospital care should focus on supporting a patent airway, effective ventilation, and adequate perfusion, regardless of cause. A complete set of vital signs, blood glucose level, and 12-lead EKG are essential. Cardiac monitoring and serial EKGs are also worthwhile. Evaluate for arrhythmias.

11. Which arrhythmias cause syncope?
    Common arrhythmias that cause syncope include severe bradycardia (less than 40 beats/minute), frequent sinus pauses, high-grade atrioventricular (AV) blocks, supraventricular tachycardia (SVT), and wide-complex tachycardia (including ventricular tachycardia).

12. What other EKG findings are important?
    Syncope associated with atrial fibrillation or flutter, a widened QRS complex ($\geq$ 120 milliseconds), or a prolonged QT interval is associated with increased risk of arrhythmia and death. ST-segment elevations or depressions and T-wave inversions are signs of cardiac ischemia. Potentially dangerous congenital cardiac syndromes, such as Brugada or Wolff-Parkinson-White, may also cause syncope.

13. Which risk factors make cardiac causes of syncope more likely?
    Age greater than 60, male sex, known heart disease, known cardiac arrhythmia, family history of early cardiac death, or an abnormal cardiac exam are all risk factors for cardiac syncope. Additionally, syncope that occurs during exertion, while supine, or with no or minimal prodromal symptoms is more likely to be from a cardiac cause.

14. What is orthostatic hypotension?
    Orthostatic hypotension occurs when blood inappropriately pools in the vessels of the lower extremities. It causes a drop in systemic blood pressure when the patient assumes a standing position, resulting in presyncope or syncope. Patients with orthostatic hypotension should be provided oral or IV fluids and remain supine.

15. How is orthostatic hypotension diagnosed?
    Orthostatic hypotension is confirmed when the patient's systolic blood pressure drops by $\geq$20 mm Hg (or $\geq$10 mm Hg diastolic) within 3 minutes of transitioning from lying to standing. It is also confirmed if the patient develops presyncope immediately after standing. A sustained heart rate increase of $\geq$30 beats/minute is also a worrisome orthostatic finding.

16. What is vasovagal syncope?
    Vasovagal syncope is a fainting episode caused by an inappropriate neurologic reflex (excess parasympathetic tone) that results in hypotension and bradycardia. It often occurs in the setting of emotional stress or prolonged standing. Patients may report preceding symptoms like nausea, dizziness, anxiety, sweating, blurred vision, and

a sensation of warmth. Vasovagal syncope is a diagnosis of exclusion, and more dangerous causes should be considered first.

17. Are there maneuvers to stop vasovagal syncope?

Yes. Patients can be instructed to perform specific countermeasures once symptoms begin. Effective maneuvers include tensing up the arm muscles, squeezing an object tightly, or crossing the legs and tensing up the muscles of the legs, buttocks, and abdomen.

18. What is hypertrophic cardiomyopathy?

Hypertrophic cardiomyopathy (HCM) is a cardiac anomaly with an abnormally thickened heart wall. It can obstruct cardiac outflow and lead to cardiovascular collapse and death. HCM frequently lies dormant and is often found only after symptoms like syncope. It has a characteristic systolic murmur at the left lower sternal border that increases in intensity with the Valsalva maneuver. Patients with HCM who experience syncope are at increased risk of death. HCM frequently requires medications, septal ablation, or surgical repair once recognized.

19. What is long QT syndrome, and how is it diagnosed?

Long QT syndrome is a disorder of cardiac repolarization characterized by a prolonged QT interval on the EKG. The primary symptoms associated with long QT syndrome include palpitations and syncope. There is an increased risk of polymorphic ventricular tachycardia (torsades de pointes) and sudden death. Diagnostic criteria include EKG findings, clinical history, and family history (see Table 24.3).

20. Are there certain medications that can lead to a prolonged QT, and what can be done to lessen the associated risk of arrhythmia in these patients?

There are numerous medications that cause QT prolongation, including antipsychotics (e.g., haloperidol, droperidol, olanzapine), certain antiarrhythmics (e.g., procainamide, amiodarone), antidepressants (e.g., amitriptyline, citalopram), antihistamines (e.g., diphenhydramine, loratadine), and certain antimicrobials (e.g., erythromycin, hydroxychloroquine). Pharmacological causes of QT prolongation are treated with ceasing the offending medication. Optimization of potassium, magnesium, and calcium is important to minimize the risk of torsades de pointes.

21. What is Wolf Parkinson White (WPW) syndrome, and how is it diagnosed and treated?

WPW syndrome is a condition in which episodes of tachycardia occur due to an abnormal accessory pathway, usually the bundle of Kent, in the conduction system of the heart. People with WPW may experience palpitations, dizziness, light-headedness, and fainting, although some people with WPW have no symptoms. The classic EKG

Table 24.3. Long QT Syndrome (LQTS) Diagnostic Criteria	
	POINTS
Electrocardiographic Findings	
QTc ≥480 ms	3
QTc 460–479	2
QTc 450–459 (in men)	1
QTc 4th minute of recovery from exercise stress test ≥480 ms	1
Torsades de pointes	2
T-wave alternans	1
Notched T wave in three leads	1
Heart rate below second percentile for age	0.5
Clinical History	
Syncope with stress	2
Syncope without stress	1
Congenital deafness	0.5
Family History	
Family members with definite LQTS	1
Unexplained sudden cardiac death younger than age 30 among immediate family members‖	0.5

Score: ≤1 point, low probability of LQTS; 1.5–3 points, intermediate probability of LQTS; ≥5 points, high probability of LQTS.

pattern for WPW is a short PR interval with a delta wave. Patients with WPW syndrome may develop supraventricular arrhythmias, and any AV nodal blocking agent, including adenosine, diltiazem, and amiodarone, may cause an adverse reaction. It is important to anticipate a lethal reentry tachycardia with administration of any AV nodal slowing agent. As always, synchronized cardioversion is indicated for the unstable tachycardic patient and may even be the optimal treatment for all WPW syndrome patients with a supraventricular arrhythmia.

22. What workup is likely to occur at the hospital?

    Hospital evaluation varies by risk assessment, which is determined by history, physical examination, known risk factors, and EKG findings. Common testing includes cardiac monitoring, an EKG, chest X-ray, and targeted blood testing. Brain imaging is generally reserved for patients with significant head injury or neurologic deficits. For high-risk patients, cardiac stress testing, cardiac ultrasound, tilt-table testing, or long-term cardiac rhythm monitoring may be performed.

KEY POINTS

- A thorough history, physical examination, and EKG interpretation are three critical elements in the evaluation of syncope.
- Patients with true syncope should have a rapid return to baseline.
- Seizures, preceding head trauma, neurologic deficits, or persistent symptoms (such as confusion, chest pain, or dyspnea) exclude a diagnosis of syncope and should raise concern for more dangerous etiologies.
- The diagnosis of orthostatic hypotension is made by measuring a systolic blood pressure drop of 20 mm Hg, or a diastolic blood pressure drop of 10 mm Hg, when the patient moves from a lying to standing position.

BIBLIOGRAPHY

Brignole M, Alboni P, Benditt D, et al. Guidelines on management (diagnosis and treatment) of syncope. *Eur Heart J.* 2001;22(15):1256-1306.

Gauer RL. Evaluation of syncope. *Am Fam Phys.* 2011;84(6):640-650.

Linzer M, Yang EH, Estes III NA, et al. Diagnosing syncope. Part 1: value of history, physical examination, and electrocardiography. Clinical Efficacy Assessment Project of the American College of Physicians. *Ann Intern Med.* 1997;126(12):989-996.

Nishijima DK, Lin AL, Weiss RE, et al. ECG predictors of cardiac arrhythmias in older adults with syncope. *Ann Emerg Med.* 2018;71(4):452-461.

Shen WK, Shelton RS, Benditt DC, et al. 2017 ACC/AHA/HRS guideline for the evaluation and management of patients with syncope: executive summary: a report of the American College of Cardiology/American Heart Association Task Force on Clinical Practice Guidelines and the Heart Rhythm Society. *Circulation.* 2017;136(5):e25-e59.

Van Dijk N, Quartieri F, Blanc JJ, et al. Effectiveness of physical counterpressure maneuvers in preventing vasovagal syncope: the Physical Counterpressure Manoeuvres Trial (PC-Trial). *J Am Coll Cardiol.* 2006;48(8):1652-1657.

Waytz J, Cifu AS, Stern SD. Evaluation and management of patients with syncope. *JAMA.* 2018;319(21):2227-2228.

CHAPTER 25

GENERAL ADULT TRAUMA PRINCIPLES AND TRIAGE

Sarah A. Gibson

QUESTIONS AND ANSWERS

1. **What is a traumatic injury?**
   A traumatic injury is a term that refers to physical injuries of sudden and onset severity. These injuries require immediate medical attention as they can sometimes be life-threatening. Trauma makes up a significant percentage of the calls to which prehospital personnel respond and is the leading cause of death for those between the ages of 1 and 44 years. After cardiovascular disease, stroke, and cancer, trauma makes up the fourth leading cause of death for all age groups.

2. **What are the kinetics of trauma and why do they matter?**
   The kinetics of trauma are important because they can give indication and high index of suspicion for traumatic injuries. Kinetic energy = ½ (mass × velocity²). The kinetic energy of a moving body depends on the weight and the speed of the body. Essentially, the heavier the weight and the faster the speed, the greater risk for injury.

3. **How does acceleration and deceleration impact injury in the trauma patient?**
   The rate at which the body increases speed is known as acceleration. Therefore, the rate at which the body decreases speed is known as deceleration. A faster change in speed results in a higher exerted force. This is why a patient traveling at a high speed and striking a tree has a higher injury pattern than someone who gradually decelerates and bumps that same tree.

4. **What are the different types of traumatic injuries and why are the mechanisms important?**
   A force applied to the body results in either blunt or penetrating trauma. Blunt trauma is a force, but no penetration from an object. Penetrating trauma produces a break in the continuity of the skin. Understanding the mechanism of injury is important because you will be able to arrive at the scene and suspect certain injuries based quickly on just your observations. The four most common mechanisms of injury include vehicle or collisions, falls, penetrating gunshots or stabbings, and explosions.

5. **What is blunt trauma?**
   Blunt trauma is an injury caused by a force without skin penetration. Vehicle collisions frequently cause blunt trauma and can create different injury patterns based on the impact location: frontal impact, rear end, lateral, rotational, or rollover. Do not forget that restraints and airbags can also cause specific injuries (Table 25.1).

6. **What are the high-risk findings in a motor vehicle collision that indicate significant traumatic injury?**
   Significant injury is suggested by the following findings:
   • Death of an occupant within the same vehicle
   • An unresponsive patient or altered mental status
   • Intrusion greater than 12 in for the occupant site including the roof or greater than 18 in anywhere to the vehicle
   • Ejection from the motor vehicle
   • Severe deformity of the vehicle or intrusion into the vehicle
   • High rate of speed
       Digital photos of the crash scene may provide valuable information to the staff and treating providers at the trauma center.

7. **What are typical injury patterns in patients involved in motorcycle and all-terrain vehicle (ATV) crashes?**
   Motorcycle and ATV collisions have three main types of impacts. The incidence of significant injury and death is greatly impacted by whether the rider is wearing a helmet.
   • Head-on impact: the motorcycle tends to tip forward and injury occurs when the rider strikes the handlebars.
   • Angular impact is typically when an object comes into contact with the rider. This can be objects such as the edges of signs or fence posts and injuries associated with that contact.
   • Ejection injuries occur if the rider clears the handlebars.
   • "Laying the bike down" is a maneuver used by the rider to avoid impending collision. These are often associated with abrasions and burns.

Table 25.1. Significant MOI in Motor Vehicle Collisions

MOI	AREA OF BODY	EFFECTS AND INJURIES
Frontal Impact		• Occupant goes either over or under the steering wheel, may strike the dashboard • Look for signs of impact on the windshield, dashboard, and steering wheel
	Abdomen	• Suspect damage to the liver and spleen
	Chest	• Suspect injuries to ribs and sternum such as fractures • Suspect injuries to the heart from shear forces including pericardial effusion, cardiac tamponade, cardiac contusion • Suspect injuries to the lungs such as pneumothorax, pulmonary contusion
	Face, head, neck	• Check for soft tissue damage, airway compromise, bleeding head wound, signs of skull fracture, mental status change • Place a c-collar on patient as soon as trauma to head suspected
	Pelvis	• Suspect pelvis fractures or posterior hip dislocations
Rear-end impact		• Head and neck are "whipped" back quickly and the body is held in place and propelled forward due to the seat belt
Lateral impact		• Check for crush injuries, especially on the side of impact
	Head and neck	• Suspect ligament injuries of the neck, temporal bone skull fractures
	Chest and abdomen	• Suspect shoulder and clavicle fractures, dislocations • Suspect rib fractures • Suspect spleen or liver injury based on the side of impact
	Pelvis	• Suspect pelvis or upper femur fractures
Rollover or rotational crash		
	Rotational injuries	• Consistent with both lateral and head-on injury patterns
	Rollover injuries	• Suspect multiple organ system injuries • Suspect ejection
Vehicle vs. pedestrian crash		• Suspect high injury, high velocity, multiorgan system injuries • Be prepared to stabilize and transport quickly
Hidden injuries from restraints		• Confirm and relay to hospital staff the use of restraints, which type (lap, shoulder belts, or both), and if there was airbag deployment
	Lab belts only	• Suspect intra-abdominal injuries, check for seat belt sign (discoloration along lower abdomen from seat belt impact)
	Shoulder belts	• Check for neck injury and airway compromise • Check for clavicle fracture
	Airbags	• Airbags deflate quickly after the accident so be sure to lift the airbag and check for steering wheel or dashboard deformities in the vehicle • Check for head, spine, eye, and facial trauma (abrasions, foreign body, corneal injury) • Elevated injury risk for geriatric patients, pediatric patients, and patients shorter than 5'2"

MOI, Mechanism of injury.

8. What are the typical injury patterns noted in falls?

Falls are extremely common, and the severity of the trauma depends on the distance, surface, and body part that impacts first. In general, the greater the distance of the fall, the more severe the injury. Have a high index of suspicion for any adult falls over than 20 ft or pediatric falls greater than 10 ft.

A feet-first landing causes energy to travel up to the skeletal system. A patient may be complaining of pain at the heels, consistent with a calcaneal fracture. But remember, spinal precautions may need to be maintained due to the high associated risk for vertebral body fracture from the transmission of the energy force.

In a headfirst fall, the pattern of injury can start at the arms or shoulders, but the head can be forcibly flexed or extended. The patient can have an injury to the skull, cervical spine, and then secondarily to the remainder of the body as it continues the downward motion.

9. What is penetrating trauma?

Penetrating trauma is classified as a force causing a break in the continuity of the skin. These can be further broken down into low-velocity injuries and medium- and high-velocity injuries. This is based on the trajectory and dissipation of energy. Low-velocity injuries often result from a knife or other object being impaled into the body. The length of the object used provides valuable information towards the underlying bodily injury.

Medium- and high-velocity injuries often result from bullets or pellets. The injury profile severity increases based on trajectory, which is the path of motion, and the dissipation of energy, which is the way energy is transferred to the human body. This is often further described by the drag, profile, cavitation, and fragmentation.

- Drag refers to the factors that slow the bullet down, such as wind resistance.
- Profile refers to the impact point of the bullet. The greater the size of the impact point, the more energy has been transferred and, therefore, higher risk of potential injury.
- Cavitation refers to the pathway of expansion that has been caused by the pressure wave of the moving bullet. The hole that has been created in the tissue can be larger than the diameter of the bullet, indicating high velocity of the traveling bullet.
- Fragmentation refers to a bullet breaking into small pieces and releasing those pieces into the body, causing damage.

10. What are the specialized injury patterns associated with blast injuries?

Blast injuries can release tremendous amounts of energy. Every explosion has five phases, and each phase causes a specific pattern of injury.

In the first phase (*primary phase*), injuries occur from the pressure of the blast. These injuries primarily affect gas-containing organs, such as the lungs, stomach, intestines, and ears. Severe damage and death can occur without any external sign of injury. These are the injuries that are most commonly missed because there is no significant external evidence of injury.

Injuries consistent with the *secondary phase* are due to flying debris propelled by the force of the blast. These injuries are obvious and are most commonly lacerations, fractures, burns, or impaled objects.

The *tertiary phase* occurs when the patient is thrown from the source. These injury patterns are consistent with injuries seen from a vehicular ejection pattern.

The *final two phases* result from structural collapse and exposure to chemicals or other related materials from the blast.

11. How do I approach the multisystem trauma patient?

The multisystem trauma patient is one that has injuries involving more than one body system. These patients statistically have a higher incidence of morbidity and mortality; therefore, the EMT needs to respond quickly. Approach the patient with basic advanced trauma life support (ATLS) guidelines of maintaining airway, breathing, circulation, disability, and exposure (Tables 25.2 and 25.3). Beware of the pitfall of distracting injuries and tunnel vision: it does not matter that the patient has an exposed femur if the airway is compromised. Address the airway first, then breathing and oxygenation. Next, as you assess circulation, you address the blood loss associated with an open femur fracture. If the patient is screaming, you know that they are oxygenating and their airway is patent therefore you can quickly address the injury.

12. What do the terms "golden period" and "platinum 10 minutes" refer to and why are they important in trauma care?

These two terms are often used in emergency care because severely injured patients have the best chance of survival when intervention occurs quickly.

The *golden period* refers to the period of care that is needed for a patient to have a good survival outcome. This is different for each patient because of the unknown underlying injuries. For example, the patient could have a bowel injury but not show significant signs until much later in the disease course. *The golden period* refers to the time of transport, intervention, and treatment prior to the patient having significant signs and symptoms.

The *platinum 10 minutes* is often referred to by EMS systems and the cases of severe trauma. Ten minutes is the maximum time the EMS team should stay on scene prior to transporting the patient for definitive care. The key is to identify life-threatening injuries, provide emergent stabilization, and prepare for rapid transport.

13. What are the special considerations that an EMS provider needs to be aware of when assessing a trauma patient?

When assessing a trauma patient, the EMT personnel first needs to worry about personal safety. Once the personnel and trauma patients are in a safe and stable environment, you can begin to follow the guidelines for field triage of an injured patient (Fig. 25.1).

Information that can be gathered at the scene and relayed at patient handoff is critical to patient outcomes. Determine the mechanism of injury (MOI) and kinetics involved, provide primary assessment, and manage

Table 25.2. Recognizing Worsening Traumatic Injury Based on Symptoms and MOI

MOI	SYMPTOMS
Head trauma	GCS $\leq$8 Repetitive or amnestic to events LOC Altered mental status Changes in speech patterns Headache, especially with nausea and vomiting
Neck trauma	Noisy or labored breathing Increased respiratory rate Swelling of the face or neck Severe neck pain Inability to move or feel extremities
Chest wall trauma	Significant chest pain Shortness of breath Increased respiratory rate Tracheal deviation Subcutaneous emphysema Presence of JVD Loss of peripheral pulses during inspiration Muffled heart sounds Absent breath sounds Asymmetrical chest wall movement Hypoxia
Abdominal trauma	Pain Vomiting Rigid or distended abdomen Seat belt sign
Extremity trauma	Weak or absent pulse Obvious deformity Active bleeding Long-bone injury
Multisystem trauma	Decreasing GCS Weak, rapid, or slow pulse Hypotension Hypoxia

GCS, Glasgow Coma Scale; JVD, jugular vein distention; LOC, level of consciousness; MOI, mechanism of injury.

Table 25.3. Glasgow Coma Scale

EYE OPENING RESPONSE		VERBAL RESPONSE		MOTOR RESPONSE	
Spontaneous	4	Oriented	5	Obeys commands	6
Verbal stimuli	3	Confused conversation	4	Purposeful movement to painful stimulus	5
Pain only	2	Inappropriate words	3	Withdraws in response to pain	4
No response	1	Incomprehensible speech	2	Flexion in response to pain (decorticate posturing)	3
		No response	1	Extension in response to pain (decerebrate posturing)	2
				No response	1

Total score: _____ **(out of 15)**
Source: https://www.cdc.gov/masstrauma/resources/gcs.pdf

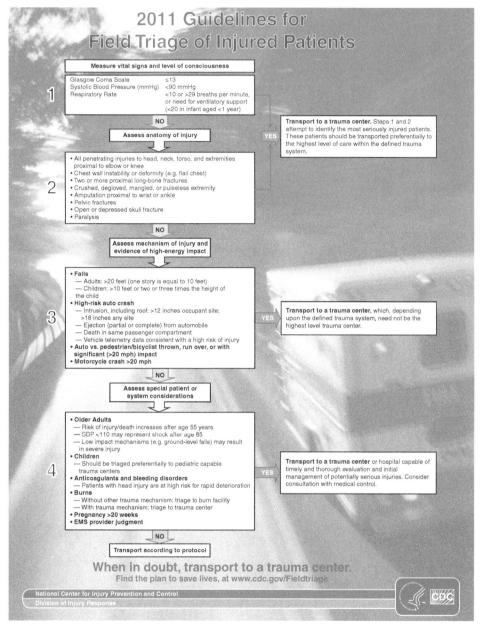

Fig. 25.1. 2011 Guidelines for field triage of an injured patient algorithm *(From Centers for Disease Control and Prevention, https://stacks.cdc.gov/view/cdc/23038.)*

immediate life threats. Take photos of the crime scene if you think it will help the hospital personnel. Maintain spinal precautions; establish and maintain a patent airway; establish and maintain adequate oxygenation; maintain normal body temperature; splint fractures when appropriate; transport critically injured patients within 10 minutes of extrication; obtain a history from the patient, relatives, or bystanders; and perform a secondary assessment to monitor any changes en route (Table 25.4).

Table 25.4. Indications for Rapid Transport and On-Scene Time of Less Than 10 Minutes

SYSTEMS	INDICATIONS
Airway	• Airway trauma, occlusion, or difficulty maintaining a patent airway
Breathing	• Respiratory rate <10 or >29 breaths per minute • Hypoxia • Respiratory distress • Flail chest • Suspected pneumothorax, hemothorax, or tension pneumothorax
Circulation	• Uncontrolled external hemorrhage • Signs and symptoms of shock • Significant blood loss, even if controlled
Disability	• Suspected skull fracture • Altered mental status or suspected brain injury • Seizure activity • Sensory or motor deficit • Suspected pelvis fracture • Crushed or significantly deformed extremity • Two or more suspected long bone fractures • Extremity amputation
Exposure	• Penetrating trauma to the head, neck, anterior or posterior chest, abdomen, and above the elbow or above the knee • Hypothermia • Burns
Special considerations	• Multisystem trauma patient • Pregnancy • Geriatric trauma • Pediatric trauma

14. How do I determine the best transport method and hospital designation for a trauma patient?
    Hospitals go through a strict certification and recertification process to maintain trauma level designations. Level 1 trauma facilities can manage all types of trauma 24 hours a day, 7 days a week. Level 4 trauma facilities are typically small community hospitals in a remote area, capable of stabilizing injured patients and then transferring them to a higher level trauma center (Table 25.5).
    EMS is an integral component of the trauma system and is critical to ensuring good patient outcomes.

KEY POINTS

• Knowing the mechanism of injury and the kinetics of the injury can provide valuable information into the injuries the patient has sustained. Take photos of the scene when possible.
• Blunt trauma is when a force is applied to the body and there is no penetration by an object.
• Penetrating trauma produces a break in the skin and has specific injury patterns associated with it.
• Vehicle collisions have typical injury patterns based on the type of impact and surrounding findings at the scene, which can be helpful information for hospital personnel at handoff.
• Blast injuries resulting from an explosion are associated with five phases of injury; the first phase injuries can be fatal, but are often missed.
• Fall injuries have patterns based on the height and direction of body impact.
• Certain MOI should cause the EMT to have a high index of suspicion for significant traumatic injuries.
• Trauma designations have been assigned to facilities with various levels of care to allow for rapid intervention of the injured patient. Follow the trauma triage criteria to stabilize an injured patient and determine the most appropriate facility for transport.
• Know the physiological criteria for rapid transport of a trauma patient.
• Know the high-risk traumatic mechanisms of injury for rapid transport.

Table 25.5. Trauma Level Designations

LEVEL	DESIGNATION	DESCRIPTION
Level I	A Level I Trauma Center is a comprehensive regional resource that is a tertiary care facility central to the trauma system. A Level I Trauma Center is capable of providing total care for every aspect of injury—from prevention through rehabilitation.	• 24-hour in-house coverage by general surgeons and prompt availability of care in specialties such as orthopedic surgery, neurosurgery, anesthesiology, emergency medicine, radiology, internal medicine, plastic surgery, oral and maxillofacial, pediatric, and critical care. • Referral resource for communities in nearby regions. • Provides leadership in prevention, public education to surrounding communities. • Provides continuing education of the trauma team members. • Incorporates a comprehensive quality assessment program. • Operates an organized teaching and research effort to help direct new innovations in trauma care. • Program for substance abuse screening and patient intervention. • Meets the minimum requirement for annual volume of severely injured patients.
Level II	A Level II Trauma Center is able to initiate definitive care for all injured patients.	• 24-hour immediate coverage by general surgeons, as well as coverage by the specialties of orthopedic surgery, neurosurgery, anesthesiology, emergency medicine, radiology, and critical care. • Tertiary care needs such as cardiac surgery, hemodialysis and microvascular surgery may be referred to a Level I Trauma Center. • Provides trauma prevention and continuing education programs for staff. • Incorporates a comprehensive quality assessment program.
Level III	A Level III Trauma Center has demonstrated an ability to provide prompt assessment, resuscitation, surgery, intensive care, and stabilization of injured patients and emergency operations.	• 24-hour immediate coverage by emergency medicine physicians and the prompt availability of general surgeons and anesthesiologists. • Incorporates a comprehensive quality assessment program. • Has developed transfer agreements for patients requiring more comprehensive care at a Level I or Level II Trauma Center. • Provides back-up care for rural and community hospitals. • Offers continued education of the nursing and allied health personnel or the trauma team. • Involved with prevention efforts and must have an active outreach program for its referring communities.
Level IV	A Level IV Trauma Center has demonstrated an ability to provide advanced trauma life support (ATLS) prior to transfer of patients to a higher level trauma center. It provides evaluation, stabilization, and diagnostic capabilities for injured patients.	• Basic emergency department facilities to implement ATLS protocols and 24-hour laboratory coverage. Available trauma nurse(s) and physicians available upon patient arrival. • May provide surgery and critical care services if available. • Has developed transfer agreements for patients requiring more comprehensive care at a Level I or Level II Trauma Center. • Incorporates a comprehensive quality assessment program. • Involved with prevention efforts and must have an active outreach program for its referring communities.

(Continued)

Table 25.5. Trauma Level Designations (*Cont.*)

LEVEL	DESIGNATION	DESCRIPTION
Level V	A Level V Trauma Center provides initial evaluation, stabilization, and diagnostic capabilities and prepares patients for transfer to higher levels of care.	• Basic emergency department facilities to implement ATLS protocols. • Available trauma nurse(s) and physicians available upon patient arrival. • After-hours activation protocols if facility is not open 24-hours a day. • May provide surgery and critical care services if available. • Has developed transfer agreements for patients requiring more comprehensive care at a Level I though III Trauma Centers.

Source: https://www.amtrauma.org/page/traumalevels

CHAPTER 26

HEAD INJURIES AND FACIAL TRAUMA

J. Elizabeth Neuman

QUESTIONS AND ANSWERS

1. What is the anatomy of the brain and pathophysiology of injury?
   Familiarity with the anatomy leads to an understanding of the pathophysiology of traumatic brain injury. The skull is a hard area with a fixed volume. Contact of the brain against the bone of the skull can cause primary injury. The fixed volume of the skull allows for little room for any type of expansion either due to bleeding or cerebral edema. Expanding volume in the skull leads to pressure on the brain and vascular structures, compromising blood flow. Treatment is geared to reducing this pressure on the brain. When the pressure within this fixed compartment becomes too great, the brain is forced downward through the skull base, and this is called herniation. Herniation of the brain compromises the regulation of heart rate and blood pressure and is typically a lethal event.

2. When I get on scene and see a patient with a potential head injury, what are the most important first steps to take?
   The initial approach to any trauma patient should still focus on **A**irway, **B**reathing, and **C**irculation. Assess whether the patient has a patent airway, if they are breathing, and if they have adequate perfusion. Remember that patients can exsanguinate from scalp wounds. The scalp is very well perfused and bleeds profusely. Hemorrhage control is critical.

3. How do I objectively assess a patient's mental status?
   Practitioners still use the Glasgow Coma Scale (GCS) to attempt a standardized method of communication regarding mental status. The 10th edition of the *Advanced Trauma Life Support Student Course Manual* reflects the revised GCS, which allows for an area that cannot be assessed.[1] Remember that a low GCS score may have other etiologies, such as acute intoxication, medication overdoses, and a low GCS does not always imply a severe brain injury.

Eye opening (E)	Spontaneous	4
	To Sound	3
	To pressure	2
	None	1
	Not testable	NT
Verbal response (V)	Oriented	5
	Confused	4
	Words	3
	Sounds	2
	None	1
	Not testable	NT
Best motor response (M)	Obeys commands	6
	Localizing	5
	Normal flexion	4
	Abnormal flexion	3
	Extension	2
	None	1
	Not testable	NT

*Normal flexion—withdrawal to pain in the original GCS.

4. Why is the GCS important?
   If the patient's GCS score is declining, this is very important. In general, intubation should be considered if the patient has a GCS score ≤8. Intubation, however, should not delay transport to the closest trauma center. If transport time is long, and there is a change in condition, online medical oversight should be advised so that the receiving facility can prepare accordingly. The more time the receiving facility has to prepare for a possible airway, and alert their neurosurgical and trauma support, the better.

5. Does the pupil exam matter?
   The pupillary exam is an important part of the physical exam. A unilateral dilated pupil is an ominous finding and, unfortunately, is an indicator of brainstem herniation. This is, however, an important finding to communicate to the receiving facility, as it will allow them to prepare accordingly as discussed previously. Remember, a unilateral dilated pupil does

not mean that the patient is herniating if they are awake and talking. Direct ocular trauma can result in a dilated pupil, and in the elderly, ocular surgery is common, and this finding may be baseline. Do not intubate a patient with a GCS score of 14 because they have a unilateral dilated pupil.

6. What is the difference between primary and secondary injury, and why does it matter?
    Primary injury is the injury that occurs at the time of the insult—intraparenchymal hemorrhage, for example. Secondary injury is the injury that occurs due to hypotension, hypoxia, decreased blood flow, and edema. This is where prehospital care and avoiding factors that can worsen secondary injury, such as hypoxia and hypotension in particular, are of critical importance. Studies have shown that increased depth and duration of hypotension are associated with increased mortality.[2]

7. Do I have to immobilize the cervical spine?
    Yes, the incidence of concomitant cervical spine injury in patients with traumatic brain injury is estimated to be between 4% and 8%.[3]

8. What is the difference between epidural and subdural hematoma, and will I be able to tell which the patient has clinically?
    a. Epidural hematoma—typically results from a direct blow to the skull, resulting in disruption of, most commonly, the middle meningeal artery. Arterial bleeding into the space between the skull and the dura is associated with more rapid declines in mental status. Patients may have initial loss of consciousness, followed by the "lucid interval" and subsequent deterioration. The lucid interval is observed only in a minority of patients.
    b. Subdural hematoma—typically results from deceleration mechanism, tearing the bridging veins between the brain and the dura. This is classically seen in elderly patients who fall, as the subdural space is larger due to brain atrophy. Clinical signs of subdural hematoma can be slow to manifest. Differentiating an epidural hematoma from a subdural hematoma in the prehospital setting is not possible. Having a high index of suspicion for either and treating to avoid secondary insult are the goals.

9. I come on scene to a patient who was in a motor vehicle collision. The patient has been extricated and immobilized and has a GCS score of 7. What do I do? What prehospital interventions can help this patient?
    a. Assess airway and breathing. Intubate if necessary, according to protocol. Hypoxia can increase secondary brain injury and should be avoided. Administer supplemental oxygen to maintain saturations >98%.
    b. If the patient is intubated, only hyperventilate if the patient has signs of herniation, or if they acutely decompensate. End-tidal CO_2 capnography should be monitored. Hypercarbia worsens secondary brain injury, but pCO_2 should be maintained around 35 mmHg. Hyperventilation leads to cerebral vasoconstriction, which decreases cerebral perfusion. Hyperventilation to pCO_2 25–30 is only a last-ditch effort to alleviate increased intracranial pressure (ICP) in the herniating patient,
    c. Even the immobilized patient can have the head elevated to 30 degrees to facilitate venous return from the brain, and potentially decrease ICP. Place the patient in reverse Trendelenburg position.
    d. Maintain sedation in the intubated patient—the endotracheal tube is painful and irritating. Every "buck" against the tube increases ICP and can worsen their condition. Analgesia and sedation should be provided according to protocol and as hemodynamics allow.
    e. Avoid hypotension. Hypotension decreases cerebral perfusion and worsens outcomes.[4] Administer volume to correct hypotension when possible.
    f. Transport according to protocol. Literature supports that patients may benefit from transport directly to a trauma center, rather than initial evaluation at a nontrauma center and subsequent interfacility transfer.[5]

10. What do I do if the patient has signs of facial trauma?
    While the anatomy, vasculature, and innervation of the face are extremely complex, the issues related to prehospital care are fairly straightforward. The face is very vascular, and injuries can result in significant hemorrhage, similar to scalp lacerations. Close attention must be paid to hemorrhage control. The complicating factors surrounding facial trauma are the potential for airway edema, hemorrhage, and even foreign bodies due to dislodged teeth. Patients with significant facial trauma should be monitored with extreme vigilance for signs of airway compromise. Facial or tongue swelling, changes in phonation, stridor, or drooling are all indications for immediate airway protection. All of these factors, however, can lead to impaired visualization, and the provider must be prepared to perform a surgical airway if needed. If transport time is long, airway protection should be given strong consideration, as should aeromedical transport. Giving as much notice to the receiving facility to allow for adequate preparation for the potentially difficult airway is critical.

11. What about ocular trauma?
    Trauma to the orbit can result in significant ocular injury. Avoid anything that could potentially increase pressure in the eye, and never apply direct pressure to the injured eye. Protect the injured eye using a rigid shield or a cup. Taping the uninjured eye can help minimize movement of the injured eye, and elevating the patient's head

to 30 degrees if there is no concern for spine injury may help decrease intraocular pressure.[1,6] Consider reverse Trendelenburg position to allow for elevation of the head and maintenance of spine precautions.

KEY POINTS

- The skull has a fixed volume, and expansion of the brain creates pressure in that space, compromising blood flow to the brain.
- Airway, breathing, and circulation are critical management interventions in the prehospital setting.
- The scalp is well perfused and can be a significant source of hemorrhage.
- The GCS is an objective way to communicate to medical command about the mental status of a patient.
- Monitoring for changes in GCS score is of critical importance particularly when transport times are long.
- Avoiding hypoxemia and hypotension is a critical action to help mitigate secondary brain injury.
- Facial trauma can result in significant hemorrhage. Attention to potential airway compromise due to bleeding, foreign bodies, or unstable facial fractures is a critical component of prehospital care.

REFERENCES

1. *Advanced Trauma Life Support Student Course Manual*. 10th ed. Chicago, IL: American College of Surgeons; 2018:102-126.
2. Spaite DW, Chengcheng H, Bobrow BJ, et al. Association of out-of-hospital hypotension depth and duration with traumatic brain injury mortality. *Ann Emerg Med*. 2017;70(4):522-530.
3. Holly LT, Kelly DF, Counelis GJ, et al. Cervical spine trauma associated with moderate and severe head injury; incidence, risk factors, and injury characteristics. *J Neurosurg Spine*. 2002;96:285291.
4. Vella MA, Crandall ML, Patel MB. Acute management of traumatic brain injury. *Surg Clin N Am*. 2017;97:1015-1030.
5. Chowdhury T, Kowalski S, Arabi Y, Dash HH. Pre-hospital and initial management of head injury patients: an update. *Saudi J Anaesth*. 2014;8(1):114-120.
6. Yeon D-Y, Yoo C, Lee T-E, Park J-H, Kim YY. Effects of head elevation on intraocular pressure in healthy subjects: raising bed head *vs* using multiple pillows. *Eye*. 2014;28(11):1328-1333.

CHAPTER 27

CERVICAL SPINE AND SPINAL CORD INJURIES

J. Elizabeth Neuman

QUESTIONS AND ANSWERS

1. How common are traumatic spine injuries (TSIs)?

   There are an estimated 12,000 injuries per year in the United States, with the majority occurring as a result of motor vehicle crashes and falls.[1]

2. Why is this subject important?

   The morbidity associated with severe TSI results in significant change in quality of life and financial costs. Patients with severe TSI have significant reductions in life expectancy, and average lifetime expenses can be in the millions of dollars for one patient with an incomplete spinal injury.[1] Over 50% of injuries are of the cervical spine, which are associated with much higher morbidity and long-term cost than injuries of the thoracic and lumbar spine.[1] The elderly constitute an at-risk population, as patients with osteoporosis and other spinal arthropathies, such as rheumatoid arthritis, are at higher risk of injury.

3. Why are we so worried about the cervical spine?

   The cervical spine consists of seven vertebrae separated by intervertebral disks and is held in place by the anterior and posterior longitudinal ligaments. The cervical spine has the greatest degree of mobility and is therefore the most vulnerable portion of the spine.[2] The cervical canal from the base of the skull to the inferior portion of C2 is fairly large but narrows at the level of C3, making injury to the spinal cord at this level and distal much more likely.[2] The cervical spinal cord is also of critical importance because the phrenic nerves that innervate the diaphragm originate at the C3–5 levels. A complete spinal cord injury in this area can as a result cause apnea and death. Extreme care must be taken to avoid converting a patient with an incomplete cord injury who can breathe to a patient with a complete cord injury who then would become apneic.

4. What do I do about extricating patients after a motor vehicle collision?

   Extrication and spinal motion restriction (SMR) should be performed according to local protocol. A recent retrospective review demonstrated that the rapid extrication maneuver (REM) and Kendrick Extrication Device (KED) appear to be equivalent in the ability to protect from further neurologic injury after motor vehicle collisions.[3]

5. What do I do about SMR in trauma?

   The latest policy statement from the American College of Emergency Physicians (ACEP) is the uniform consensus of ACEP, the American College of Surgeons Committee on Trauma (ACS-COT), and the National Association of EMS Physicians (NAEMSP).[4] Main excerpts from the statement follow, and the full statement can be found online.

   Points of consensus
   - Unstable spinal column injuries can progress to severe neurological injuries in the presence of excessive movement of the injured spine.
   - While current techniques limit or reduce undesired motion of the spine, they do not provide true spinal immobilization. For this reason, the term "spinal motion restriction (SMR)" has gained favor over "spinal immobilization," although both terms refer to the same concept. The goal of both SMR and spinal immobilization in the trauma patient is to minimize unwanted movement of the potentially injured spine.
   - While backboards have historically been used to attempt spinal immobilization, SMR may also be achieved by use of a scoop stretcher, vacuum splint, ambulance cot, or other similar device to which a patient is safely secured.
   - Indications for SMR following blunt trauma include:
     - Acutely altered level of consciousness (e.g., Glasgow Coma Scale [GCS] score <15, evidence of intoxication)
     - Midline neck or back pain and/or tenderness
     - Focal neurologic signs and/or symptoms (e.g., numbness or motor weakness)
     - Anatomic deformity of the spine
     - Distracting circumstances or injury (e.g., long bone fracture, degloving or crush injuries, large burns, emotional distress, communication barrier, etc.) or any similar injury that impairs the patient's ability to contribute to a reliable examination
   - SMR, when indicated, should apply to the entire spine due to the risk of noncontiguous injuries. An appropriately sized cervical collar is a critical component of SMR and should be used to limit movement of the cervical spine

whenever SMR is employed. The remainder of the spine should be stabilized by keeping the head, neck, and torso in alignment. This can be accomplished by placing the patient on a long backboard, a scoop stretcher, a vacuum mattress, or an ambulance cot. If elevation of the head is required, the device used to stabilize the spine should be elevated at the head while maintaining alignment of the neck and torso. SMR cannot be properly performed with a patient in a sitting position.

- All patient transfers create potential for unwanted displacement of an unstable spine injury. Particular attention should be focused on patient transfers from one surface to another including, for example, ground to ambulance cot. A long spine board, a scoop stretcher, or a vacuum mattress is recommended to assist with patient transfers in order to minimize flexion, extension, or rotation of the possibly injured spine.
- There is no role for SMR in penetrating trauma.
- For SMR in children, age alone should not be a factor in decision-making for prehospital spinal care, both for the young child and the child who can reliably provide a history. Young children pose communication barriers, but this should not mandate SMR purely based on age. Based on the best available pediatric evidence from studies that have been conducted through the Pediatric Emergency Care Applied Research Network (PECARN), a cervical collar should be applied if the patient has any of the following:
  - Complaint of neck pain;
  - Torticollis;
  - Neurologic deficit;
  - Altered mental status, including a GCS score <15, intoxication, and other signs (agitation, apnea, hypopnea, somnolence, etc.); and
  - Involvement in a high-risk motor vehicle collision, high-impact diving injury, or has substantial torso injury.
- There is no evidence supporting a high risk/incidence for noncontiguous multilevel spinal injury in children. The rate of contiguous multilevel injury in children is extremely low at 1%. The rate of noncontiguous multilevel injury in children is thought to be equally as low.
- Minimize the time on backboards with consideration for use of a vacuum mattress or padding as adjuncts to minimize the risk of pain and pressure ulcers if this time is to be prolonged.
- Because of the variation in the head size to body ratio in young children relative to adults, additional padding under the shoulders is often necessary to avoid excessive cervical spine flexion with SMR.

6. If a patient is ambulatory at the scene, do I have to place them in SMR?
   Yes. A recent study cited that 8% of patients who were ambulatory at the scene had spinal injuries, the most common being vertebral fracture.[5]

7. Why can cervical collars be harmful in penetrating trauma?
   If there are no signs of spinal cord injury, cervical collars should not be applied in patients with penetrating trauma, in particular isolated gunshot wounds (GSWs) to the head. Studies have shown that prehospital immobilization is associated with increased mortality. In one study, the number needed to harm and potentially cause one death was 66, as opposed to the number needed to potentially benefit (>1030).[5] This is thought to be related to the extra time that is required on scene, delaying transport to definitive care.[5,6] The increase in morbidity and mortality is also likely related to the cervical collar itself that can obscure physical findings such as tracheal deviation, expanding hematoma, subcutaneous emphysema, and other signs that would require emergent airway intervention.[5]

8. What do I need to know about airway management?
   The debate surrounding endotracheal intubation vs. supraglottic airway insertion continues and is beyond the scope of this chapter. If the patient requires airway intervention, this should be performed according to local protocols. If a difficult airway is anticipated, however, serious consideration should be given to the use of a supraglottic airway to avoid delay to transport, risk of misplaced endotracheal tube (ETT), and potential traumatization of the airway that could complicate further attempts at intubation. Special considerations are related to the potential movement of the cervical spine during intubation, and the limitation of placement into optimal position due to the concerns for spinal injury. Sawin et al. studied movement of the cervical spine during intubation; they found that laryngoscope blade elevation caused significant extension at all segments of the cervical spine, in particular at the atlanto-occipital and atlanto-axial joints.[7] The standard approach to airway management should be utilized, with close attention paid to protecting the cervical spine.
- Maintain inline stabilization of the spine.
- Preoxygenate as much as possible; utilize the oropharyngeal airway when needed.
- Use sedatives and paralytics per protocol.
- Remove the anterior portion of the cervical collar for intubation.
- Perform intubation with direct visualization of the ETT passage through the vocal cords.
- Confirm placement of the ETT with auscultation and end-tidal capnometry.
- Replace the anterior portion of the cervical collar for transport.

9. My patient is hypotensive. Is this neurogenic shock?

Neurogenic shock results from loss of sympathetic tone to the vasculature. Hypotension without tachycardia is the hallmark sign. Hypotension in the trauma patient, however, should be assumed to be hemorrhagic until proven otherwise. Resuscitate the patient accordingly.

10. What else can I do to help patients with potential traumatic spinal cord injuries (TSCIs)?

Similar to traumatic brain injury, the spinal cord is subject to not only the primary injury but also to secondary injury that results from a complex cascade of processes that are not fully understood. Hypoxia and hypotension have been shown to worsen outcomes in TSCI. Maintaining oxygen saturations and mean arterial pressures >85 help to minimize spinal cord ischemia and secondary insult.[8]

11. Should I give methylprednisolone for TSCI?

Studies have been and continue to be conflicting. Discussion with online medical oversight in accordance with local protocols is encouraged.

KEY POINTS

- TSIs are common and are associated with significant morbidity and mortality.
- Prehospital extrication and SMR are critical procedures that can affect primary and secondary injury of the spinal cord.
- There is a consensus agreement regarding indications for SMR in blunt and penetrating trauma.
- Airway and blood pressure management is a critical factor in helping to mitigate secondary spinal cord injury.

REFERENCES

1. Stein DM, Knight WA. Emergency neurological life support: traumatic spine injury. *Neurocrit Care*. 2017;27:S170-S180.
2. *Advanced Trauma Life Support Student Course Manual*. 10th ed. Chicago, IL: American College of Surgeons; 2018:129-145.
3. Misasi A, Ward JG, Dong F, et al. Prehospital extrication techniques: neurological outcomes associated with the rapid extrication method and the Kendrick Extrication Device. *Am Surgeon*. 2018;84(2):248-253.
4. A joint policy statement of the American College of Emergency Physicians, the American College of Surgeons Committee on Trauma, and the National Association of EMS Physicians. 2018. https://www.acep.org/globalassets/new-pdfs/policy-statements/spinal-motion-restriction-in-the-trauma-patient.pdf.
5. McCoy CE, Loza-Gomez AL, Puckett JL, et al. Quantifying the risk of spinal injury in motor vehicle collisions according to ambulatory status: a prospective analytical study. *J Emerg Med*. 2016;32(2):151-159.
6. Haut ER, Kalish BT, Efron DT, et al. Spine immobilization in penetrating trauma: more harm than good? *J Trauma*. 2010;68(1):115-121.
7. Sawin PD, Todd MM, Traynelis VC, et al. Cervical spine motion with direct laryngoscopy and orotracheal intubation. An in vivo cinefluoroscopic study of subjects without cervical abnormality. *Anesthesiology*. 1996;85:26-36.
8. Catapano JS, Hawryluk GWJ, Whetsone W, et al. Higher mean arterial pressure values correlate with neurologic improvement in patients with initially complete spinal cord injuries. *World Neurosurg*. 2016;96:72-79.

CHAPTER 28

CHEST, ABDOMINAL, AND PELVIC INJURIES

Kian Preston-Suni and Bradley Chappell

QUESTIONS AND ANSWERS

1. How should chest trauma be evaluated?

   Patients suffering from significant chest trauma may complain of chest pain, shortness of breath, back or flank discomfort, or abdominal pain. Significant injuries may be accompanied by tachycardia, tachypnea, hypotension, and hypoxia. The first step is visual inspection of the patient. How is the work of breathing—is there any splinting or flail chest? Further inspection should evaluate for any obvious signs of injury including bruising, abrasions (such as a seat belt sign), and penetrating wounds. Palpation can detect crepitus from a pneumothorax, point tenderness suggesting a rib fracture, and instability, which may be present with multiple rib fractures. Diminished breath sounds may be present in hemothorax or pneumothorax, but normal breath sounds do not rule out these conditions. The mechanism of injury provides a framework to help determine the risk of sustaining serious injuries. Extensive vehicle damage, passenger space intrusion, prolonged extrication, air bag deployment, and steering wheel damage are all risk factors for significant injury.

2. How should chest trauma be managed in the prehospital setting?

   First, ensure that the patient is maintaining their airway. Obstruction may be relieved with jaw thrust or oral airway placement in the comatose patient, with care taken to minimize cervical spine movement. In a patient with an intact gag reflex, a nasopharyngeal airway may be beneficial. For those who are unresponsive, an oropharyngeal airway, laryngeal mask airway (LMA), or endotracheal tube can be used. Failure to protect the airway is an indication for intubation, which is guided by local prehospital protocols. Supplemental oxygen should be administered for hypoxia, which is generally considered <93% oxygen saturation in a critically ill adult. Always evaluate the patient for tension pneumothorax, and if present, perform needle decompression.

3. What is flail chest and how should it be treated?

   Fractures of two or more ribs in two locations, including anterior costochondral separation, can result in a segment of chest that moves independent of the surrounding chest wall (Fig. 28.1). This results in paradoxical movement of the injured segment of chest wall, with inward movement during inhalation and outward movement

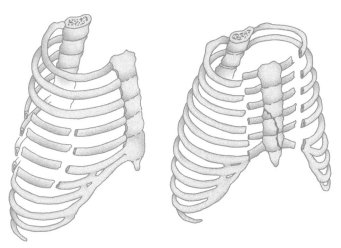

Fig. 28.1. Flail chest. *(From Raja AS. Thoracic trauma. In: Walls RM, Hockberger RS, Gausche-Hill M, eds.* Rosen's Emergency Medicine Concepts and Clinical Practice. *9th ed. Philadelphia: Elsevier; 2018.)*

on exhalation, causing impairing ventilation. It is usually accompanied by pulmonary contusion, which may cause hypoxia. Historically, these injuries were managed with splinting, but this is no longer recommended as splinting impairs ventilation and may lead to further atelectasis and potential pneumonia. Upright positioning, pain management, and supplemental oxygen may help. Patients with flail chest often require mechanical ventilation.

4. What is a pulmonary contusion?

Significant blunt trauma to the chest that displaces the chest wall inward may bruise the underlying lung. Injury to capillaries causes blood and fluid to accumulate in the airspaces, impairing oxygenation and ventilation. Supplemental oxygen can be used to treat hypoxia, but significant hypoxia and increased work of breathing may require positive pressure ventilation. Excessive fluid resuscitation can worsen airspace disease and hypoxia in pulmonary contusions, so IV fluids should be administered only if necessary.

5. What is a pneumothorax?

A pneumothorax is collapse of the lung with escape of air into the thorax surrounding the lung (Fig. 28.2). It can be caused by both penetrating and blunt trauma. In penetrating trauma, the chest wall or lung is directly injured, whereas blunt injuries most often cause a rib fracture, which punctures the lung and causes air to escape into the chest cavity. Presentations may include chest pain, dyspnea, tachypnea, and subcutaneous emphysema. If the patient is intubated before the pneumothorax is treated, the positive pressure may cause conversion to a tension pneumothorax. Therefore, if the patient requires emergent airway management, a needle decompression of the pneumothorax should be performed prior to intubation.

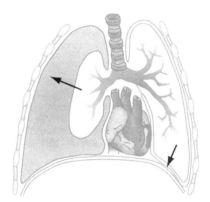

Fig. 28.2. Pneumothorax. Air escapes *(arrows)* from the right lung into the thoracic cavity through an injury to the visceral pleura. *(From Raja AS. Thoracic trauma. In: Walls RM, Hockberger RS, Gausche-Hill M, eds. Rosen's Emergency Medicine Concepts and Clinical Practice. 9th ed. Philadelphia: Elsevier; 2018.)*

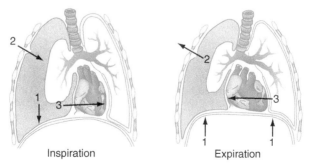

Inspiration   Expiration

Fig. 28.3. Open pneumothorax. Inspiration *(left)*: The diaphragm contracts, causing negative intrathoracic pressure *(arrow 1)* that draws air through the sucking chest wound in the pleural cavity *(arrow 2)* and causing the mediastinal structures to shift to the patient's left *(arrow 3)*. Expiration *(right)*: The diaphragm recoils *(arrow 1)*, causing air to exit the chest *(arrow 2)* and allowing the mediastinum to shift back to normal position *(arrow 3)*. The collapsed lung paradoxically shrinks on inspiration and expands on expiration. *(From Raja AS. Thoracic trauma. In: Walls RM, Hockberger RS, Gausche-Hill M, eds. Rosen's Emergency Medicine Concepts and Clinical Practice. 9th ed. Philadelphia: Elsevier; 2018.)*

6. **What is an open pneumothorax?**
   An open pneumothorax is an injury with free communication between the chest cavity and the external environ-ment (Fig. 28.3). Most commonly associated with gunshot injuries, these wounds present with sucking sounds from air entry into the chest during inspiration. Large wounds may impair ventilation as air preferentially enters the chest defect rather than through the airway. Open pneumothoraces should be covered using a partially oc-clusive dressing sealed on three sides or with a vented chest seal to prevent the pneumothorax from increasing in size with each respiration. These dressings are designed to allow air to exit the wound during exhalation. Complete occlusion of the wound can cause conversion to a tension pneumothorax.

7. **What is a tension pneumothorax?**
   A tension pneumothorax forms when air enters the hemithorax and cannot escape, as in a one-way valve. The point of entry can be from an injury to the visceral pleura, tracheobronchial tree, or the chest wall itself. As air enters the chest cavity, the intrathoracic pressure rises. This impairs ventilation, decreases venous return to the heart, and causes hypotension and distention of the neck veins. As intrathoracic pressure builds further still, the tension pneumothorax pushes the mediastinum toward the contralateral chest, causing deviation of the trachea and cardiovascular collapse. If left untreated, a tension pneumothorax may lead to respiratory and cardiac arrest. The previous classic features may be absent, and more frequently, patients present with a combination of tachy-pnea, respiratory distress, or hypoxia. Other signs and symptoms of tension pneumothorax include dyspnea, chest pain, and absence of unilateral breath sounds.

8. **How should needle decompression of tension pneumothorax be performed?**
   Placement of a needle thoracostomy is a potentially life-saving procedure for a patient suffering from a tension pneumothorax. The needle and catheter should be advanced in the 4th or 5th rib interspace, just over the rib and anterior to the midaxillary line. Placement in this location may be more likely to achieve decompression than in the midclavicular line. The needle is removed with the catheter left in place, allowing for decompression and convert-ing it to a simple pneumothorax. Serial reassessment is required as the catheter may become kinked or dislodged, causing the return of tension physiology. To increase the likelihood of adequate decompression, an angiocatheter at least 5 cm in length should be used as shorter needles are less likely to be successful.

9. **What is a hemothorax?**
   Penetrating and blunt trauma can cause lacerations of the intercostal arteries, thoracic great vessels, or the lung itself, leading to an accumulation of blood in the hemithorax. Signs and symptoms can include chest pain, dyspnea, diminished breath sounds, dullness to percussion, hypotension, and tachycardia. Tube thoracostomy for hemothorax is generally performed in the emergency department but may be performed in the field in special cir-cumstances according to local protocols. Caution to ensure adequate use of personal protective equipment should always be used when placing a chest tube. Additionally, always clamp or manually kink the end of the chest tube until it is attached to suction.

10. **What is cardiac tamponade?**
    Tamponade results from a collection of fluid around the heart that increases pressure inside the pericardium, preventing filling during diastole and resulting in increased venous pressures and decreased cardiac output. Cardiac tamponade may present with dyspnea, chest pain, tachycardia, hypotension, tachypnea, and distended neck veins. Tamponade may result from a penetrating injury to the heart or, more rarely, from blunt trauma causing aortic injury.

11. **How should cardiac tamponade be treated in the prehospital setting?**
    Tamponade, like tension pneumothorax, is a form of obstructive shock. A proximal, large-bore IV should be placed with rapid infusion of IV fluids.

12. **What is a cardiac contusion?**
    Blunt injuries to chest, often from rapid deceleration or steering wheel impact, may push the ribs toward the ver-tebral bodies, compressing the heart. This can lead to bruising of the myocardium, with varying effects including life-threatening arrhythmias, reduced cardiac output, and cardiogenic shock. Patients at risk of cardiac contusion should receive an IV and cardiac monitoring. Arrhythmias should be treated per standard Advanced Cardiovascular Life Support (ACLS) protocol.

13. **How should abdominal trauma be evaluated in the prehospital setting?**
    Symptoms of abdominal injury may include pain, vomiting, nausea, or light headedness. The abdomen should be inspected for signs of injury including abrasions, bruising (including seat belt sign), or wounds from penetrat-ing injuries. The abdomen should be palpated as tenderness may be a finding of intra-abdominal hemorrhage or intestinal injury. Bleeding in the abdomen may present with signs of shock, including hypotension, tachycardia, pallor, altered mental status, diaphoresis, or tachypnea.

14. How should abdominal trauma be managed?

    Patients with any signs or symptoms of abdominal injury should have a large-bore IV placed in a proximal location. Hypotension or other signs of shock should be treated with an IV bolus of crystalloid solution. Penetrating abdominal wounds and any herniated viscera should be covered with saline-soaked gauze to prevent contamination.

15. How is pelvic trauma evaluated?

    Most commonly caused by motor vehicle accidents, crush injuries, and falls, significant pelvic fractures can rapidly cause life-threatening bleeding and shock. Symptoms of pelvic fracture can include pain and the inability to ambulate. Signs of pelvic fracture include widening of the pubic symphysis, pelvic instability, and blood at the urethral meatus. Leg length discrepancy and internal/external rotation of the lower leg often indicate proximal femur fracture. Care must be taken when examining the pelvis to avoid rocking or significant manipulation as these maneuvers can increase bleeding.

16. How is pelvic trauma managed?

    Patients at risk for pelvic fracture should receive an IV with fluid bolus administration if hypotension or other signs of shock are present. Pelvic binding using either a wrapped sheet with towel clamps or a commercially available pelvic binder is effective in reducing pelvic volume in the setting of certain pelvic fractures. It also stabilizes bone fragments and allows for clot formation, potentially reducing hemorrhage. Care must be taken to apply the binder centered over the greater trochanters, as placement too high over the iliac crests can worsen pelvic disruption. If blood pressure worsens after application of a binder, consider discontinuing its use.

17. How should hypotension in the setting of chest or abdominal trauma be managed?

    Due to the significant number of large vessels in the thoracoabdominal cavity, traumatic injuries can lead to rapid loss of high volumes of blood. In the prehospital setting, IV fluids should be used to maintain a systolic blood pressure greater than 90 mm Hg. If tranexamic acid (TXA) is available, this should be given as soon as possible in the setting of suspected hemorrhage. Likewise, if packed red blood cells are available in the field, they should be transfused if the patient remains hypotensive after 1 L of IV fluid.

KEY POINTS

- Manage the airway according to local protocols. This may include jaw thrust, oral airway placement, or endotracheal intubation. Provide supplemental oxygen for patients with hypoxia (<93%).
- Place a large-bore, proximal IV for any patient at risk of serious injury. Give a bolus of crystalloid fluid for patients with hypotension or signs of shock.
- Evaluate for life-threatening conditions that can be treated in the prehospital setting. These include tension pneumothorax and open pneumothorax.
- If a patient with pneumothorax requires emergent airway management, a needle decompression of the pneumothorax should be performed prior to intubation.

BIBLIOGRAPHY

American College of Surgeons Committee on Trauma. *Advanced Trauma Life Support for Doctors: Student Course Manual.* 10th ed. Chicago, IL: American College of Surgeons; 2018.

Ball CG, Wyrzykowski AD, Kirkpatrick AW, et al. Thoracic needle decompression for tension pneumothorax: clinical correlation with catheter length. *Can J Surg.* 2010;53:184-188.

Cotton BA, Jerome R, Collier BR, et al. Guidelines for prehospital fluid resuscitation in the injured patient. *J Trauma Acute Care Surg.* 2009;67:389-402.

Cullinane DC, Schiller HJ, Zielinski MD, et al. Eastern Association for the Surgery of Trauma practice management guidelines for hemorrhage in pelvic fracture—update and systematic review. *J Trauma Acute Care Surg.* 2011;71:1850-1868.

Leech C, Porter K, Steyn R, et al. The pre-hospital management of life-threatening chest injuries: a consensus statement from the Faculty of Pre-Hospital Care, Royal College of Surgeons of Edinburgh. *Trauma.* 2017;19:54-62.

Roberts DJ, Leigh-Smith S, Faris PD, et al. Clinical presentation of patients with tension pneumothorax: a systematic review. *Annals Surg.* 2015;261:1068-1078.

Scott I, Porter K, Laird C, Greaves I, Bloch M. The prehospital management of pelvic fractures: initial consensus statement. *Trauma.* 2015;17:151-154.

Siemieniuk RA, Chu DK, Kim LH-Y, et al. Oxygen therapy for acutely ill medical patients: a clinical practice guideline. *BMJ.* 2018;363.

CHAPTER 29

EXTREMITY INJURIES

Brett Campbell and Matthew R. Garner

QUESTIONS AND ANSWERS

1. You are called to the scene of a 78-year-old male who was involved in a motor vehicle collision after he ran a red light. He is reporting pain in his right wrist and left leg. Describe the initial evaluation of the patient's extremities after completion of the initial Basic Life Support (BLS) assessment.
   Once basic life support has been completed, a secondary survey can be performed. The advanced trauma life support (ATLS) training outlines the secondary survey to include[1] gross inspection and palpation of both upper and lower extremities for signs of injury, assessment of vascular status by checking peripheral pulses in all four extremities, assessment of pelvis for evidence of instability or associated hemorrhage, and assessment of motor and sensory function of arms and legs.

2. A 22-year-old female loses control of her motorcycle while going around a sharp turn. She is noted to have a large laceration over the back of her knee with pulsatile bleeding. What are you concerned about and how will you initially manage this patient before she can get to the hospital?
   A primary concern for this patient is active arterial bleeding from injury to the popliteal artery. First, dress the wound and apply direct pressure. A tourniquet can be considered, but note that they are not benign and should be used with caution. A tourniquet can be used in situations where there is extreme life-threatening limb hemorrhage, hemorrhage not controlled by direct pressure, and/or a multiple casualty event with lack of resources to maintain simple hemorrhage control with direct pressure.[2] The principles of tourniquet application include applying at least 5 cm proximal to the injury, applying directly onto skin to avoid slippage, and evaluating for successful use by cessation of external hemorrhage and loss of distal pulses. Document the time the tourniquet was applied. Complications associated with tourniquet use include creation of an ischemic limb resulting in nerve, muscle, vascular, or skin compromise if left on for prolonged time periods, risk of reperfusion injury after the tourniquet is removed, incorrect application that may occlude venous return without occluding arterial flow, and pain generation requiring higher levels of analgesia.

3. A 31-year-old female slips and falls down a grassy hill while intoxicated. Her foot is externally rotated and she is in a lot of pain. What is the benefit of splinting this patient's ankle while you are transporting her to the hospital?
   You have identified that the patient likely has an ankle fracture. The next step is to immobilize the extremity. The benefits of immobilization include improved pain control, reduced motion at the fracture site, prevention of further soft tissue injury, and promotion of the tamponade effect of muscle to control bleeding.

4. A 6-year-old girl falls off the slide and is reporting pain in her left forearm. You notice an obvious deformity of the arm. What is the likely diagnosis and initial treatment?
   The patient likely has an acute fracture, and therefore, your next step would be immobilization of the injured extremity. Various types of splints are available, including air splints, vacuum splints, rigid splints, slings, and traction splints.[3] Use what you have available. Current guidelines recommend splinting in the position the patient is found. Document and relay any areas of skin lacerations or abrasions that will be covered by the splint.

5. A 36-year-old male working at a saw mill accidentally sticks his right hand under the saw and sustains traumatic amputations of the index and long fingers. What do you do with the amputated digits?
   Once you have recovered the digits, wrap them in a saline-moistened gauze, place them in a sealed plastic bag, and submerge in an ice/saline mixture at approximately 4 °C.[4] Your goal is to minimize warm ischemia time but avoid freezing or direct immersion in fluid to maximize the patient's chances for replantation of the digit.

6. You are covering a college football game when a 21-year-old takes a hard hit in the backfield and is noted to have a deformity of his right shoulder with significant pain. Describe one method for reducing a dislocated shoulder.
   Controversy exists about whether or not EMS providers should reduce shoulders in the field, so follow your specific guidelines when approaching this patient. There are over 20 different techniques that can be employed to reduce an anterior shoulder dislocation; a few are listed here.[5] X-rays should always be taken after reduction to confirm successful reduction and ensure no fractures are present (Fig. 29.1).
   a. Milch maneuver—Abduct the arm to overhead and externally rotate to 90 degrees while pushing humeral head superiorly and laterally (Fig. 29.2).
   b. Janecki's maneuver—Apply traction and gradual forward elevation of the arm with the arm externally rotated and then abduct the arm while holding traction.

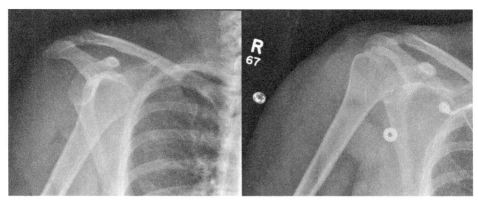

Fig. 29.1. X-ray of a shoulder dislocation before and after successful reduction.

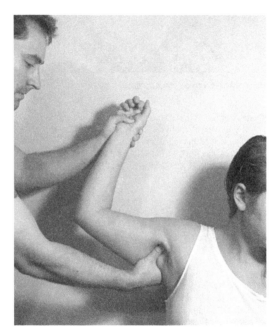

Fig. 29.2. Milch technique for shoulder reduction.

    c. Hanging arm technique—The patient is prone with the arm hanging over the side of the table. Apply gentle traction, abduction and then forward flexion and internal rotation of the arm.

        Keep in mind that although the most common direction of a shoulder dislocation is anterior, it is possible for the humeral head to dislocate posteriorly or inferiorly as well.

7. A 57-year-old male gets his forearm caught in an industrial printing press while at work. You determine that there are some superficial abrasions without any obvious deformities, but the forearm is very swollen. He is continuing to have worsening pain with tiny movements of his hand and wrist despite pain medications and is endorsing some numbness in his hand as well. What are you concerned is happening to this patient and what is the urgency of this diagnosis?

    This is an acute compartment syndrome and it is a surgical emergency. This condition is due to increased tissue pressure within a limited space that is compromising capillary perfusion to the tissues and limiting blood flow to the muscles.[6] Signs and symptoms include a swollen, tense compartment, pain out of proportion to the injury, pain with passive stretch of the fingers (most sensitive finding), sensory deficits, motor deficits, increasing analgesic requirements, and coolness of the extremity beyond the zone of injury. Of note, the patient may still have strong pulses when diagnosed with an acute compartment syndrome.

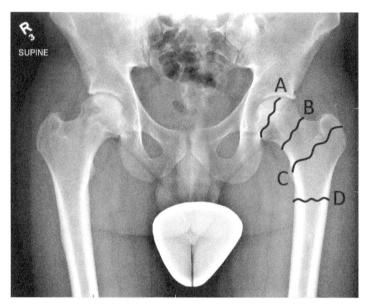

Fig. 29.3. X-ray demonstrating different types of proximal femur fractures.

8. An 18-year-old male was running from the police and jumped from a second-story window and sustained an injury to his left leg. When you arrive, you immediately notice a large opening in the shin with exposed bone. What is the injury and how should it be initially managed?
   This patient has sustained an open tibia fracture. Look out for associated injuries of the head, spine, and abdomen. Be sure to assess the vascular and neurological status of the extremity. The wound needs to be dressed with a clean bandage and the leg splinted.

9. You receive a call about an 82-year-old female who fell at her nursing home and is complaining of left-sided groin pain and inability to walk. You suspect a fracture. List the different types of proximal femur fractures (Fig. 29.3).
   Femoral head fracture, femoral neck fracture, intertrochanteric femur fracture, and subtrochanteric femur fracture.[7]

10. A 24-year-old male was setting off fireworks for 4th of July when one accidentally goes off next to him, and he sustains large burns to his left anterior thigh, right arm, and the front of his abdomen. What percentage of the patient's body surface is affected by the burns?
    This patient would have an estimated burn area of 27%. The Wallace rule of nines can be used to estimate the extent of the patient's body surface that is affected.[8] The body is divided into areas each representing 9% and include head, each arm, front and back of the chest, front and back of the abdomen, front of each leg, and back of each leg (Fig. 29.4).

11. A 4-year-old boy falls while riding a scooter and is noted to have a right wrist deformity. While at the hospital, you overhear that three other children have also been brought to the hospital for broken bones. What are the five most common fractures in the pediatric population?
    Distal forearm fractures, clavicle fractures, finger and toe fractures, ankle fractures, and supracondylar humerus fractures (distal humerus).[9]

12. A 52-year-old male involved in a high-speed motor vehicle collision is reporting significant bilateral hip and groin pain and is noted to be hypotensive and tachycardic. What is the most likely diagnosis and the initial treatment?
    The patient likely has a pelvic ring fracture or disruption contributing to hemodynamic instability. A pelvic binder can be applied in this situation and should be applied at the level of the greater trochanters. The goal of this device is to reduce intrapelvic volume to tamponade the bleeding vessels. The most commonly injured vessels are the presacral venous plexus. The most common error is placing the binder too high, at the level of the iliac crest.

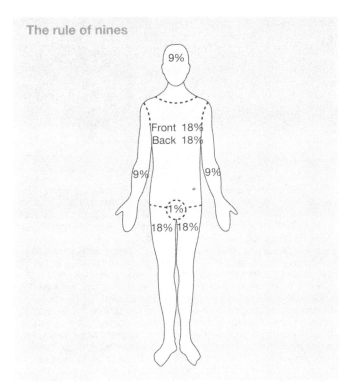

Fig. 29.4. Diagram of Wallace Rule of Nines for estimating the extent of skin surface involved. *(From Quick CRG, Biers SM, Arulampalam THA. Soft tissue injuries and burns. In: Quick CRG, Biers SM, Arulampalam THA, eds.* Essential Surgery: Problems, Diagnosis and Management. *6th ed. Oxford, UK: Elsevier Ltd.; 2020:260-271.)*

KEY POINTS

- Up to 39% of trauma patients will have a missed injury after initial evaluation. Help reduce this number by performing a thorough secondary survey in the field and in the emergency department.[3]
- Tourniquets can be a very effective method for achieving hemostasis in trauma patients but are not without risk; know when and how to properly use them to avoid unnecessary complications.[4]
- Splinting or otherwise immobilizing an extremity with a fracture can provide significant pain relief for the patient and is an important temporizing tool for the emergency care provider.[10]

REFERENCES

1. Galvagno SM, Nahmias JT, Young DA. Advanced trauma life support update 2019: management and applications for adults and special populations. *Anesthesiol Clin.* 2019;37(1):13-32.
2. Lee C, Porter KM, Hodgetts TJ. Tourniquet use in the civilian prehospital setting. *Emerg Med J.* 2007;24(8):584-587.
3. Pfeifer R, Pape HC. Missed injuries in trauma patients: a literature review. *Patient Saf Surg.* 2008;2:20.
4. Maricevich M, Carlsen B, Mardini S, Moran S. Upper extremity and digital replantation. *Hand (N Y).* 2011;6(4):356-363.
5. Singh S, Yong CK, Mariapan S. Closed reduction techniques in acute anterior shoulder dislocation: modified Milch technique compared with traction-countertraction technique. *J Shoulder Elbow Surg.* 2012;21(12):1706-1711.
6. Chandraprakasam T, Kumar RA. Acute compartment syndrome of forearm and hand. *Indian J Plast Surg.* 2011;44(2):212-218.
7. Parker M, Johansen A. Hip fracture. *BMJ.* 2006;333(7557):27-30.
8. Quick CRG, Biers SM, Arulampalam THA. Soft tissue injuries and burns. In: Quick CRG, Biers SM, Arulampalam THA, eds. *Essential Surgery: Problems, Diagnosis and Management.* 6th ed. Oxford UK: Elsevier Ltd.; 2020:260-271.
9. Hedström EM, Svensson O, Bergström U, Michno P. Epidemiology of fractures in children and adolescents. *Acta Orthop.* 2010;81(1):148-153.
10. Powell RA, Weir AJ. EMS, bone immobilization. StatPearls [Internet]. Treasure Island, FL: StatPearls Publishing; January 2019. Updated February 28, 2019. Available at: https://www.ncbi.nlm.nih.gov/books/NBK507778/.

CHAPTER 30

THERMAL BURNS AND INHALATIONAL INJURIES

Elizabeth Barrall Werley

QUESTIONS AND ANSWERS

1. What characteristics describe the various degrees of burns?

The historical classification of burns was first established almost 200 years ago and was based on the depth of the burn and is still utilized today. First-degree burns are superficial. Second-degree burns are partial-thickness. Third-degree burns are full-thickness. Although less frequently utilized, higher-grade burn descriptions also exist. Fourth-degree burns extend into the underlying soft tissue. Fifth-degree burns extend beyond muscle and to the level of bone, and sixth-degree burns actually involve the bone.[1]

Superficial burn is now the preferred terminology instead of first-degree burns. There is no involvement of the epithelium and the damage is isolated to the epidermal later. The injured area is erythematous but without blistering or other skin changes. After several days, the skin may desquamate, or peel, as the cells regenerate; it will typically heal on its own within a few days, not requiring anything more than supportive therapy and rarely leaving a scar. The classic example of this type of burn is a sunburn.[1,2]

Partial-thickness burns are subcategorized into *superficial partial-thickness* or *deep partial-thickness*. Superficial partial-thickness burns are characterized by intact sensation, including light touch and proprioception, as well as pain; associated pain may be quite severe. These burns blanch and weeping and blistering are common, typically involving serous fluid. These burn wounds take longer to heal, up to 2 or 3 weeks. Fortunately, these burns are infrequently associated with contractures or hypertrophic scarring; therefore, surgical excision or skin grafting is not typically required.[1,2] Deep partial-thickness burns have variable sensation. Sensation to light touch may remain intact, as well as vibration and various forms of pressure as well as stretch; however, sensation to pain is typically diminished or absent. These burn wounds may appear pink or white due to underlying vascular damage, and they will either blanch poorly or not at all.[1,2]

Full-thickness burns penetrate beyond the dermis and into the subcutaneous tissue. Dermal tissue is permanently destroyed and therefore cannot be regenerated. Nerve endings are also destroyed, so these wounds are insensate, and therefore painless. Wounds can vary in appearance from white to pink to brown and leathery or black eschar.[2]

2. What degrees of burns are included when estimating the body surface area involved?

Superficial or first-degree burns should not be included in the measurement of estimated total body surface area (TBSA). All higher degrees of burn are incorporated into the estimated TBSA. As noted earlier, superficial or first-degree burns do not extend beyond the epidermal layer; therefore, none of the pathophysiologic responses seen with deeper burns occurs since the epithelial layer and deeper structures are not damaged. Overestimating TBSA can lead to overutilization of resources, overaggressive intravenous fluid resuscitation, and unnecessary transport to a burn center when a closer facility may have been appropriate, factors all relevant to the prehospital setting.[2]

It is also important to ensure that soot, dirt, and other debris are cleansed from the patient, if possible, so as to not incorporate this into the estimate.[3]

3. How can you estimate the percentage body surface area involved in adult burn patients?

There is a "Rule of Nines" used to estimate TBSA for burn injuries in adults.[1-4] This is perhaps the easiest estimate and works well for large contiguous areas. All major sections of the body are multiples of nine, except for the perineum:

- Head—anterior and posterior = 9%
- Right upper extremity—anterior and posterior = 9%
- Left upper extremity—anterior and posterior = 9%
- Right lower extremity—anterior = 9%, posterior = 9%, or total = 18%
- Left lower extremity—anterior = 9%, posterior = 9%, or total = 18%
- Torso—anterior = 18%
- Torso—posterior = 18%
- Perineum = 1%

4. When should the "Rule of Nines" be adjusted?

Pediatric patients have a different body surface area than adults. In particular, their heads are larger and their legs are smaller relative to the remainder of the body. This must be accounted for when estimating TBSA.[3]

When estimating TBSA in children, especially those younger than age 3, the perineum remains at 1%. The head estimate is increased to 18%, each arm is increased slightly to 10%, and each leg is decreased to 14%. The anterior torso and posterior torso are decreased slightly to 16% each.

In obese patients with a body mass index >35, the "Rule of Nines" is adapted to a "Rule of Sevens." The head remains estimated at 9% and the perineum remains at 1%. The anterior torso and posterior torso are increased to 28% each. Each upper extremity (anterior and posterior) is decreased to 7%, and each lower extremity (anterior and posterior) is decreased to 14%.[2]

5. Are there any other ways to estimate percentage body surface area involved in burn victims?

The patient's own hand (palm plus fingers) can be used to estimate TBSA. Each "hand" equals approximately 1% TBSA. This estimate works well for smaller and/or noncontiguous burns.[1–3]

There is also a more complex system, the Lund-Browder chart, that is more accurate in estimating TBSA according to various ages. However, this can be very time intensive and is more frequently utilized at burn treatment centers and less commonly utilized by nonburn centers or in the prehospital setting.[1–3]

6. What are the main factors that drive the decision to refer a patient to a burn center?

Prehospital diversion or hospital transfer to a burn center is typically determined based on estimated TBSA, depth of burns, and specific locations.[1–4]

The American Burn Association lists specific criteria for referral to burn centers[3,4]:
- Partial-thickness burns >10% TBSA
- Full-thickness burns, regardless of age
- Burns to specific body locations: face, hands, feet, genitalia, perineum, major joints
- Electrical burns (including lightning injuries)
- Chemical burns
- Inhalational burns
- Comorbidities that could compromise treatment and recovery or increase mortality
- Patients with concomitant trauma:
  - Transfer to burn center if the burn places the patient at greatest risk
  - May be stabilized at a trauma center if other traumatic injuries pose a greater initial risk
- Burned pediatric patients if personnel and equipment are not qualified to care for children
- Those patients who may need specialized support in terms of their social, emotional, or rehabilitative needs
- High-risk patients
  - Younger than 10 years of age
  - Older than 50 years of age

7. What are the goals of prehospital burn management?

The first step in management of burn patients is to ensure that the patient is removed from the burning environment, with any active burning to be stopped. A primary survey of the patient consisting of assessment of airway, breathing, and circulation is of utmost importance, with special attention to a detailed airway assessment and securing of the airway if compromised or potentially compromised. Following this, a more detailed top-to-bottom secondary assessment should follow. Clothing should be removed at this stage, as well as any circumferential accessories (i.e., belts, jewelry, etc.), which may cause a tourniquet-like effect should edema develop and may retain heat depending on composition. Intravenous access should be established with ideally two large-bore intravenous catheters in nonburned portions of extremities.[5] Intravenous fluid resuscitation and analgesia should be provided, followed by application of wound dressings. Transport to an appropriate facility must then follow.[3]

8. How does one provide analgesia to burn patients?

In the hospital, the goals of care surrounding analgesia are threefold: baseline pain control, analgesia for breakthrough pain, and then pain control during any relevant procedures. In the prehospital setting, analgesia will primarily focus on acute pain, equivalent to breakthrough pain. "Treatment strategies should be individualized and multimodal in nature, including the use of analgesics, sedatives, and anxiolytics."[2] Burns are very painful, with superficial partial-thickness being the worst. Analgesia is typically provided parenterally, and opioids are an appropriate choice for initial treatment.[3] Subcutaneous and intramuscular administration of medications should be avoided if possible.[5]

9. Are there specific recommendations for intravenous fluids in burn patients?

Burns and the tissue damage that results generate a profound inflammatory response within the body, which can lead to capillary leak. Patients may be hypotensive with ongoing hypoperfusion. The most well-known formula for intravenous fluid resuscitation in burn patients is the Parkland formula, which incorporates weight-based fluid administration based on the percentage of TBSA involved. This formula guides the fluid resuscitation over the first 24 hours. The Parkland formula promotes the use of lactated Ringer's solution as the resuscitative fluid of choice.[1] However, in the prehospital setting, if lactated Ringer's is not routinely available, other isotonic crystalloid fluids should be used.[6] Additionally, in the prehospital setting, fluid administration may be guided by the patient's vital signs, cardiac and pulmonary status, and urine output.[3] It is not uncommon to overresuscitate a patient in terms of intravenous fluids, so large-volume resuscitation is not always needed. Fluids should be adjusted according to the patient's status, and the type and amount of fluids administered should be accurately documented and provided to the receiving facility.[3]

10. Are inhalational injuries common?

Inhalational injuries make up only a small percentage of burns; however, of the subgroup of burn victims who eventually succumb to their injuries, inhalational injuries are noted in a large percentage.[7] "Inhalational injuries are commonly seen in tandem with burn injuries and are known to increase mortality in burned patients. Smoke inhalation is present in as many as 35% of hospitalized burn patients and may triple the hospital stay compared to isolated burn injuries. Mortality for inhalation injury has been reported to be as high as 25%, with this increasing to 50% in patients with ≥20% TBSA burns."[1] Because of improved treatment of shock and sepsis in burn patients, inhalation injury is now a leading cause of mortality.[3]

Inhalation injuries take two forms. The first form is typically more of an upper airway issue and results from a direct thermal injury to the upper airway tissue. This can result in the rapid formation of edema.[1,3] Occasionally, thermal injury can reach below the vocal cords in the setting of steam exposure.[3] Edema to the airway from direct thermal injury is typically worst within the first 24 to 48 hours.[1] The second form of inhalation injury affects the lower respiratory tract more and is a direct result of exposure to products of combustion.[1,3] The inhaled gases serve as "tissue asphyxiants, pulmonary irritants, and systemic toxins."[3] The lower respiratory tract becomes injured, which causes an inflammatory process with resulting edema, bronchoconstriction, and obstruction.[1,3]

11. Are there specific chemicals of concern associated with inhalation injuries?

Carbon monoxide poisoning is a major concern in burn victims, particularly to those with obvious burns to the face and upper torso, as well as burns in an enclosed space.[1,3,6,7] Carbon monoxide levels may be measured in the prehospital setting as an estimate. Due to the possibility of carbon monoxide poisoning and resulting tissue hypoxia, all patients should be placed on 100% oxygen while in transport.[3,5,6] Arterial oxygen saturation and carboxyhemoglobin levels should be measured as early as possible upon arriving to a hospital.[3,6] High-flow oxygen should be given to patients with suspected carbon monoxide poisoning.

Cyanide poisoning may be a concern given the environment in which the burn occurred. "Hydrogen cyanide is formed by the combustion of nitrogen-containing polymers such as wool, silk, polyurethane, and vinyl." The end result of cyanide poisoning is also profound tissue hypoxia. Specific treatments may be necessary.[3] One available treatment, hydroxocobalamin, has been used in Europe since 1980, but there are little data on the prevalence of its availability, use, and outcomes in North American prehospital settings.[8]

12. What are the indications for intubation in burn victims?

If the airway is potentially compromised, physicians in the hospital setting can directly assess the airway with a nasopharyngeal scope or a bronchoscope.[3,7] This is not a tool that is readily available in the prehospital setting. Signs of smoke inhalation include facial burns, singed nasal hairs, soot in the nose or oropharynx, hoarseness, wheezing, and carbonaceous sputum.[3]

Therefore, there are clear indications for intubation for airway protection[3,5,6]:

- Deep/full-thickness burns to the face, perioral region, or neck
- Circumferential burns to the neck
- Acute respiratory distress or worsening air hunger
- Progressive hoarseness
- Respiratory depression or altered mental status

It is important to stress the need for early intubation due to the rapid progression in which edema can occur.[5,6] Due to the potential for a difficult airway with obscured landmarks, intubation should be performed by the most experienced provider available.[5]

KEY POINTS

- Superficial burns, superficial partial-thickness, deep partial-thickness, and full-thickness are the preferred terms used in describing burns.
- Accurate estimation of the TBSA involved helps dictate appropriate management of the burned patient.
- Inhalation injury can be associated with upper airway structures, lower airway structures, or both. If there is any clinical concern for airway involvement, it is better to secure the airway via intubation early.
- Burns and inhalation injuries may also expose patients to carbon monoxide and hydrogen cyanide toxicity.

REFERENCES

1. Anderson JH, Mandell SP, Gibran NS. Burns. In: Brunicardi F, Anderson DK, Billiar TR, et al., eds. *Schwartz's Principles of Surgery, 11e.* New York, NY: McGraw-Hill; 2019.
2. Collier ZJ, Pham C, Carey JN, Gillenwater TJ. Burn wound management. In: Hamm RL, ed. *Text and Atlas of Wound Diagnosis and Treatment.* 2nd ed. New York, NY: McGraw-Hill; 2019.
3. DeKoning EP. Thermal burns. In: Tintinalli JE, Ma O, Yealy DM, et al., eds. *Tintinalli's Emergency Medicine: A Comprehensive Study Guide.* 9th ed. New York, NY: McGraw-Hill; 2019.
4. American Burn Association. Burn center referral criteria. http://ameriburn.org/public-resources/burn-center-referral-criteria/.
5. Milcak RP, Buffalo C, Jimenez CJ. Prehospital management, transportation, and emergency care. In: Herndon DN, ed. *Total Burn Care.* 5th ed. Galveston, TX: Elsevier; 2018:58-65e1.
6. Demling RH. Burns & other thermal injuries. In: Doherty GM, ed. *Current Diagnosis & Treatment: Surgery, 14e.* New York, NY: McGraw-Hill; 2019.
7. Levi B, Wang S. Burns. In: Kang S, Amagai M, Bruckner AL, et al., eds. *Fitzpatrick's Dermatology, 9e.* New York, NY: McGraw-Hill; 2019.
8. Purvis MV, Rooks H, Young Lee J, Longerich S, Kahn SA. Prehospital hydroxocobalamin for inhalation injury and cyanide toxicity in the United States—analysis of a database and survey of ems providers. *Ann Burns Fire Disasters.* 2017;30(2):126-128.

CHAPTER 31

CARE OF THE ENTRAPPED PATIENT INCLUDING CRUSH INJURIES

Bradley Chappell

QUESTIONS AND ANSWERS

1. Why is scene safety so important?

   There are a variety of scenarios to which EMS providers will be called. When discussing patient extrications, the majority will be from severe motor vehicle accidents. There are also many possible industrial and agricultural accidents, as well as the rare but catastrophic natural disasters and acts of terrorism. Extreme caution must be used to avoid secondary injury to first responders—having a keen awareness of potential chemical leaks and the structural integrity of buildings after a fire, bombing, tornado, hurricane, or earthquake. With the increase in mass shootings, first responders must be aware of the possibility of a secondary shooter targeting EMS responders. As an EMS responder, you are no good to the patient if you become injured or incapacitated.

2. How can I protect myself when responding to an emergency?

   Situational awareness (understanding your surroundings) is paramount to ensuring your own safety. Personal protective gear such as gloves, helmet, and a high-visibility reflective vest should always be used along with emergency lighting when parked on a road or other potentially dangerous scene. Larger vehicles such as fire engines should be parked diagonally across the roadway ahead of the accident as an impact barrier to keep the primary accident scene safe. EMS providers must be cognizant of potential fuel or other hazardous material spills and wait for fire/hazmat to clear the scene. Medical vehicles should be close to the patient for quick access to supplies and ease of transport.

3. What are the components of a systematic approach to rescue trapped patients?

   a. Scene assessment: Approximately 10% of motor vehicle accident patients are trapped for more than 30 minutes prior to extrication. The incident commander must assess the scene and rapidly identify immediate hazards, the number of victims, and possible rescue strategies. It is important to activate all possible resources in a timely manner; it is better to turn away resources than to delay care because they are not on scene.

   b. Hazard management: The key components are donning personal protective equipment and controlling traffic flow.

   c. Gaining initial access: This allows initial triage of the involved patients and prioritization of resources. Glass in windows can be taped in a crisscross pattern before it is broken to minimize the pieces that fall into the car onto the patient. A fire blanket can provide soft protection.

   d. Creating space: This is staging for patient extrication. Perform immediate medical care (ABCs)—supplemental oxygen, cardiac monitoring, maintaining c-spine precautions, and establishing intravenous (IV)/intraosseous (IO) access or administration of intramuscular (IM) or intranasal medications. Without a clear egress pathway, extrication may result in further injury to the patient. Providing rapid, aggressive treatment prior to extrication may make the difference between life and death.

   e. Getting full access: It is important to shield both the patient and rescuers from falling objects, glass fragments, rescue tools, bare metal edges, and noise as to not further injure the patient by efforts of the rescue team.

   f. Patient extrication: Appropriate analgesia and sedation will often facilitate an extrication. During the process of extrication, care should be taken to minimize movement of the spine to prevent worsening of any possible injuries. Caution should be used to maximize patient immobilization and prevent dislodgement of fractures, hematomas, and existing lines and tubes. The Kendrick Extrication Device (KED) may be helpful in safely moving the patient to a long board for easier transport.

4. What types of tools might be used to extricate a patient?

   In the event of a fire, explosion, or earthquake, EMS providers should not enter a structure until its integrity can be verified. Any structure involved should be stabilized. A variety of methods may be used, including wood block cribbing, pneumatic airbags, and strut systems. EMS personnel must be familiar with the equipment used by their agency and be comfortable with deploying it. Wide full access is achieved by systematic dismantling of the object or vehicle around the patient. The Halligan bar, which combines a blade, claw, and tapered pick, along with hydraulic tools, such as spreaders and cutters, commonly referred to as the "jaws of life," is often used. A gap can be created between the door and frame near the handle with a Halligan bar or other similar tool. Hydraulic spreaders can then be inserted into the gap and used to spread the door from the frame.

5. What are some important mechanical considerations when extricating a patient from a vehicle?

One of the first steps is to disconnect the battery. Airbags that have not deployed with the initial impact may deploy during the extrication attempt, causing severe injury to the patient or providers. A rescuer should never place themselves between a loaded airbag and the patient. Front seats can be reclined or moved backward to maximize space. In some situations, a car may need to be disassembled to extricate a patient. This is performed in a stepwise manner. The windows are first removed, starting away from the patient to allow immediate access to cover the patient before breaking windows close to them. Next, the metal support posts between the windows are cut. If necessary for roof removal, the front and rear posts can then be cut and the roof lifted off the car. Alternately, the front two to four posts can be cut, and the roof can be folded up and backward.

6. How can I address the ABCs with limited access to the patient?

Patients may be trapped for a significant portion of the critical first hour of trauma care. EMS providers should provide whatever care they can safely render to the entrapped patient.

- Airway: Maintain c-spine precautions with a cervical collar; depending on the level of alertness, adjuncts such as a nasopharyngeal or an oropharyngeal tube can be used. If completely unresponsive, devices such as a laryngeal mask airway (LMA), i-gel, King airway, or Combitube may be used.
- Breathing: Options include a simple nasal cannula, nonrebreather mask, high-flow oxygen, continuous positive airway pressure, and manual bag-valve mask. Be aware that positive pressure ventilation can rapidly worsen a pneumothorax and lead to tension pneumothorax. If there is high suspicion for pneumothorax in the setting of a prolonged extrication, needle decompression may be warranted.
- Circulation: The first priority should be to stop any bleeding. This can be achieved through direct pressure (augmented by combat gauze impregnated with a hemostatic agent), compression of arterial pressure points, tourniquets, and splints. It is important to document the time a tourniquet is initiated. Although medications may be given intranasally or intramuscularly, patients will often need IV fluids or blood products, so IV or IO access proximal to the level of a bleeding injury is critical. If the patient is actively bleeding and tranexamic acid (TXA) is available, it should be given as soon as feasible but no later than 3 hours after the onset of injury. It is important to keep the patient as warm as possible—keep the head and body covered and warm fluids as much as possible prior to administration. If a prolonged extrication is expected, and there has been a massive exsanguination, blood transfusion at the scene may be indicated and can be organized through medical control.

7. How can I treat pain if I do not have IV access?

Fentanyl is a good choice as it has minimal effect on blood pressure. The dose should be approximately 1 mcg/kg IM or IO or 2 mcg/kg if given intranasally. Ketamine is another great option as it can actually increase the blood pressure while maintaining the patient's respiratory drive. If given IM, the dose should be 4–5 mg/kg, or 1–2 mg/kg if given IO. When using an IO, it is important to initially infuse 40 mg of cardiac lidocaine followed by 20 mg as needed for local pain at the infusion site (maximum of 300 mg).

8. What is crush syndrome?

Crush syndrome occurs when there is high pressure applied directly to soft tissues over a prolonged period of time, often resulting in increased compartment pressure and subsequent limb ischemia. The crushing force causes direct mechanical injury to the muscle cell, leading to sodium and calcium release with a subsequent influx of water. This causes hypotension, leading to hypoperfusion and tissue hypoxia. The result is anaerobic metabolism with systemic lactic acidosis.

9. Why does reperfusion syndrome occur?

The longer a victim is trapped, an increasing amount of toxins is contained distal to the crush injury. Once the compressive force is released, these toxic substances are rapidly released into the systemic circulation, which can lead to rapid hypotension and cardiac arrest. The major detrimental components released during crush injury are potassium and myoglobin. Potassium leaking from damaged cells will increase intravascular potassium, potentially leading to fatal dysrhythmias. Myoglobin is deposited in the kidney more rapidly than it can be excreted, leading to acute renal failure. Examples of other chemicals released include histamine (causes vasodilation), nitric oxide (leads to further vasodilation), and thromboplastin (can cause increased bleeding and disseminated intravascular coagulation).

10. How do I treat crush and reperfusion syndromes in the prehospital environment?

The most important treatment is initiation of an IV. If intubation is required, avoid the use of succinylcholine as it may potentiate hyperkalemia. Immediately prior to the release of a crush injury, consider the use of a proximal tourniquet to limit the abrupt systemic release of toxins. It is also good to empirically give calcium and sodium bicarbonate. Lastly, be prepared to respond to hyperkalemia and hypovolemic shock.

11. How can I treat hyperkalemia?

As soon as possible, the cardiac rhythm should be monitored. With any signs of hyperkalemia such as peaked T-waves, first-degree AV block, a widened QRS interval, or other arrhythmia, the patient should immediately be given 1 g of calcium chloride (or 3 g of calcium gluconate) until the rhythm has normalized. To assist in shifting the potassium intracellularly, albuterol, and sodium bicarbonate may also be given. Use caution with the administration of insulin as its clearance may be slowed due to reduced renal function.

12. What can I do to prevent kidney injury?

Crush-induced rhabdomyolysis is the most frequent secondary cause of death after earthquakes. Delay in fluid resuscitation can increase incidence of renal failure up to 50%, so aggressive fluid resuscitation is critical. Generally, 1–2 L per hour should be given with a target of 200 mL/hour of urine output.

13. How is compartment syndrome related to crush injuries?

Approximately 80% of crush syndrome patients die, and 10% develop compartment syndrome. Compartment syndrome occurs when the tissue pressure within a closed muscle compartment exceeds the perfusion pressure, leading to muscle death and nerve damage. This can be caused by acute fractures with swelling, postcasting, hemorrhage (exacerbated by anticoagulation), burns, and IV drug use or IV extravasation. Compartment pressures greater than 30 mm Hg for 4–6 hours can result in irreversible nerve and muscle damage. Roughly 40% of compartment syndrome cases involve tibia/fibula fractures.

14. What are the 6 P's of compartment syndrome?

- Pain is the most common finding and is often disproportionate to the expected level (severe and refractory);
- Passive range of motion causes pain;
- Paresthesia—numbness or tingling sensation;
- Pressure is noted by tight compartments to palpation and may be measured using commercial devices in the hospital setting;
- Poikilothermia is an altered temperature sensation; and
- Pulseless is a very late finding.

15. How is compartment syndrome treated?

It is critical to notify the hospital when there is concern for compartment syndrome to allow time for mobilizing the necessary resources. The definitive treatment is fasciotomy, which is rarely performed in the field.

16. How should I prepare an amputated body part for transportation?

Rinse the part off with sterile water, cover it with sterile gauze that has been moistened with sterile saline, place the part in a sterile bag, seal the bag, and place it on ice. Mangled extremities typically cannot be reimplanted, but this decision should be made by a reimplantation surgeon.

17. What are the criteria for field amputation?

In extreme circumstances, a patient may require a field amputation as a last resort to extricate a patient who would otherwise die. This is typically performed by a physician-led hospital emergency response team (HERT) that is dispatched to the scene.

18. What items are needed for a field amputation?

- Airway: endotracheal intubations supplies and a surgical airway kit
- Breathing: needle decompression kit
- Circulation: IO, IV fluids, blood products, TXA, Combat gauze, tourniquets
- Medications: ketamine, rocuronium, midazolam, morphine, ondansetron
- Amputation: scalpel, battery-powered electrocautery, Gigli saw, bone saw
- Transport: Ziploc bags, gauze, ice

KEY POINTS

- If unable to obtain IV access during a prolonged field extrication, consider placing an IO device or administering IM/intranasal analgesics, such as fentanyl and ketamine.
- The most important prehospital treatment for crush syndrome is aggressive IV hydration.
- Prior to releasing a crushed/entrapped limb, consider applying a tourniquet to limit the rapid systemic release of toxins. The patient should have continuous cardiac monitoring, and consider giving calcium and bicarbonate immediately before freeing the crushed limb to prevent hyperkalemia.
- Post extrication, anticipate and aggressively treat hypovolemic shock.

BIBLIOGRAPHY

Bono MJ, Halpern P. Bomb, blast, and crush injuries. In: Tintinalli JE, Stapczynski J, Ma OJ, Yealy D, Meckler G, Cline D, eds. *Tintinalli's Emergency Medicine: A Comprehensive Study Guide.* 8th ed. New York, NY: McGraw-Hill; 2015.

Bunyasaranand J, Espino E, Rummings KA, Christiansen GM. Management of an entrapped patient with a field amputation. *J Emerg Med.* 2018;54:90-95.

ProlongedFieldCare.org. Crush syndrome from a prolonged field care perspective. August 23, 2016. https://prolongedfieldcare. org/2016/08/23/crush-syndrome-from-a-prolonged-field-care-perspective/.

Ginglen JG, Tong H. EMS, gaining access and extrication. In: StatPearls. Treasure Island, FL: StatPearls Publishing; 2019. *https://www. ncbi.nlm.nih.gov/books/NBK482471/*.

Haller PR. Compartment syndrome. In: Tintinalli JE, Stapczynski J, Ma OJ, Yealy D, Meckler G, Cline D. eds. *Tintinalli's Emergency Medicine: A Comprehensive Study Guide*. 8th ed. New York, New York: McGraw-Hill; 2015.

Henry S. *Advanced Trauma Life Support for Doctors: Student Course Manual*. 10th ed. Chicago, IL: American College of Surgeons; 2018.

Parrish A, Tagore A, Ariyaprakai N, Hohbein JL, DiCorpo JE, Merlin MA. Managing the toxic chemical release that occurs during a crush injury. *JEMS*. October 22, 2018. https://www.jems.com/2018/10/22/managing-the-toxic-chemical-release-that-occurs-during-a-crush-injury/.

Mackenzie R, Sutcliffe MA. Pre-hospital care: the trapped patient. *J R Army Med Corps*. 2000;146:39-46. doi: 10.1136/jramc-146-01-09.

CHAPTER 32

PREHOSPITAL PHYSICAL ASSESSMENT AND CRITICAL INTERPRETATION OF VITAL SIGNS

Lilia Reyes

QUESTIONS AND ANSWERS

1. Why is it important to have a systematic approach to the evaluation of a seriously ill or injured child?
   It is important because it will help the provider quickly recognize clear signs of respiratory distress, respiratory failure, and shock, as well as immediately provide lifesaving procedures once these signs are identified.

2. According to the American Heart Association (AHA) Pediatric Advanced Life Support (PALS), how should you initially evaluate a patient to help you identify quickly what type of physiologic problem the patient is having?
   Your initial impression should include the patient's appearance (tone, ability to interact, consolability, look/gaze, speech/cry), circulation (see question 4), and work of breathing (abnormal breath sounds, abnormal positioning, retractions, nasal flaring). This is otherwise known as the Pediatric Assessment Triangle (PAT). The PAT will help the provider quickly identify if the problem is respiratory, circulatory, or neurologic, as well determine the urgency of treatment and transportation.

3. If the child's condition is identified as life threatening, what are the next steps that should be followed?
   You should start life support interventions. For example, in a patient that is unresponsive with agonal breaths with pulse less than 60/min, it is imperative that the provider start cardiopulmonary resuscitation (CPR) immediately, starting with chest compressions.

4. You are at a cross-country race when a 15-year-old male athlete crosses the finish line. He immediately falls to the ground. During your assessment, you note that he is conscious but not able to answer in full sentences. You note that he has nasal flaring along with suprasternal retractions. What is the third part of the Pediatric Assessment Tool (PAT) tool that should be used to assess this patient?
   The third part of the PAT is to assess the child's overall circulatory status. This consists of evaluating the patient's skin color, noting for signs of compromised perfusion such as pallor, mottling, or cyanosis. Another skin finding that can be abnormal is flushing, as this can be seen in distributive shock. Petechiae or purpura, which is are purplish discolorations of the skin, are signs of possible infection.

5. You are dispatched to a call for a 12-month-old poorly responsive patient. What continuous sequence does the AHA PALS recommend you use when caring for a seriously ill or injured child?
   The AHA PALS recommends that providers use the evaluate-identify-intervene sequence (Fig. 32.1) to help determine the best course of action or treatment through your care of the patient.

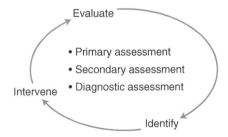

Fig. 32.1. Evaluate-identify-intervene sequence for the initial assessment of an ill or injured pediatric patient.

6. You are called to the home for a 15-month-old female with respiratory distress. The mother reports that the patient is healthy overall and has had mild upper respiratory symptoms of cough and nasal congestion in the last 2 days but this morning awoke with difficulty breathing and is making a weird noise when breathing. What would your primary assessment consist of for this patient?

   Your primary assessment should follow an active ABCDE approach along with vital signs. The ABCDE approach consists of Airway, Breathing, Circulation, Disability, and Exposure.

7. You evaluate the patient (from question 6) and note the following vital signs: respiratory rate of 55, heart rate of 150, blood pressure of 90/55, and oxygen saturation of 86% in room air. What is considered normal for this age group?

   According to the AHA PALS, a 15-month-old could be considered a toddler. For the toddler age, the normal respiratory range is 22–37. The normal heart rate range when awake is 98–140 bpm and 80–120 bpm when sleeping. In addition, the toddler range for systolic blood pressure is 86–106 mm Hg, for diastolic blood pressure is 42–63 mm Hg, and for mean arterial pressure is 49–62 mm Hg. If you are concerned for hypotension, a quick way to estimate the lowest systolic blood pressure for age is as follows: <70 + (age in years × 2) for children 1–10 years of age. Over the age of 10 years, the minimum systolic blood pressure is 90 mm Hg.

8. You have identified that our patient from questions 6 and 7 has abnormal vital signs. On your exam, there is a patent airway, notable grunting, and intercostal retraction with expiratory wheeze. What is your next step in management?

   You have identified that this patient has a patent airway and is in respiratory distress along with hypoxia. The first step should be to provide supplemental oxygen via nasal cannula. Grunting in this patient means that the child is trying to keep the small airways and alveolar sacs in the lungs open. Given that the patient does not have a history of wheezing but is currently is wheezing in the setting of a Upper Respiratory Infection (URI) this could indicate that this patient likely has bronchiolitis. One cannot make the diagnosis of reactive airway at this time.

9. Your team is called to the home of a 12-year-old female patient with altered mental status. Upon your arrival, you perform your ABCDE primary assessment, noting that the patient has a patent airway, equal breath sounds, bounding pulses, and capillary refill of 2 seconds; responds to verbal stimuli; and on exposure is not noted to have any evidence of trauma, but does have diffusely flushed skin. While your partner is performing vital signs you conduct a secondary assessment. What information are you expecting to obtain for your secondary assessment?

   The secondary assessment consists of the focused history, focused physical examination, and ongoing reassessment. The focused history can be remembered by using the pneumonic SAMPLE.
   S: signs and symptoms at the onset of illness
   A: allergies
   M: medications
   P: past medical history
   L: last meal
   E: events leading to the current illness or injury
   The focused physical should include meticulous evaluation of the main area of concern of the illness or injury. Ongoing reassessment of the patient is needed to assess whether the patient is responding to treatment and to track any progression of physiologic or anatomic issues that may arise from the illness or trauma.

10. Your partner obtained the following vital signs for the patient in the previous question: heart rate of 120 bpm, blood pressure of 86/50 mm Hg, respiratory rate of 23, and oxygen saturation of 96% in room air. Keeping in mind your primary assessment on this patient, what is the next step in management for this patient?

    This patient has bounding pulses with flushed skin and altered mental status. You have also identified that the patient is tachycardic and hypotensive. These findings suggest that the patient is in uncompensated shock. It is likely warm shock given the bounding pulses and flushed skin. The immediate first step is providing crystalloid fluids. AHA PALS recommends giving the patient a 20 cc/kg isotonic fluid bolus (maximum of 1000 mL) as a first step. Provide ongoing reassessment of the patient to assess response to isotonic fluid bolus. AHA PALS recommends giving three isotonic fluid boluses, and if this is not effective, consider a vasopressor(s).

KEY POINTS

- It is important to have a systematic approach to the evaluation of critically ill or seriously injured child because it will help the provider quickly recognize clear signs of respiratory distress, respiratory failure, and shock, as well as immediately provide lifesaving procedures once these signs are identified.
- A primary assessment should follow an active ABCDE (Airway, Breathing, Circulation, Disability, and Exposure) approach along with vital signs.
- A secondary assessment consists of the focused history, focused physical examination, and ongoing reassessment. The focused history can be remembered by using the pneumonic SAMPLE.
- If there is concern for hypotension, a quick way to estimate the lowest systolic blood pressure for age is as follows: <70 + (age in years × 2) for children 1–10 years of age. Over the age of 10 years, the minimum systolic blood pressure is 90 mm Hg.
- The AHA PALS recommends giving the patient a 20 cc/kg isotonic fluid bolus (max of 1000 mL) as a first step to address hypotension. Provide ongoing reassessment of patient to assess response to isotonic fluid bolus(es). If the patient does not respond to three isotonic fluid boluses to address their hypotension, it is recommended that a vasopressor be used in the patient with isotonic fluid refractory shock.

BIBLIOGRAPHY

American Heart Association *Pediatric Advanced Life Support*. Dallas, TX: American Heart Association; 2016.

CHAPTER 33

CARDIAC ARREST AND ARRHYTHMIAS

Derya Caglar and Richard Kwun

QUESTIONS AND ANSWERS

1. What is the most common cause of cardiac arrest in children?
   Respiratory failure. In sharp contrast to adults, cardiopulmonary arrest in infants and children is most often associated with hypoxia, respiratory failure, and respiratory arrest. While arrest in adults is often triggered by myocardial ischemia and dysrhythmias, children typically have no primary cardiac dysfunction. A child in cardiac arrest must be supported with immediate bag-mask ventilation with high concentrations of oxygen and high-quality cardiopulmonary resuscitation (CPR). Reversible causes of cardiopulmonary arrest in children can be seen in Table 33.1.

2. What are the most common initial arrhythmias seen in children in cardiac arrest?
   Most episodes of cardiac arrest in infants and children are associated with a terminal rhythm of bradycardia or pulseless electrical activity (PEA), which, if untreated, progresses to asystole. As a child becomes more and more hypoxic, the heart slows down and becomes bradycardic until no pulse is felt and the child is in cardiac arrest.

3. What is the exception to the arrhythmia progression outlined in the previous question?
   Apparent sudden cardiac collapse.

4. How does the initial action for a solo responder for an unresponsive child differ from that for an adult?
   If you are alone and find an unresponsive child under 8 years old, provide 1 minute of CPR first before calling for additional emergency services.

5. How do you define high-quality CPR?
   Push hard ($\geq 1/3$ of anteroposterior diameter of the chest) and fast (100–120 compressions/minute), allowing complete chest recoil. Minimize interruptions in compressions. Avoid excessive ventilation. Rotate compressor every 2 minutes, or sooner if fatigued. If no advanced airway, 15:2 compression-ventilation ratio.

6. What factors are important to consider when assessing a pediatric patient's heart rate?
   - Patient age
   - History of congenital heart disease or cardiac surgery. These patients may have underlying conduction abnormalities and heart rate should be evaluated with regard to their baseline heart rate and rhythm.
   - Level of activity
   - Body temperature
     Normal heart rates in children can be found in Table 33.2.

7. Where do you check for pulses in infants and children?
   Brachial artery in infants to 12 months of age, which is located inside the upper arm midway between the elbow and shoulder. Carotid or femoral artery in children over 1 year of age.

8. What rhythm "abnormalities" can be normal in children?
   15%–25% of children can have sinus arrhythmia, ectopic atrial rhythm, wandering pacemaker, and junctional rhythm.

Table 33.1. Normal Pulse Rates in Children

AGE	AWAKE RATE (BEATS/MINUTE)	ASLEEP RATE (BEATS/MINUTE)
Neonate (0 to 1 month)	100–205	90–160
Infant (1 month to 1 year)	100–180	90–160
Toddler (1 to 2 years)	98–140	80–120
Preschooler (3 to 5 years)	80–120	65–100
School-age child (6 to 12 years)	75–118	58–90
Adolescent	60–100	58–90

Table 33.2. Reversible Causes of Cardiopulmonary Arrest in Children

Hypovolemia	Tension pneumothorax
Hypoxia	Tamponade, cardiac
Hydrogen ion (acidosis)	Toxins
Hypoglycemia	Thrombosis, pulmonary
Hypo-/hyperkalemia	Thrombosis, coronary
Hypothermia	

9. How is bradycardia defined in neonatal and pediatric patients?
   Pediatric Advanced Life Support defines bradycardia as a heart rate less than 60 beats per minute.

10. What is symptomatic bradycardia?
    Bradycardia with one or more of the following: poor pulses, inadequate perfusion, hypotension, or abnormal respirations.

11. What are some reversible causes of bradycardia in children?
    - Hypoxia
    - Hydrogen excess (acidosis)
    - Hyperkalemia
    - Hypothermia
    - Heart block. May be seen in children with a history of cardiac surgery
    - Toxic exposures. Includes organophosphates (nerve agents, pesticides), calcium channel blockers, beta-blockers, clonidine, opioids
    - Trauma, particularly with significant head injury and increased intracranial pressure

12. In symptomatic bradycardia, what is the preferred initial medication for treatment?
    Epinephrine at a dose of 0.01 mg/kg intraosseously or intravenously, repeated every 3–5 minutes. Endotracheal dose is 0.1 mg/kg.

13. When should you give atropine first in symptomatic bradycardia?
    When bradycardia is suspected to be of vagal origin (e.g., deep suctioning, intubation), primary atrioventricular (AV) block, or cholinergic drug toxicity.

14. When should you consider transcutaneous pacing?
    Pacing may be considered in patients with complete heart block or sinus node dysfunction with underlying congenital heart disease or history of cardiac surgery who present with symptomatic bradycardia refractory to initial treatment with medications.

15. What is the most common cause of sudden cardiac death in adolescents?
    Hypertrophic cardiomyopathy.

16. What is hypertrophic cardiomyopathy and how does it cause sudden cardiac death?
    Hypertrophic cardiomyopathy is an inherited disease that leads to abnormal thickening of the cardiac muscle, causing outflow obstruction. Electrocardiogram (EKG) is abnormal in 90% of patients. Patients are at high risk for the development of ventricular dysrhythmias, often ventricular fibrillation (VF), which can lead to sudden cardiac death.

17. What percentage of children who suffer sudden cardiac death have a history of syncope?
    25%

18. How is tachycardia defined in pediatric patients?
    When the heart rate exceeds the upper limit of normal for a child's age. See Table 33.1 for normal resting heart rates in children.

19. What is the most frequent narrow-complex tachydysrhythmia requiring treatment in children?
    Supraventricular tachycardia (SVT).

20. What is the heart rate for children in SVT?
In infants, heart rates are usually between 220 and 300 beats per minute, while older children may present with heart rates above 180.

21. What are the clinical features of infants and children in SVT?
An infant in SVT may present with poor feeding, fussiness, irritability, lethargy, or "not acting right." Older children may report nausea, palpitations, dizziness, chest pain, or shortness of breath.

22. How is SVT treated?
   • If hemodynamically unstable, the patient should have synchronized cardioversion at a dose of 0.5–1 J/kg.
   • If stable, vagal stimulation may be attempted with ice to the face or directing the child to perform Valsalva maneuvers. Additionally, intravenous (IV) adenosine at a dose of 0.1 mg/kg can be given via fast push once IV access has been established.

23. What is long QT syndrome?
Long QT syndrome (LQTS) is a disorder of ventricular myocardial repolarization in which patients have a prolonged QT interval that can lead to ventricular arrhythmias, particularly torsades de pointes, and subsequent sudden cardiac death. Many patients will have a family history of cardiac disease or of sudden cardiac death in a close family member in adolescence or young adulthood.

24. Define QT prolongation.
A corrected QT interval greater than 440 milliseconds.

25. What is torsades de pointes?
A polymorphic ventricular tachycardia (VT) with rapid, irregular QRS complexes that appear to "twist" around a baseline. This may evolve into VF.

26. With what symptoms is QT prolongation associated?
Most patients remain asymptomatic their entire lives. Symptomatic patients may present with syncope, seizure, or cardiac arrest following strong emotions and/or exercise.

27. What can cause acquired (noninherited) QT prolongation?
   • Medications: antiarrhythmics, psychotropics, and antibiotics (macrolides, fluoroquinolones, antifungals), cancer treatments
   • Hypomagnesemia
   • Hypokalemia
   • Anorexia nervosa

28. What is the most frequent wide-complex tachydysrhythmia requiring treatment in children?
Ventricular tachycardia.

29. How do you define wide-complex tachycardia?
Tachycardia with a QRS complex greater than 0.09 seconds.

30. What causes VT?
Most children with VT have underlying structural heart disease, prolonged QT syndrome, myocarditis, or cardiomyopathy. Other causes include electrolyte abnormalities (e.g., hyperkalemia, hypokalemia, hypocalcemia), metabolic abnormalities, drug toxicity, cardiac tumors, acquired heart disease, and idiopathic causes.

31. What percentage of pediatric patients with myocarditis develop a significant arrhythmia?
45%. Significant arrhythmias include SVT, high-grade ventricular ectopy, VT or VF, and high-grade AV block (e.g., Mobitz type II or complete heart block).

32. How is VT treated?
   • If hemodynamically unstable with a pulse, synchronized cardioversion at a dose of 0.5–1 J/kg, increasing to 2 J/kg if needed.
   • If hemodynamically unstable without a pulse, defibrillate at 2 J/kg with an additional 4 J/kg if no response.
   • If stable, give amiodarone 5 mg/kg IV/IO over 20–60 minutes or procainamide 15 mg/kg IV/IO over 30–60 minutes in consultation with a pediatric cardiologist.

33. What size electrode pads should you use, and where do you place them?

Use child pads for patients up to 8 years of age, otherwise use adult pads. Place one pad to the right upper chest below the clavicle, and the other left of the nipple in the anterior axillary line. You can also use the anterior-posterior orientation, which is recommended if your patient is an infant and you only have adult pads.

34. What is commotio cordis?

Commotio cordis refers to VF and sudden death triggered by blunt trauma to the chest. In children less than 15 years of age, the most common causes result from sporting injuries, e.g., projectiles to the chest (mostly baseballs, softballs, lacrosse balls, or hockey pucks), or blunt contact with other athletes.

35. How is VF treated?

Defibrillate at 2 J/kg with an additional 4 J/kg if no response. See Table 33.2 for reversible causes of cardiac arrest.

KEY POINTS

- Cardiac arrest in children is most often due to respiratory failure.
- In cases of VF or pulseless VT, rapid defibrillation is key.
- Children 9–17 years of age have a similar prevalence of shockable rhythms and automated external defibrillator (AED) use when compared to adults.

BIBLIOGRAPHY

American Heart Association. *Pediatric Advanced Life Support*. Dallas, TX: American Heart Association; 2016.

Doniger SJ, Sharieff GQ. Pediatric dysrhythmias. *Pediatr Clin N Am*. 2006;53:85-105.

Drago F, Battipaglia I, Di Mambro C. Neonatal and pediatric arrhythmias: clinical and electrocardiographic aspects. *Card Electrophysiol Clin*. 2018;19:397-412.

Johnson MA, Grahan BJH, Haukoos JH, et al. Demographics, bystander CPR and AED use in out-of-hospital pediatric arrests. *Resuscitation*. 2014;85:920-926.

Maron BJ, Estes NAM. Commotio cordis. *N Engl J Med*. 2010;362:917-927.

Miyake CY, Teele SA, Chen L, et al. In-hospital arrhythmia development and outcomes in pediatric patient with acute myocarditis. *Am J Cardiol*. 2014;113:535-540.

SHOCK

John Park

CHAPTER 34

QUESTIONS AND ANSWERS

1. What is shock?
   Shock is inadequate blood flow (and therefore oxygen delivery) to meet tissue demands.

2. Why is early recognition and treatment of shock important?
   Early recognition and treatment of shock are associated with improved outcomes, with decreased morbidity and mortality. As shock progresses, it often becomes more refractory to treatment.

3. What is the difference between compensated and uncompensated shock?
   Blood pressure is maintained by compensatory mechanisms (increasing heart rate, increased cardiac stroke volume, vasoconstriction) in compensated shock. These mechanisms are overwhelmed in uncompensated shock, resulting in hypotension.

4. What determines blood pressure?
   Peripheral vascular resistance and cardiac output

5. What determines cardiac output?
   Heart rate and cardiac stroke volume

6. What determines cardiac stroke volume?
   Preload—degree of filling of the heart before contraction
   Afterload—resistance to flow out of the heart
   Contractility—how hard or deeply the heart contracts

7. What are the lower limits for systolic blood pressure in children (i.e., below what number is a child considered hypotensive)?
   See Table 34.1.

8. Describe the signs and symptoms of compensated shock.
   Tachycardia for age, cool extremities, increased capillary refill time. Of note, initially, tachycardia may be the only finding in compensated shock in pediatric patients.

9. Describe the signs and symptoms of uncompensated shock.
   Tachycardia for age, hypotension for age, mottled/cool extremities, increased capillary refill time, decreased urine output

10. What are the upper limits for heart rate in children (i.e., above what number is a child considered tachycardic)?
    See Chapter 34, Table 34.2.

11. Describe the four main types of shock.
    Hypovolemic
    - When circulating intravascular volume is decreased
    - Occurs from blood loss, emesis and diarrhea, "third spacing," or any other condition in which intravascular fluid loss exceeds intake for long enough

Table 34.1. Lower Limits for Systolic Blood Pressure in Children

AGE	SYSTOLIC BLOOD PRESSURE IN MM HG
Neonates	60
Infants	70
Children 1–10 years	70 + (2 × age in years)
Adolescent >10 years	90

Table 34.2. Treatment of Shock Based on Subtype

SEPTIC	ANAPHYLACTIC	NEUROGENIC
Broad spectrum antibiotics	Intramuscular epinephrine:	Fluid resuscitation
Aggressive fluid resuscitation	>30 kg: 0.3 mg	Early infusion of peripheral vaso-
Vasoactive infusions	<30 kg: 0.15 mg	constrictor (epinephrine)
Cold shock: epinephrine	Corticosteroids	
Warm shock: norepinephrine	Antihistamines	
	Inhaled beta agonists	

- Symptoms include dry mucous membranes, decreased tears, increased capillary refill time, poor skin turgor, and sunken fontanel/eyes.

Cardiogenic
- When cardiac dysfunction leads to inadequate cardiac output
- Occurs from myocarditis, cardiomyopathy, dysrhythmias, congenital heart disease, etc.
- Symptoms include lung crackles, respiratory distress, edema, and hepatomegaly.

Obstructive
- When blood flow is obstructed
- Blockage of venous return: tension pneumothorax, cardiac tamponade
- Blockage of arterial flow: aortic stenosis, aortic coarctation
- Symptoms include:
  Tension pneumothorax: tracheal deviation and unilateral diminished breath sounds
  Cardiac tamponade: muffled heart sounds
  Aortic stenosis: systolic murmur
  Aortic coarctation: diminished lower extremity pulses

Distributive
- When peripheral vasculature is dilated, decreasing peripheral vascular resistance
- Often with associated capillary leakage causing "third spacing"
- Occurs from infections causing a systemic inflammatory response (septic shock), anaphylaxis (anaphylactic shock), and loss of sympathetic tone (neurogenic shock)
- Symptoms include:
  Anaphylaxis: angioedema, stridor, wheezing, abdominal pain, vomiting
  Neurogenic shock: flushed skin, wide pulse pressure, presence of central nervous system injury
  Septic: fever
  Early "warm shock"—flushed skin, wide pulse pressure
  Late "cold shock"—cool, mottled skin

12. What are warm and cold septic shocks?
   In some instances, there may be an initial phase of "warm shock" with rapid or "flash" capillary refill, widened pulse pressures, and bounding pulses caused by peripheral vasodilation. Untreated, this progresses to "cold shock," with more typical signs of poor perfusion.

13. Does shock require advanced life support (ALS) transport to the hospital setting?
   Treatment of shock is best managed by ALS-trained emergency medical services (EMS) crews as, although this varies by location, they are most often able to provide services that can begin the treatment of shock in the field. This being said, the definitive treatment of shock necessitates emergency department and hospital care and transport via the most expeditious route should be considered.

14. How is shock treated by EMS in the prehospital setting?
   Treatment varies somewhat by type of shock, but in general, treatment of shock is focused on increasing tissue oxygen delivery without delaying delivery to definitive care in an emergency department/hospital setting. Patients should be placed supine or in reverse Trendelenburg position. 100% oxygen should be administered by, at a minimum, a nonrebreather mask even if oxygen saturation levels are within normal limits. Intravenous vascular (IV) access should be obtained, and age-appropriate bolus isotonic crystalloid fluids such as normal saline or lactated Ringer's solution delivered. The underlying causes of shock should be treated whenever possible, and online medical control when available should generally be consulted as well. Depending on practice area, some EMS crews may have access to broad-spectrum antibiotics and have the ability to draw labs and blood cultures when obtaining IV access, and this may be performed when available as well. Blood culture should always be obtained prior to administration of antibiotics when possible. If available, vasoactive infusions may be needed for shock that does not respond to fluid resuscitation and other initial measures.

15. Does treatment of shock vary by subtype?

    As each type of shock has a different underlying cause, treatment will vary somewhat (Table 34.2).

16. How is hypovolemic shock treated?

    Fluid resuscitation forms the core of treatment. The amount required is guided by the degree of fluid deficit and severity of shock. Initial management should include isotonic fluid boluses. Multiple boluses may be required. After administration of each bolus, effect and volume status should be carefully reassessed. Fluid resuscitation should continue until vital signs, perfusion, and urine output are normalized but should be stopped if there is evidence of volume overload.

    In the setting of trauma, stopping or at least slowing any ongoing bleeding is a priority and may be accomplished by use of tamponade with direct pressure, tourniquets, and/or procoagulant agents such as combat gauze where appropriate. When there is suspicion of pelvic or intraabdominal injury, a pelvic binder should be placed. Similarly, traction splinting of the lower extremity should be used if there is strong suspicion of displaced femur fracture.

    Isotonic crystalloid is typically administered initially in pediatric trauma/hemorrhage; this varies from recommendations in adult care. Excessive administration of crystalloid fluids can have a dilutional effect on red blood cells in bleeding patients and should be avoided.

    The use of vasoactive infusions can result in end organ ischemia via peripheral vasoconstriction or theoretically increase any ongoing blood loss and thus should be avoided when possible in hypovolemic shock.

17. How much fluid is in a pediatric IV fluid bolus?

    In general, 20 mL/kg to a maximum of 1 L per bolus. This may be reduced to 10 mL/kg in fluid-sensitive conditions such as cardiogenic shock and heart or renal failure. Patient weight may be estimated by use of a Broselow tape or similar instrument as scales are rarely available in the prehospital setting.

18. How is cardiogenic shock treated?

    When due to decreased myocardial contractility or "pump failure" the mainstay of treatment in cardiogenic shock is the use of vasoactive infusions. In particular, those with inotropic (increasing myocardial contractility) and vasodilator (reduce afterload) effects. This typically means the use of dobutamine and milrinone, although these may not be available in the prehospital setting.

    Gentle fluid resuscitation may increase preload and thus may increase contractility due to the Starling effect. Cardiogenic shock and congestive heart failure are tied together, making these patients predisposed to relative volume overload. 5–10 mL/kg of isotonic crystalloid may be administered over 10–20 minutes, carefully watching for signs of volume overload, such as crackles on lung auscultation, a palpable liver edge, or any edema.

    Arrhythmias can also lead to cardiogenic shock and should be treated according to pediatric advanced life support guidelines.

19. How is obstructive shock treated?

    Careful examination for possible etiologies of obstructive shock should be performed. If present, tension pneumothorax should be treated with needle decompression, cardiac tamponade with pericardiocentesis. These procedures should be performed only if they fall within a provider's scope of practice.

20. How is distributive shock treated?

    Distributive shock may be further subclassified and treatment varies by type.

KEY POINTS

- Shock is inadequate delivery of blood flow to meet tissue needs.
- Shock becomes uncompensated when it results in hypotension.
- The four types of shock are hypovolemic, cardiogenic, distributive, and obstructive.
- A crystalloid fluid bolus in pediatric patients is generally 20 mL/kg to a maximum of 1 L per bolus. This may be reduced to 10 mL/kg in fluid-sensitive conditions such as cardiogenic shock and heart or renal failure.
- Expeditious transport, vascular access with fluid administration, and supplemental oxygen delivery are the mainstays of prehospital treatment of shock.

BIBLIOGRAPHY

Mendelson J. Emergency department management of pediatric shock. *Emerg Med Clin North Am*. 2018 May;36(2):427-440.
Silverman AM. Septic shock: recognizing and managing this life-threatening condition in pediatric patients. *Pediatr Emerg Med Pract.*. 2015 Apr;12(4):1-25.

CHAPTER 35

ALTERED MENTAL STATUS

Jennifer Dunnick and Angelica Mazzarini

QUESTIONS AND ANSWERS

1. What does altered mental status (AMS) mean?

   AMS is synonymous with an altered level of consciousness. It encompasses the spectrum of responsiveness between a patient's baseline level of consciousness and a comatose state. It alerts the provider that an underlying condition is causing the patient to act in an abnormal or altered way.

2. What terms should be used to describe altered mentation?

   In pediatrics, we have various ways of labeling children with AMS. A child with "decreased activity level" describes a child that is awake and alert, but the parents report that they are not as playful or active during the day. A child who is "obtunded" describes a child who can remain awake but may not be oriented. A child who is "lethargic" describes a nonawake, nonalert child who can awaken briefly with verbal or painful stimuli but then the child returns to being nonresponsive. However, a more objective way to describe the mental status of a child is the Glasgow Coma Scale (GCS) or AVPU (for alert, verbal, pain, and unresponsive).

3. What tools can be utilized to quantify a child's mental status?

   Similar to adults, the GCS can be used to discuss mental status in a standardized way. Since GCS uses verbal response as part of the scoring system, a separate scale has been developed for your youngest patients. AVPU can also be used in pediatrics (Fig. 35.1).

4. AMS can be caused by any number of medical problems. How can you remember the main categories?

   There is a mnemonic for that! AEIOU TIPS (Fig. 35.2) can help you remember the common causes of AMS in your pediatric patients.

5. What are signs of AMS in infants and young children?

   In patients who are not yet verbal, it can be very difficult to decide if they are altered. Infants and young children may present with inconsolability, lethargy, or poor feeding. Parents are an important resource here, as they can tell you how their child is acting compared to usual.

Table 35.1. Glasgow Coma Scale (GCS) for Infants and Children

	SCORE	INFANT	CHILD
Eye opening	4	Spontaneous	Spontaneous
	3	To speech	To speech
	2	To pain	To pain
	1	None	None
Verbal response	5	Coos and babbles	Oriented, appropriate
	4	Irritable, cries	Confused
	3	Cries in response to pain	Inappropriate words
	2	Moans in response to pain	Incomprehensible sounds
	1	None	None
Motor response	6	Spontaneous and purposeful	Obeys commands
	5	Withdraws to touch	Localizes painful stimulus
	4	Withdraws to pain	Withdraws to pain
	3	Abnormal flexion to pain	Flexion in response to pain
	2	Abnormal extension to pain	Extension in response to pain
	1	None	None

> A: Alert
> V: Response to verbal stimuli
> P: Response to painful stimuli
> U: Unresponsive

Fig. 35.1. AVPU mnemonic.

> A: Alcohol, Abuse of substances
> E: Epilepsy, Encephalopathy, Electrolytes
> I: Infection, Intussusception, Ischemia
> O: Overdose, Oxygen deficiency
> U: Uremia
> T: Trauma, Temperature abnormality, Tumor
> I: Infection, Increased intracranial pressure, Insulin-related problems
> P: Poisoning, Psychiatric conditions, blood Pressure
> S: Shock, Stroke, Space-occupying lesions, Shunt problems

Fig. 35.2. AEIOU TIPS mnemonic.

6. What historical features are important when assessing a patient who appears altered?
   Think back to AEIOU TIPS (see Fig. 35.2) and ask focused questions based on these common etiologies. Again, most of these questions will be asked of the parents or caregivers. What medications are in the home? Did you see any abnormal movements? Have they had recent sick symptoms? Has the child suffered any traumas, especially head injuries? Does the child have a known history of a seizure disorder or diabetes? These basic but focused questions will help guide the remaining questions and management.

7. What physical findings are important?
   It might not be as easy as noting rhythmic movements or a large scalp hematoma; some important physical exam findings will be more subtle. Look closely at the child's pupils, as many of the common causes of AMS will affect the size and reaction of the pupils. For instance, pinpoint pupils may make you more concerned about an opioid ingestion, whereas fixed and dilated pupils are worrisome for increased intracranial pressure. Assessing the skin can reveal a delayed capillary refill or mottling, which would indicate poor perfusion seen in shock. Additional important exam findings are located in the paragraphs below.

8. What should the examination include if someone has a head injury?
   The physical exam of the head should include looking for areas of abrasion, contusion, hematoma, depression of the skull, or penetrating injuries. Asymmetry of the pupils should be noted as this is an indicator of impending herniation. Periorbital contusions or contusions behind the ears could indicate skull fractures. Nonaccidental (abusive) head trauma may present with only subtle bruising on the body or no physical exam findings. Remember that impact to the head also means that the spine could be affected. Strongly consider using cervical spine or full spine precautions in patients with an exam concerning for head trauma.

9. How is a seizure patient with AMS evaluated?
   A quick physical exam can lead to clues about a possible seizure. The eyes should be checked to see if they are deviated to the left or right side. The mouth should be examined to see if the patient bit their tongue or had frothing at the mouth during the seizure. Check to see if the patient lost bowel or bladder control during the event. If the patient is diapered, then there is no reliable way to gather this information. A patient who has had a seizure will have a slow return to their normal mentation, usually over several hours.

10. How are diabetic patients evaluated?
    When considering the diagnosis of diabetes, it is helpful to look for medical alert bands or insulin pumps located on the abdomen. Pediatric diabetic patients may have the sweet smell of acetone on their breath or they may show signs of Kussmaul breathing, which is described as deep breaths at a rapid rate. Parents may report that they were complaining of abdominal pain or vomiting prior to becoming altered, which is a sign of diabetic

ketoacidosis (DKA). Glucose should be checked immediately, and the value will be high if the patient's symptoms are from uncontrolled diabetes. It is also important to keep the opposite in mind; too much insulin causes hypoglycemia, another etiology for AMS.

11. If opiate ingestion is suspected, what specific treatment can be used?
First, you have to know when you should suspect an ingestion. If the child's mental status declined suddenly, without preceding symptoms or injuries, have a high suspicion for a toxic ingestion. Ask the caregivers what medications are in the home. Next, the exam can help you distinguish what type of medications you should be thinking about. While many ingestions have antidotes, the most readily available in the field is naloxone (Narcan). Pinpoint pupils with slow respiratory and heart rates are signs concerning for an opiate intoxication and should make you think about administering naloxone.

12. How can temperature extremes change mental status?
Pediatric patients are unique because their surface area is larger than their body mass, which unfortunately makes them more susceptible to heat loss. They also have fewer compensatory mechanisms to help maintain their temperature. Pediatric patients who have prolonged exposure to environments that are exceedingly warm or cold will have changes in their mental status. Hypothermia is defined in a child as a temperature $<35\ °C$ (95 °F) and hyperthermia is defined as a temperature $>39\ °C$ (102.2 °F). Treatment is focused on bringing the body's temperature back toward baseline.

13. What is field treatment for someone with AMS?
As always, the priority is airway, breathing, circulation (ABC). A full set of vital signs should be obtained. Children who present with AMS should be placed on 100% oxygen via a nonrebreather mask to maximize oxygen delivery throughout their bodies. Depending on your capabilities, an electrocardiogram (EKG) or rhythm strip may be useful. Rapid glucose testing should be performed. If possible, obtain intravenous (IV) access since many of these patients may need IV medications during their course. Most importantly, children with AMS need rapid transport to the nearest emergency department.

14. What laboratory studies should be obtained by all children who are altered?
In the field, your laboratory capabilities are limited. However, this does not mean that you are without useful tests. Every child who has AMS should have immediate blood glucose testing. Correcting a low glucose will likely improve mental status significantly. Recognizing a high glucose level helps you narrow your differential diagnosis to a metabolic cause, most often diabetes.

KEY POINTS

- The GCS is different for infants compared to children and adults, especially for verbal response.
- Utilize parents as a resource to determine if an infant or young child's mental status is baseline.
- Have a high index of suspicion for toxic ingestion in a child who had a rapid decline in mental status without preceding symptoms.
- Every child who has AMS should have immediate blood glucose testing.

BIBLIOGRAPHY

Avner JR. Altered state of consciousness. *Pediatr Rev.* 2006;27:331.
Cone D, Brice JH, Delbridge TR, Myers JB. *Emergency Medical Services: Clinical Practice and Systems Oversight.* 2nd ed. Hoboken, NJ, USA: Wiley and Sons, Ltd.; 2015.
Dunnick J, Herman B, Rose JA. Pediatric emergencies presenting to urgent care centers. In: Olympia R, O'Neill R, Silvis M, eds. *Urgent Care Medicine Secrets.* Philadelphia, PA, USA: Elsevier; 2018:328-337.
Fleisher GR, Ludwig S, Henretig FM. *Textbook of Pediatric Emergency Medicine.* 7th ed. Philadelphia: Lippincott Williams & Wilkins; 2010.

CHAPTER 36

CHEST PAIN AND SYNCOPE

Kayla Stiffler

QUESTIONS AND ANSWERS

CHEST PAIN

Case: You are called to evaluate a 12-year-old boy with no medical history who has been complaining of chest pain over the last few hours. He reports the pain as central, sharp, and worse with deep inspiration. He denies any additional symptoms. He reports that he helped his father over the weekend move some firewood but denies any other increased physical activity or trauma to his chest. His exam is benign with regular heart rate (HR) and rhythm, no murmurs, pulses brisk bilateral. Lungs are clear to auscultation. He endorses pain when you push on his chest. His vital signs are blood pressure (BP) 110/74, HR 71, respiratory rate (RR) 16, SpO_2 100%, and temperature (T) 37.2 °C.

1. Given what he has told you, what is the most likely cause of his chest pain?

   Musculoskeletal pain and/or costochondritis is the most common cause of chest pain in the pediatric population. The boy in this scenario had sharp pain, worsened with inspiration and palpation. His vital signs were all stable. He had recently been lifting firewood, which likely caused some irritation to his chest wall.

2. What are other common causes of benign chest pain in the pediatric population?

   Psychogenic: Up to one-third of emergency room (ER) visits for chest pain will be related to some form of anxiety, panic attack, or somatization.

   Respiratory: Children may complain of chest pain with pneumonia, pleuritis, or while having an asthma exacerbation.

   Gastrointestinal: Children may complain of chest pain in the setting of reflux or esophageal spasm. More common in the pediatric population are foreign bodies—be sure to ask about choking or the possibility of a younger child putting something (i.e., toy, coin, battery, etc.) in their mouth.

   Precordial catch: This is a nonserious condition of unknown exact etiology that elicits sharp, stabbing pain, usually in a small area along the left sternal border, which is worse with breathing. The episodes of pain are usually sudden onset and brief and have no other associated symptoms.

   Idiopathic: There are some cases of chest pain in children in which we are unable to identify a specific cause.

Case: You arrive to a local high school to evaluate a 16-year-old boy who is complaining of chest pain. He was walking to class when he had sudden onset of pain. While sitting in class, he continued to have a dull ache along his left chest and subjective shortness of breath. On exam, he is very tall and thin. He is tachycardic and tachypneic and appears to be taking short, shallow breaths. Upon auscultation, he has diminished breath sounds along his left upper lung fields. RR is 24 and SpO_2 is 91%.

3. What are you concerned about as the cause of his chest pain?

   You should be most suspicious for a spontaneous pneumothorax given his age, physique, and physical exam. Serious causes of chest pain such as a pneumothorax will make up about 6% of ER visits. These may also include acute chest in a sickle-cell patient, pulmonary embolism, pneumomediastinum, asthma, and less commonly, aortic dissection in patients with collagen vascular disease such as Ehlers-Danlos, Turners, or Marfans syndrome. Congenital cardiac disorders, cardiomyopathies, myocarditis, pericarditis, and pulmonary hypertension should also be ruled out.

4. What questions should be part of your history taking when caring for a child with chest pain?

   A good history and physical are usually enough to determine the likely cause of chest pain. Sample questions you should ask include the following: What does the pain feel like? Where is it located? How long have you had it? Is it constant or intermittent? How frequent is the pain? What were you doing when it started? Any associated symptoms? What makes it feel better/worse? Have you had this before? Have you been ill leading up to this?

   Medical history. Ask about past medical history and what medications they are taking.

   Personal history of cardiac disease, pulmonary disease, Kawasaki disease, sickle cell, cancer, coagulopathy, collagen vascular disease, diabetes, hypertension, hyperlipidemia, rheumatologic disease, and history of recent infection all have increased risk of chest pain caused by more serious etiology.

   Family history. Ask if family members have had cardiac disorders at a young age, sudden death, syncope, or prolonged QT syndrome.

   Social history. Ask about smoking or drug use (cigarette smoking, vaping, bath salts, cocaine, amphetamines, synthetic cannabis, and cough medicines); recent travel, trauma, surgeries, or periods of immobilization; sexual activity/possibility of pregnancy.

5. What are red flags indicating a potentially more serious cause of chest pain?
    History: Crushing/pressure-type pain; radiation of pain (mainly jaw, arm, neck and back); constant, worsening pain; exertional pain; associated symptoms such as dizziness, syncope, shortness of breath, and hemoptysis.
    Examination: Murmurs, gallop, rub, jugular venous distention, peripheral edema, abnormal breath sounds, shortness of breath, unstable vital signs, or abnormal electrocardiogram (EKG) findings (see Chapter 33).

6. What interventions should you perform for a child with chest pain?
    The two most important interventions you will need to perform are obtaining vital signs and an EKG. Vital signs should be performed as soon as possible. An EKG will also help identify if there is an emergent cardiac condition causing the pain.
    Treatment should be deferred until a more formal evaluation is performed but will be focused toward the etiology. Nonsteroidal anti-inflammatory drugs (NSAIDs) and rest are recommended for chest wall or muscular injuries. Nebulizers, oxygen, and steroids are often used for upper respiratory infections and asthma exacerbations. Reassurance, not only to the patient but to the parents as well, is a key factor in treating children with chest pain.

SYNCOPE

Case: You arrive at a church where a 14-year-old girl reportedly fainted during choir practice. She fainted into another child, who helped lower her to the ground. She initially complained of a headache but upon your arrival has no symptoms and seems to be back to baseline per choir director. She states she saw black spots and felt sick to her stomach prior to fainting. Vitals are BP 118/65, HR 76, RR 18, and SpO_2 100%.

1. What is the most common cause of her syncopal episode?
    The most common cause of syncope in children is vasovagal syncope. This occurs when the body reacts to certain stressors by suddenly lowering the BP and HR, which subsequently decreases perfusion to the brain. Triggers such as standing for a prolonged period of time, such as in this scenario, as well as pain, fear, bearing down, the sight of blood, and heat exposure can cause vasovagal syncope.

2. What are other common causes of benign syncope?
    Dysautonomia is a dysfunction of the autonomic nervous system that can cause orthostatic hypotension and fainting upon standing. In younger children, breath-holding spells can commonly lead a child to faint. This occurs when the child stops breathing and loses consciousness immediately following an emotional, painful, or frightening stressor. Older children may also play games in which they purposefully hold their breath.

3. If the patient in the earlier scenario would have instead been running at track practice and said, "It's okay, everyone in my family passes out," would this change your impression of the etiology of her syncope?
    Yes —you would be more concerned about long QT syndrome, which can be hereditary. This is an arrhythmia that can cause fast, erratic beats leading to fainting. It can also be caused by medications and other medical conditions.

4. What are other serious causes of syncope?
    Cardiac disorders such as hypertrophic obstructive cardiomyopathy, Wolfe-Parkinson-White syndrome, coronary anomalies, third-degree AV block, as well as seizures, intracranial hemorrhage, drug ingestions, and carbon monoxide poisoning are more serious causes of syncope.

5. What are important history questions that you should ask when caring for a child with syncope?
    Were there any prodromal symptoms? What were the events leading up to the syncope? Has this occurred before? If the patient is altered, you want to be sure to evaluate further with AEIOU TIPS (see Chapter 35).
    Family history: Ask about family members with sudden death, syncope, single car accidents, cardiac disorder.
    Social history: Ask about smoking or drug use, recent travel or trauma, recent surgeries or periods or immobilization, and sexual activity/possibility of pregnancy.
    Medical history: Ask about past medical history and what medications they are taking.

6. What are concerning signs/symptoms that could indicate a more serious etiology of syncope?
    History: Occurred during exercise/exertion, occurred while laying down, preceded with loud noise, no prodrome/warning signs, associated chest pain, palpitations, shortness of breath, family history.
    Examination: Not back to baseline, cyanosis, murmur, abnormal vital signs.

Case: You are called to transport a 7-year-old female to the ER who passed out at the local pharmacy. Her mother is worried, however, that her daughter had a seizure because when she was waking up, "her arms and legs were shaking." The patient does not recall what happened but states she feels fine. The pharmacist states the patient went limp right after receiving her flu shot.

7. How do you determine if this was a syncopal episode versus a seizure?

Seizures can be precipitated by an aura. Patients can have preloss of consciousness jerks, stiffness, tongue biting, and bowel/bladder incontinence. They generally have some form of a postictal state following a seizure. Patients who suffered from a syncopal episode, however, usually have no aura and are pale and flaccid when the event occurs. They can have postloss of consciousness jerks but generally recover quickly. In this scenario, the patient did not have any warning or aura. She had postloss of consciousness jerks and the pharmacist reports the patient being flaccid. She is currently back to baseline and therefore likely had a vasovagal episode in response to her flu shot.

8. What interventions will you perform on the child in the previous scenario?

A full set of vital signs should obtained, as well as an EKG to screen for arrhythmia. A blood glucose test should be performed to rule out hypoglycemia. Other interventions may include urine pregnancy test, orthostatic vitals, and intravenous fluids. If the patient had a head injury, be sure to follow c-spine precautions.

KEY POINTS

Chest Pain

- Chest pain in the pediatric population is usually benign, with chest wall pain/costochondritis being the most common cause.
- A thorough history and physical exam will often help you determine if the etiology of chest pain is concerning or benign.
- Interventions will be focused toward the cause of chest pain.
- Obtain vital signs and EKG as soon as possible.

Syncope

- The most common cause of syncope in children is a vasovagal response, which can have several triggers.
- A thorough history and physical can usually indicate the cause.
- Know the differences between seizure and syncope.

BIBLIOGRAPHY

Cava JR, Sayger PL. Chest pain in children and adolescents. *Pediatr Clin North Am.* 2004;51:1553.
Evangelista JA, Parsons M, Renneburg AK. Chest pain in children: diagnosis through history and physical examination. *J Pediatr Health Care.* 2000;14:3.
Dimario Jr FJ, Wheeler Castillo CS. Clinical categorization of childhood syncope. *J Child Neurol.* 2011;26:548.
Friedman KG, Alexander ME. Chest pain and syncope in children: a practical approach to the diagnosis of cardiac disease. *J Pediatr.* 2013;163:896.
Massin MM, Bourguignont A, Coremans C, et al. Syncope in pediatric patients presenting to an emergency department. *J Pediatr.* 2004;145:223.
Strieper MJ. Distinguishing benign syncope from life-threatening cardiac causes of syncope. *Semin Pediatr Neurol.* 2005;12:32.

CHAPTER 37

RESPIRATORY DISTRESS EMERGENCIES

Lydia R. Younger

QUESTIONS AND ANSWERS

PNEUMONIA

1. You are called to the house of a 7-year-old male. His mother tells you that he has been coughing for about a week. Yesterday, he developed a fever up to 103°F and today he began coughing more and seemed to be struggling to breathe. What are the first steps in assessing this child?
   You should always use the Pediatric Assessment Triangle (PAT), which includes the components of appearance, circulation, and work of breathing. For appearance, you are assessing level of consciousness (awake, responsive, sleepy, lethargic, and so forth). Circulation can be assessed by checking capillary refill and noting the child's skin tone (i.e., pallor, cyanosis, mottling). Work of breathing can be assessed with respiratory rate, presence of retractions, and any abnormal lung sounds (see Chapter 32).

2. You note that the child seems slightly pale and has a respiratory rate of 36 and subcostal retractions. When you listen to his lungs, you note that he has decreased breath sounds and crackles on the right. What do you suspect is causing his symptoms?
   The presence of cough, fever, and crackles is suggestive of pneumonia. Community-acquired pneumonia is a common childhood condition.

3. What are the common etiologies and the recommended treatment for community-acquired pneumonia in the pediatric population?
   In addition to respiratory support (anything from supplement oxygen to intubation, depending on the level of respiratory distress) and supporting hydration (whether with oral [PO] or intravenous [IV] fluids), antibiotics should be given if you suspect a bacterial etiology (Table 37.1).

4. What are indications for admission in the pediatric patient with pneumonia?
   Hypoxia, dehydration, respiratory distress, comorbidities, complications like empyema or abscess, and failure of outpatient treatment with oral antibiotics.

Table 37.1. Common Etiologies of Pneumonia in Children and Their Recommended Treatments

AGE GROUP	ETIOLOGIES FOR COMMUNITY-ACQUIRED PNEUMONIA	RECOMMENDED TREATMENTS
Children less than 5 years old	• Viral infections including RSV and influenza • Most common bacterial cause: *Streptococcus pneumoniae* • Other bacterial causes: *Haemophilus influenzae*, *Moraxella catthara-lis*, *Staphylococcus aureus*, and *Streptococcus pyogenes*	• Viral: supportive care • Bacterial: amoxicillin (80–90 mg/kg/day PO in two divided doses, adolescent dosing typically maximizes at 875 mg BID, typically for 7–10 days)
Children over 5 years old	• Most common bacterial cause: *S. pneumoniae* • Atypical bacterial causes are also common, including *Mycoplasma pneumoniae* and *Chlamydia pneumoniae*	• For typical bacterial pathogens: amoxicillin (dosing as noted earlier) • For atypical bacterial pathogens, use macrolides (for example, azithromycin 10 mg/kg PO on day 1 with maximum of 500 mg/dose, then 5 mg/kg PO on days 2–5 with a maximum of 250 mg/dose)

RSV, Respiratory syncytial virus.

CROUP

1. You take a call for a 2-year-old male with trouble breathing. He has had cough, congestion, and fever up to 101°F for several days. His coughing and his trouble breathing worsened tonight. Upon assessment, you notice that he has intercostal retractions. His cheeks appear flushed and there is no cyanosis. You also notice that he has a barky hoarse cough and stridor, especially with agitation. What diagnosis do you suspect?
   Croup is a common pediatric condition that affects the upper airway. It is most common in children under 6 years old, due to the smaller size of their airways. It is characterized by a hoarse and barky cough and can also be accompanied by nasal congestion and fever. Croup is caused by viral infections, most commonly by the parainfluenza viruses.

2. What signs and symptoms should you be looking for in order to assess the severity of this child's croup?
   Noting the work of breathing, the frequency and severity of the cough, and the presence of stridor at rest versus only with agitation will help determine how severe their croup is. You should also assess their hydration status—children with croup may have decreased oral intake due to difficulty breathing and the presence of fever may also increase their chance of dehydration.

3. The mother of your patient asks if there is anything you can do to help her son's coughing and trouble breathing. What treatments can you initiate to help with his symptoms?
   Dexamethasone helps decrease the upper airway inflammation associated with croup and should be given for mild to severe croup. For moderate or severe croup, nebulized racemic epinephrine is rapid acting and will give temporary relief of the upper airway swelling while the steroids start to work (Table 37.2). Some children will need repeated doses of the racemic epinephrine, requiring admission for observation and further treatment.

4. You take another call to the home of a 3-year-old female. The mom reports that the girl was playing in the living room while she was cooking dinner. The girl suddenly developed a hoarse cough and stridor. The mom does say that her daughter has had some nasal congestion over the last few days but this is the first time she is noticing the coughing and trouble breathing. What is another diagnosis besides croup that you should consider?
   You should always consider an airway foreign body in a patient with stridor. Croup is classically accompanied by other viral symptoms like nasal congestion and fever. In patients with airway foreign bodies, the stridor will typically not improve with the typical croup treatment (steroids and racemic epinephrine). In patients with a known or possible airway foreign body, attempt to keep them calm and support their respiratory status until you are in position so that you could secure an advanced airway if needed. Minimize agitation by avoiding invasive or painful procedures such as placing an IV unless the clinical scenario absolutely requires it.

BRONCHIOLITIS

1. You arrive on the scene and are asked to assess a 9-month-old female who is having cough, congestion, fever, and trouble breathing. She is crying but consolable. She has moderate retractions and copious amounts of rhinorrhea. She has a respiratory rate of 60 and an oxygen saturation of 95% on room air. When you listen to her lungs, you hear coarse breath sounds and a mild expiratory wheeze bilaterally. What diagnosis do you suspect?
   Bronchiolitis is a common diagnosis in children under 2 years old. It is a viral infection that affects the lower airways and causes increased mucous production leading to coughing and increased work of breathing and can cause both rales and wheezing. It typically begins with symptoms of an upper respiratory infection (i.e., nasal congestion, coughing) before progressing to more significant lower airway involvement. It can be accompanied by fever.

2. As you transport the child to the hospital, the mother asks whether you think that her child will be getting an x-ray at the hospital and whether you think she will need antibiotics. What is the appropriate response?
   Bronchiolitis is caused by a viral infection—the two most common viruses are respiratory syncytial virus (RSV) and rhinovirus. A chest x-ray is not needed to make the diagnosis of bronchiolitis, but it can be obtained if there is a clinical concern for pneumonia. Since bronchiolitis is caused by a viral infection, antibiotics are not indicated. The

Table 37.2. Treatment of Croup by Severity	
TYPE OF CROUP	**TREATMENT**
Mild croup (occasional cough and minimal retractions)	Dexamethasone 0.6 mg/kg (maximum 10 mg) PO
Moderate or severe croup (stridor at rest, moderate to severe increased work of breathing)	Dexamethasone 0.6 mg/kg (maximum 10 mg) PO or IM Nebulized racemic epinephrine, typically 0.5 mL of a 2.25% solution

primary issue with bronchiolitis is increased mucus in the lower airways and so the mainstay of treatment is frequent suctioning; other supportive measures include supporting hydration (either PO or IV fluids) and providing symptomatic relief with antipyretics. Albuterol and steroids have not been proven to be effective in bronchiolitis treatment. Some children with significant respiratory distress will require respiratory support with high-flow nasal cannula.

ASTHMA

1. You respond to a call for a 12-year-old male with trouble breathing. He seems anxious and is having subcostal and intercostal retractions, as well as nasal flaring. He has a respiratory rate of 32 and has an oxygen saturation of 92% on room air. He is only able to speak in brief phrases at a time. When you listen to his lungs, you appreciate diffuse expiratory wheezing and a prolonged expiratory phase. What diagnosis do you suspect?

   This patient is likely experiencing an asthma exacerbation. Asthma is a disease of the lower airways. The wheezing, coughing, and shortness of breath are due to bronchoconstriction. Asthma exacerbations have a variety of triggers that are unique to each patient. Viral upper respiratory infections and environmental allergens are common triggers.

2. The father of your patient is getting very anxious and asks what treatment you are going to start for his child. What medications would you consider giving this patient?

   Since the primary issue with an asthma exacerbation is constriction of the lower airways, your first step in treating this patient should include a bronchodilator, which will open up the lower airways. Albuterol (a beta-agonist) with or without ipratropium (an anticholinergic medication) should be the first choice in a patient like this with signs of a significant asthma exacerbation (Table 37.3). Patients will also require steroids, either PO or IV depending on their clinical condition. Patients will typically require 3–10 days of burst of steroids to help control the inflammation in conjunction with frequent albuterol treatments (either nebulized or via a metered-dose inhaler). In an acute exacerbation, patients will commonly require several bronchodilator treatments before their symptoms improve. Others will require continuous nebulized albuterol and will need admission to the hospital. For severe exacerbations and in situations where you are worried about respiratory failure, intramuscular epinephrine, magnesium sulfate, and terbutaline can be used in addition to bronchodilators and oxygen supplementation. Seek expert consultation when using these interventions.

ANAPHYLAXIS

1. You arrive on the scene and immediately begin to assess a 3-year-old female. The mom says that she just tried cashews for the first time and immediately developed hives and coughing. She has vomited once. Upon exam, she is alert and tearful. You note the presence of diffuse urticaria and flushed cheeks. Her lips seem swollen and she is having retractions and coughing. When you listen to her lungs, you notice diffuse expiratory wheezing. What is this patient experiencing?

   This patient is having an anaphylactic reaction, most likely to the cashews she just consumed. Food, medications, and insect stings are common allergy triggers. Allergic reactions can be categorized based on how many body systems they involve. A simple allergic reaction involves only one body system—for example, having only hives would constitute a simple allergic reaction. Your patient has involvement of the gastrointestinal (vomiting),

Table 37.3. Treatment of Acute Asthma in Children

MEDICATION		DOSAGE	
Albuterol (nebu-lized)	0.15 mg/kg (minimum 2.5 mg and maximum 5 mg per dose), can give repeated doses every 20–30 minutes for three doses and then hourly thereafter	Continuous dosing: 0.5 mg/kg per hour with maximum of 20 mg/hour	MDI (90 mcg/puff): four to eight puffs with spacer given every 20 minutes for three doses and then every 1–4 hours thereafter
Ipratropium	<20 kg—250 mcg/dose ≥20 kg—500 mcg/dose	Can give repeated doses every 20 minutes for a total of three doses	
Steroids	Methylprednisolone 1-2 mg/kg IV divided 1-2 times daily (maximum 80 mg/day)	Prednisolone or prednisone 1-2 mg/kg PO divided 1-2 times daily (maximum 60 mg/day for <12 years, 80 mg/day for 12 years and older)	Dexamethasone 0.6 mg/kg (maximum 16 mg/dose) IV, IM, or PO

MDI, Metered dose inhaler.

Table 37.4. Treatment of Anaphylaxis in Children

MEDICATION	DOSAGE		
Epinephrine	0.01 mg/kg IM, administered in the outer thigh	Maximum for prepubertal child: 0.3 mg Maximum for adolescent: 0.5 mg. Can repeat dose in 5-15 minutes if needed	Autoinjectors: the smaller size is typically 0.15 mg, appropriate for patients <30 kg. The larger size is usually 0.3 mg, appropriate for a patient ≥30 kg.
Fluids	20 mL/kg bolus of normal saline	Maximum 1000 mL/bolus	
H1 antihistamines (diphenhydramine)	1–2 mg/kg IV or PO	Maximum 50 mg/dose	
H2 antihistamines (ranitidine)	1 mg/kg IV	Maximum 50 mg/dose	
Steroids	Methylprednisolone 1-2 mg/kg IV divided 1-2 times daily (maximum 80 mg/day)	Prednisolone or prednisone 1-2 mg/kg PO divided 1-2 times daily (maximum 60 mg/day for <12 years, 80 mg/day for 12 years and older)	
Albuterol (if wheezing)	0.15 mg/kg nebulizer in 3 mL of normal saline	Minimum of 2.5 mg/dose, maximum 5 mg/dose	May require repeated doses given every 20–30 minutes

IM, Intramuscular; *IV,* intravenous; *PO,* by mouth.

respiratory (wheezing), and mucocutaneous (lip swelling and hives) systems. Having more than one body system involved constitutes an anaphylactic reaction. An anaphylactic reaction is serious and can quickly progress to shock. In addition, angioedema can occur in the airway and can rapidly progress to respiratory distress and failure.

2. What treatment should you immediately initiate with this patient?
The first treatment that you should initiate is intramuscular epinephrine. Additional medications are outlined in Table 37.4. Your patient should be monitored closely for response to treatment. Additionally, provide respiratory support such as a supplemental oxygen if needed. If there is impending respiratory failure or airway compromise that is not responding to other measures, you must consider intubation, ideally in a situation with expert consultation. Patients who require epinephrine will require several hours of observation to monitor for recurrence of symptoms.

KEY POINTS

- Always consider the possibility of an airway foreign body when evaluating a child with stridor.
- Treat severe croup with nebulized racemic epinephrine and steroids to relieve the upper airway inflammation.
- Bronchiolitis is a viral infection and the mainstays of treatment are nasal suction and respiratory support—antibiotics, steroids, and albuterol are not indicated.
- Common triggers for asthma exacerbations include viral respiratory infections and environmental allergens. In an acute exacerbation, the bronchoconstriction is treated with albuterol and steroids.
- Anaphylaxis can present with wheezing and respiratory distress—this systemic allergic response is treated with IM epinephrine.

BIBLIOGRAPHY

Auerbach M. Pediatric resuscitation technique: general assessment, primary assessment, secondary assessment. Pediatric resuscitation technique: general assessment, primary assessment, secondary assessment. Medscape. April 17, 2016. https://emedicine.medscape.com/article/1948389-technique.

Barson W. Pneumonia in children: epidemiology, pathogenesis, and etiology. UpToDate. November 1, 2018. https://www.uptodate.com/contents/pneumonia-in-children-epidemiology-pathogenesis-and-etiology?search=pneumonia&topicRef=5986&source=see_link#H10.

Barson W. Pneumonia in children: inpatient treatment. UpToDate. February 6, 2019. https://www.uptodate.com/contents/pneumonia-in-children-inpatient-treatment?search=pneumonia%2Bpediatric&source=search_result&selectedTitle=2~150&usage_type=default&display_rank=2#H3.

Campbell R, Kelso J, Feldweg A. Anaphylaxis: Acute diagnosis. UpToDate. January 8, 2019. https://www.uptodate.com/contents/anaphylaxis-acute-diagnosis?search=anaphylaxis%2Bchildren&topicRef=392&source=see_link.

Campbell R, Kelso J, Feldweg A. Anaphylaxis: emergency treatment. UpToDate. November 14, 2018. https://www.uptodate.com/contents/anaphylaxis-emergency-treatment?search=anaphylaxis%2Bchildren&source=search_result&selectedTitle=2~150&usage_type=default&display_rank=2#H38.

Expert Panel Report 3: Guidelines for the Diagnosis and Management of Asthma. 2007. https://www.nhlbi.nih.gov/files/docs/guidelines/asthgdln.pdf.

Piedra P, Stark A. Bronchiolitis in infants and children: clinical features and diagnosis. UpToDate. September 19, 2019. https://www.uptodate.com/contents/bronchiolitis-in-infants-and-children-clinical-features-and-diagnosis?search=bronchiolitis&source=search_result&selectedTitle=2~150&usage_type=default&display_rank=2.

Scarfone R, TePas E. Acute asthma exacerbations in children younger than 12 years: emergency department management. UpToDate. November 5, 2018. https://www.uptodate.com/contents/acute-asthma-exacerbations-in-children-younger-than-12-years-emergency-department-management?search=asthma%2Bexacerbation%2Bin%2Bchildren&source=search_result&selectedTitle=1~150&usage_type=default&display_rank=1.

Woods CR. Croup: clinical features, evaluation, and diagnosis. UpToDate. June 15, 2018. https://www.uptodate.com/contents/croup-clinical-features-evaluation-and-diagnosis?search=croup&topicRef=6004&source=see_link.

Woods C, Armsby C. Management of croup. UpToDate. October 16, 2019. https://www.uptodate.com/contents/management-of-croup?search=croup&source=search_result&selectedTitle=1~73&usage_type=default&display_rank=1.

CHAPTER 38

SEIZURES

Karen Y. Kwan

QUESTIONS AND ANSWERS

1. What is the definition of a seizure?
   Sudden occurrence of signs and/or symptoms causing change in motor, sensory, behavioral activity, or consciousness due to abnormal neuronal electrical activity in the brain. Seizures account for about 1% of all emergency department (ED) visits for children <18 years old.

2. What is an unprovoked seizure?
   Seizures that occur due to unknown etiology or no immediate factor.

3. What is epilepsy?
   Defined by recurrent unprovoked seizures.

4. What is a provoked seizure?
   Seizures occurring with an acute preceding cause, such as:
   • Trauma
   • Toxin (drugs, alcohol, isoniazide)
   • Electrolytes/metabolic abnormality (low glucose, sodium)
   • Fever
   • Central nervous system (CNS) infection (meningitis, encephalitis, abscess) or brain mass/lesion

5. What is the definition of status epilepticus?
   Status epilepticus—continuous unremitting or reoccurring seizure activity >30 minutes; status epilepticus is a medical emergency with a high mortality rate in both children and adults.

6. What symptoms are consistent with true seizures?
   • Rhythmic twitching or jerking of head/body/extremities
   • Eye deviation, abnormal eye movements
   • Blank stare, behavioral arrest
   • Lip smacking, teeth clenching
   • Sudden fall
   • Loss of tone or stiffening of extremities
   • Drooling or frothing
   • Increased heart rate (HR) and blood pressure (BP), desaturations, or cyanosis

7. What is the most common pediatric seizure?
   Febrile seizures are the most common seizure event, occurring in 2%–5% of children
   • Most common cause of provoked seizures.
   • No evidence of a CNS infection or acute neurological illness.
   • Usually occurs within the first 24 hours of a febrile illness in an otherwise normal child.
   • There may/may not be a family history of febrile seizures/epilepsy.
   • If the seizure is prolonged >15 minutes, first-line antiepileptic medication should be given.

8. An 18-month male has been actively seizing for the past 5 minutes. The patient's eyes are deviated upward with whole-body stiffening and rhythmic jerking movements of lower and upper extremities. He is maintaining his airway and color remains pink with minimal secretions. He feels very warm. What is your first step in stabilizing this patient?
   ABCs—Stabilize airway, breathing, circulation, and disability. Airway is the first priority in a seizing patient. Respiratory support may include:
   • Initial jaw thrust.
   • Give oxygen support via nasal cannula/mask/bag-valve-mask or intubation if respiratory assistance needed.

9. The 18-month-old has been seizing for 7 minutes, what is your next step in stabilization?
   - Time seizure from its onset.
   - Monitor vital signs.
   - Initiate electrocardiogram (ECG) monitoring.
   - Collect fingerstick blood glucose; if glucose <60 mg/dL then intravenous (IV) access—give IV push: 5 mL/kg of D10W or 10 mL/kg of D5W

10. The febrile previously healthy 18-month-old patient has now been seizing for approximately 10 minutes, with stable airway and vitals. What is the initial treatment and when do you give anticonvulsant medication?
    If you suspect febrile seizure and the patient is stable, initiate cooling measures and monitor the patient for a total of 15 minutes. If the patient continues to seize >15 minutes, immediately administer anticonvulsant rescue medication.

11. What are cooling measures for a febrile seizure?
    - Rectal antipyretics (acetaminophen 10–15 mg/kg)
    - Removing blankets and clothing
    - Sponging/cool mist

12. What is the first-line anticonvulsant medication and what form/dose do you give a pediatric patient?
    First-line: Benzodiazepine is the initial therapy of choice (Table 38.1).

13. What is the definition of a pediatric febrile seizure?
    - Fever at or above 100.4°F or 38°C by any method
    - Generalized tonic clonic seizure activity <5 minutes
    - Ages 6 months–5 years (median, 18 months–22 months)
    - Single seizure within 24 hours

14. What is a complex febrile seizure?
    Less common and accounts for 25% of febrile seizures:
    - Focal
    - Prolonged >15 minutes
    - Recurs within 24 hours

15. What is the prognosis of febrile seizures?
    - Excellent prognosis
    - 30%–50% risk of recurrence
    - Risk of epilepsy increases from 1%–> 2%

Table 38.1. Treatment of Prolonged Seizures in Children

DRUG	ROUTE	DOSE
Choose one of the following		
Lorazepam	IV	0.1 mg/kg Max single dose: 4 mg May repeat dose once in 5-10 min prn
Midazolam	IM	0.2 mg/kg (10 mg for > 40 kg, 5 mg for 13-40 kg) Max single dose: 10 mg
Diazepam	IV	0.15–0.2 mg/kg/dose >5 years Max single dose: 10 mg 30 days-5 years Max single dose: 5mg May repeat once
If none of the three previous options are available, choose one of following		
Midazolam	IN	0.2–0.3 mg/kg Max single dose: 10 mg
Diazepam	Rectal	Age 2–5 years: 0.5 mg/kg Age 6–11 years: 0.3 mg/kg Age >12 years: 0.2 mg/kg Max single dose: 20 mg May repeat once
Phenobarbital	IV	15 mg/kg/dose single dose

IM, Intramuscular; *IN*, intranasal; *IV*, intravenous.

Derived from Glauser T, Shinnar S, Gloss D, Evidence-based guideline: treatment of convulsive status epilepticus in children and adults: report of the Guideline Committee of the American Epilepsy Society. *Epilepsy Curr.* 2016;16(1):48-61 and Conway S, Horton E. Emergent Treatment of Status Epilepticus in Children. US Pharm. 2015;40(5):HS35-HS31.

16. How do you distinguish breath-holding spells from seizures?
    - Breath-holding spells happen from 6 months to 6 years old.
    - Trigger that upsets the child followed by crying, pallor, and a brief syncopal episode (due to decreased cerebral blood flow).
    - Recovery is rapid without postictal phase.
    - May have history of iron deficiency anemia.

17. What are psychogenic nonepileptic seizures (PNES) vs. true seizures?
    PNES or pseudoseizures are seizure mimics, characterized by:
    - Side-to-side head, leg, or arm movements with closed eyes
    - Eyes open, appear normal, not deviated
    - Bicycling of legs suggestive of PNES
    - Suppressible by holding extremity and activity reduced with distraction
    - Usually inciting event (emotional triggers, stress, etc.)
    - Common in the adolescent population (young pediatric patients do not know how to simulate seizure activity)

18. How to distinguish syncope vs. seizure?
    Loss of consciousness always precedes seizure-like activity with syncope.
    - Brief twitching episodes without true tonic-clonic seizure.
    - Recovery is usually rapid.

19. What is an infantile spasm?
    Childhood epilepsy disorder of developing nervous system associated with mental retardation.
    - Begins in the first year of life, most common between 4 and 8 months of age
    - Clusters of flexion jerks of neck, trunk, or extremities lasting 1–2 seconds
    - Subtle head drop
    - Occurs on awakening or after a nap

20. What is Todd's paralysis?
    - Temporary paralysis after a seizure
    - Partial or complete usually one side of body
    - Lasts 30 minutes to 36 hours (average 15 hours)
    - Resolves completely without treatment

21. When should you give pyridoxine for seizures?
    - If the patient not responding to first-line/second-line anticonvulsants.
    - Consider accidental ingestion/suicide attempt.
    - Ask parents about isoniazid availability in household.
    - Isoniazid overdose causes intractable seizures resistant to conventional anticonvulsants.
    - Pyridoxine is the antidote:
      Child: 70 mg/kg IV Max dose 5g; administer rate 0.5 to 1g/min. May repeat every 5 to 10 min.
      Known acute ingestion amount: A total dose of pyridoxine = amount isoniazid

22. What is the main concern for an infant having seizures or altered mental status?
    - Hyponatremic seizure due to free water given.
    - Infants <6 months are at risk for hyponatremia from excessive dilution of formula or free water.
    - A temperature <36.5°C is a predictor of hyponatremic seizures.
    - Child is seizing with Na <125 mEq/L.
    - Treatment: 3% hypertonic saline:
      2 mL/kg IV every 5 minutes up to three doses (reassess after each dose)

23. What is the dose of intravenous dextrose for hypoglycemic seizure in children?
    - 5 mL/kg of D10W

KEY POINTS

- Stabilize the patient (airway, breathing, circulation, disability/neurological exam), monitor vital signs, and time seizure from onset.
- Allow <15-minute seizure activity before giving a benzodiazepine while providing adequate airway support and oxygenation.
- If unable to obtain IV access, you can use intramuscular, intranasal, or rectal anticonvulsant medication to stop a seizure.
- Differentiate between seizure and other causes using history and physical exam.

BIBLIOGRAPHY

American Academy of Pediatrics. Seizures Overview. Available at: 7. https://www.aap.org/en-us/Documents/echo_session%201_ seizures_overview.pdf.

Berg CD, Schumann H. An evidence-based approach to pediatric seizures in the emergency department. *EB Med*. 2009;6(2):1-26.

Clinical Practice Guideline–Subcommittee on Febrile Seizures Guideline for the neurodiagnostic evaluation of the child with a simple febrile seizure. *Pediatrics*. 2011:127.

Conway S, Horton E. Emergent Treatment of Status Epilepticus in Children. US Pharm. 2015;40(5):HS35-HS31.

Csanyi B, Hoffman RJ. Seizure and status epilepticus. In: Fleischer, Ludwig, *5-Minute Pediatric Emergency Medicine Consult*. eds. Hoffmn, RJ, Wang VJ. Philadelphia: Wolters Kluwer/Lippincott Williams & Wilkins; 2012:842-843. 870-871.

De Leon-Crutchlow D, Lord K. UpToDate. Diagnostic approach to hypoglycemia in infants and children. Jul 08, 2021. Available at: https://www.uptodate.com/contents/diagnostic-approach-to-hypoglycemia-in-infants-and-children?csi=6d57a530-528e-4b80-80e6-c48b98433266&source=contentShare.

Glauser T, Shinnar S, Gloss D. Evidence-based guideline: treatment of convulsive status epilepticus in children and adults: report of the Guideline Committee of the American Epilepsy Society. *Epilepsy Curr*. 2016;16(1):48-61.

Joseph J, Betts M, Gruzman D, Olsen D, Chang C. Pediatric EM. Management of pediatric seizures. EM Resident. Available at: https://www.emra.org/emresident/article/pediatric-seizure/.

National Institute of Neurological Disorders and Stroke. Todd's Paralysis Information Page. Available at: https://www.ninds.nih.gov/Disorders/All-Disorders/Todds-Paralysis-Information-Page.

Shields WD. Infantile spasms: little seizures, BIG consequences. *Epilepsy Curr*. 2006;6(3):63-69.

Somers M, Traum A. Hyponatremia in children: Evaluation and management. UpToDate. Mar 29, 2021. Available at: https://www.uptodate.com/contents/hyponatremia-in-children-evaluation-and-management?search=hyponatremia%20in%20children&source=search_result&selectedTitle=1~150&usage_type=default&display_rank=1#H654027018.

CHAPTER 39

TECHNOLOGY-DEPENDENT CHILDREN

Munaza Batool Rizvi and Daniel M. Fein

QUESTIONS AND ANSWERS

1. What is the definition of a "technologically-dependent child?"
   Technology-dependent children are those who are reliant on a medical device to augment (or completely replace) a vital bodily function to sustain life.

2. What are the most common classes of technologies used by technology-dependent children?
   Respiratory support, nutritional support, indwelling venous catheters, cerebrospinal fluid shunts.

Case: You respond to a call at a chronic care facility where a 5-year-old male with a tracheostomy is having difficulty breathing and intermittent oxygen desaturations.

3. What are common indications for a tracheostomy?
   a. Acquired respiratory dysfunction (e.g., prolonged mechanical ventilation)
   b. Congenital respiratory dysfunction (e.g., bronchopulmonary dysplasia)
   c. Acquired neurological problems (e.g., hypoxic-ischemic encephalopathy)
   d. Chronic neurological problems (e.g., central hypoventilation)
   e. Anatomic airway obstruction (e.g., subglottic stenosis)

4. What are the parts of a tracheostomy tube?
   Tracheostomy tubes contain several parts (Fig. 39.1). All tracheostomy tubes contain an **outer cannula**, which serves to hold the tracheostomy open, and a **neck plate** (flange) that sits on the child's neck and contains two holes for a tie that wraps around the neck to secure the tracheostomy in place. The outer cannula may or may not have a **cuff** that can be filled with water or air. There may be an **inner cannula** that fits snugly inside the outer cannula and can be removed to facilitate the cleaning of the tracheostomy tube. An **obturator** is a small rigid stylet that fits inside the tracheostomy tube to help guide the tube into place during insertion. The obturator must be removed after insertion so that the child can breathe through the tracheostomy tube.

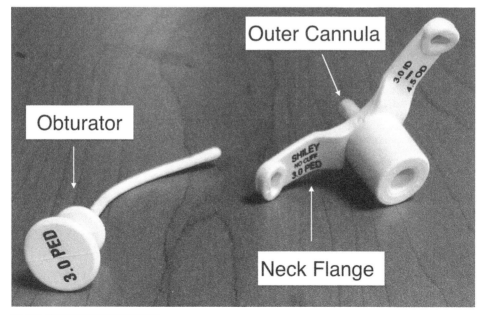

Fig. 39.1. Tracheostomy with labeled parts.

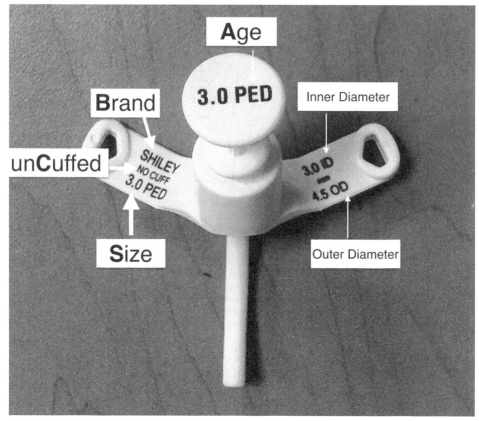

Fig. 39.2. Tracheostomy neck plate with identifying information.

5. What information is necessary when identifying a tracheostomy tube?

There are several variables relating to pediatric tracheostomy tubes, and it is crucial to be specific when requesting a tube. Variables include the **A**ge range (PEDiatric or NEOnatal), **B**rand (e.g., Shiley), **C**uffed vs. uncuffed, and **S**ize (the diameter of the outer cannula)—otherwise known as the **ABCs**. This information is typically printed on the neck plate of the tracheostomy tube (Fig. 39.2).

6. What supplies are necessary for an emergent tracheostomy tube change?
   a. Oxygen and appropriate delivery system (stoma mask and face mask)
   b. Bag-valve mask
   c. Suction
   d. Tracheostomy tubes (anticipated size and one size smaller)
   e. Sterile lubricant
   f. Syringe (for a cuffed tracheostomy tube)

7. What is the first step in evaluating an obstructed tracheostomy tube?

The first step is to attempt to suction the tracheostomy tube. If there is an inner cannula, this can be removed to facilitate suctioning. If symptoms resolve after suctioning of the tube, there is no need for tracheostomy tube replacement.

8. How is a tracheostomy tube replaced?

Changing a tracheostomy tube is a two-person procedure:
   i. The child is placed supine with support under the shoulders to facilitate access to the neck.
   ii. The new tracheostomy tube is lubricated, and the obturator is inserted before removal of the old tube.
   iii. Provider 1 holds the old tracheostomy tube in place by the neck plate while provider 2 removes the trach ties and deflates the cuff (if applicable).

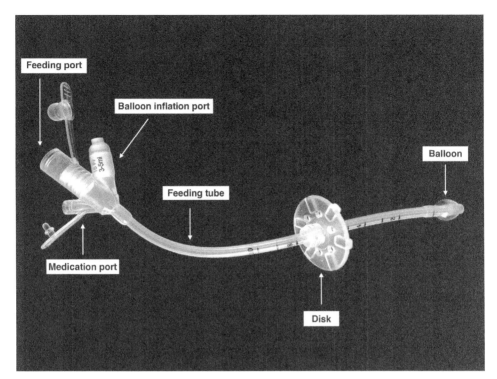

Fig. 39.3. Gastrostomy tube with labeled parts.

    iv. In a coordinated fashion, provider 1 removes the old tracheostomy tube by pulling it in an **anterior-caudal** direction out of the stoma.

    v. Provider 2 inserts the new tracheostomy tube with gentle inward pressure in a **posterior-caudal** direction into the stoma.

    vi. Provider 2 holds the new tracheostomy tube flush against the neck with one hand and removes the obturator with the other.

    vii. Provider 1 will then inflate the cuff (if applicable) and secures the tracheostomy tube.

9. What should be done if a tracheostomy tube change fails?

In the event of a difficult replacement of a tracheostomy tube, the first step is to ensure optimal positioning of the child. An attempt can be made with a smaller sized tracheostomy tube. Care should be maintained to provide supplemental oxygen in between replacement attempts. Ultimately, if recannulation fails, cover the stoma and provide bag-mask ventilation until further help with the airway can be obtained.

Case: You are called to the home of a 3-year-old who has short bowel syndrome and both a gastrostomy tube and an indwelling central venous catheter. Upon arrival, you find the gastrostomy tube is dislodged.

10. What are the indications for placement of a gastrostomy tube?

The indications for a gastrostomy tube (Fig. 39.3) include prolonged failure of adequate caloric intake, inability to swallow (anatomical or functional), certain chronic medical problems (e.g., short bowel syndrome), and recurrent aspirations.

11. Children with a gastrostomy tube are at risk for what complications?

Dislodgement of the tube, local cellulitis, and potentially deeper-seated infections such as peritonitis, peritoneal abscess, and fasciitis.

12. What should be done if a gastrostomy tube is dislodged?

The tract around the tube is fully formed 6 weeks after placement. If the dislodgement occurs before that time, reinsertion should **not** be attempted outside the hospital setting due to the higher risk of creating a false tract. The stoma should be covered and the patient transported to the hospital as quickly as possible. For patients with a gastrostomy tube for more than 6 weeks, reinsertion can be attempted with a replacement tube by lubricating the tube and placing gentle pressure down toward the gastrostomy. If the tube advances, the balloon should be inflated to secure the tube. If any resistance is met, attempts at reinsertion should cease, and transportation to the hospital should occur.

13. What are the complications of an indwelling central venous catheter?
The most common complications of an indwelling central venous catheter are mechanical (e.g., occlusion due to a clot or a broken catheter) and infection.

14. How would a central venous catheter infection present clinically?
Indwelling central venous catheters are at significant risk to be infected, and bacteremia can quickly follow. The range of presentation varies from a well-appearing child with a fever to florid sepsis.

Case: *You are called to the home of a teenager with a history of hydrocephalus and a ventriculoperitoneal shunt who has been vomiting and complaining of a severe headache. His vital signs include a heart rate of 42 beats per minute, respiratory rate of 14 breaths per minute, and blood pressure of 152/100 mm Hg. He is lethargic but otherwise has a normal physical exam.*

15. What is a ventriculoperitoneal shunt?
A ventriculoperitoneal shunt, also known as cerebral shunt, is a permanent catheter inserted subcutaneously to drain excess cerebrospinal fluid into the abdominal cavity for reabsorption.

16. What are the different components of a ventriculoperitoneal shunt?
A ventriculoperitoneal shunt consists of three parts (Fig. 39.4). The **ventricular catheter** (inflow catheter) has its tip in one of the ventricles in the brain. This catheter drains the cerebrospinal fluid and exits the cranium through a small hole in the skull. A one-way **valve** is connected to the catheter and lies between the scalp and the skull, typically behind an ear. This valve regulates the pressure in the brain and the rate of cerebrospinal fluid flow through the shunt. There is also a small **reservoir** of cerebrospinal fluid around the area of the valve. The **peritoneal catheter** (outflow catheter) runs under the skin and transports the cerebrospinal from the valve to the peritoneal cavity.

17. What are the indications for a ventriculoperitoneal shunt?
A ventriculoperitoneal shunt is indicated in the setting of congenital hydrocephalus or when the flow of cerebrospinal fluid is obstructed, causing increased intracranial pressure. This can be due to tumors, congenital variants (e.g., aqueductal stenosis, Dandy-Walker malformation), arachnoid cysts, or development of a Chiari malformation.

18. What are the complications of a ventriculoperitoneal shunt?
Complications include shunt malfunction, infection, and overdrainage (resulting in low intracranial pressure).

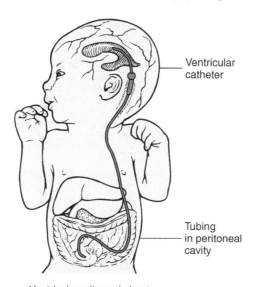

Ventricular catheter

Tubing in peritoneal cavity

Ventriculoperitoneal shunt

Fig. 39.4. Schematic of a ventriculoperitoneal shunt. *(From Frazier MS, Fuqua T: Essentials of Human Diseases and Condition, ed 7. St. Louis: Elsevier, 2020.)*

19. What are the symptoms of a ventriculoperitoneal shunt malfunction?

The symptoms of shunt malfunction are the same as that of symptoms of increased intracranial pressure and vary based on age. Nonspecific symptoms such as vomiting, irritability, and sleepiness, as well as swelling along the shunt tract, can be present in all age groups.

Specific symptoms are as follows:

1. **Infants:** Fontanel fullness or a tense fontanel, prominent scalp veins, sudden increase in head circumference and downward deviation of the eyes (i.e., "sunsetting sign"). Additionally, vocal cord paralysis due to a palsy of the vagus nerve can cause stridor, which may mimic croup.
2. **Toddlers**: Enlargement of the head (prior to fontanel closure), headache, loss of sensory or motor milestones.
3. **Adolescents:** Headache, vision problems, loss of coordination or balance, change in gait. Additionally, more nonspecific symptoms of personality changes and a decline in academic performance can occur.

20. What is "Cushing triad?"

Cushing triad is a triad of hypertension, bradycardia, and irregular decreased respiration that occurs in the setting of increased intracranial pressure.

21. What is the treatment of a ventriculoperitoneal shunt malfunction?

Treatment depends on which part of the shunt has malfunctioned. If the shunt has broken distal to the reservoir, a ventriculoperitoneal shunt tap can be performed as a temporizing measure to remove excessive cerebrospinal fluid until surgery can be performed. If the shunt has broken proximal to the reservoir, surgery is needed as soon as possible.

22. What temporizing measures can be taken to reduce increased intracranial pressure?

Ultimately, surgery is required in this setting; however, several actions may help decrease the intracranial pressure:

i. The head of the bed should be elevated to 30 degrees and the neck of the patient should be kept midline to facilitate cerebral venous drainage.
ii. Maintain normothermia, normocarbia, and normal oxygenation levels.
iii. Maintain euvolemia and avoid hypotension.
iv. Use of mannitol or hypertonic saline (hyperosmotic agents) may also result in decreasing intracranial pressure.
v. Avoid deep suctioning as this may cause a vagal response and a temporary reduction in the mean arterial pressure.
vi. If the patient is showing signs of impending herniation, hyperventilation can be performed transiently to increase the pH of the blood. This leads to temporary cerebral vasoconstriction and reduced cerebral blood flow.
vii. If endotracheal intubation is needed, preadminister lidocaine to blunt any vagal response during intubation.
viii. Administer antiepileptic drugs if the patient has a seizure.

23. What are the signs and symptoms of a ventriculoperitoneal shunt infection?

Presence of a wound infection in the area of the shunt can be suggestive of an underlying shunt infection. However, there may be a shunt infection without any overlying skin changes. Fever, irritability, mental status changes, vomiting, and abdominal pain can all be associated with a ventriculoperitoneal shunt infection.

KEY POINTS

- If there is difficulty replacing a dislodged tracheostomy tube, the tracheostomy site can be occluded, and bag-mask ventilation can be attempted over the mouth and nose while awaiting further assistance.
- Children with an indwelling central venous catheter who have sepsis may be extremely well-appearing.
- A gastrostomy tube placed within 6 weeks, if dislodged, should not be replaced outside of the hospital setting.
- Presentation of a ventriculoperitoneal shunt malfunction will vary based on the age of the child.

BIBLIOGRAPHY

El-Matary W. Percutaneous endoscopic gastrostomy in children [review]. *Can J Gastroenterol*. 2008;22(12):993-998.

Glader LJ, Palfrey JS. Care of the child assisted by technology [review]. *Pediatr Rev*. 2009;30(11):439-444; quiz 445.

McPherson ML, Shekerdemian L, Goldsworthy M, et al. A decade of pediatric tracheostomies: Indications, outcomes, and long-term prognosis. *Pediatr Pulmonol*. 2017;52(7):946-953.

Pinto VL, Tadi P, Adeyinka A. Increased intracranial pressure [review]. 2021. In: StatPearls [Internet]. Treasure Island (FL): StatPearls Publishing; 2021.

U.S. Congress, Office of Technology Assessment. *Technology-Dependent Children: Hospital v. Home Care—A Technical Memorandum, OTA-TM-H-38*. Washington, DC: U.S. Government Printing Office; May 1987.

Vella MA, Crandall ML, Patel MB. Acute management of traumatic brain injury [review]. *Surg Clin North Am*. 2017;97(5):1015-1030.

CHAPTER 40

GENERAL PEDIATRIC TRAUMA PRINCIPLES AND TRIAGE

Anthony Tsai

QUESTIONS AND ANSWERS

Case: Your healthcare unit is sent to a farm to see a child who has fallen through a hay hole. You find a 7-year-old boy lying on the grass near a barn. His mother tells you that she saw him fall from the second floor of the barn through the hay hole down about 12 feet. Initial assessment shows that the boy is responding only to painful stimuli. Breathing is superficial with audible snoring. The skin is pale, with mild cyanosis. Respiratory rate is 12 breaths per minute; heart rate is 130 beats per minute. The skin is cold, radial pulse is weak, and capillary refill is > 3 seconds. Pupils are equally dilated and are reactive to light. Air influx cannot be detected through auscultation in the right hemithorax and is diminished in the left. Oxygen saturation is 82%. He has broken teeth and a swollen nose, with moderate hemorrhage. The abdomen is stiff on palpation. The right leg is swollen, with evident deformity to the femur.

1. How often do blunt injuries occur in the pediatric population compared to penetrating injuries?
   While the prevalence of blunt pediatric injuries varies by geography and region, blunt injury accounts for approximately 90% of all pediatric traumas. When blunt force is applied to a child's small body, multisystem trauma occurs frequently, although the majority of injuries are mild to moderate in severity.

2. What are the typical patterns of injury in pediatric patients?
   Falls account for the majority of all pediatric injuries, the majority of which are not fatal. Most common causes of death from injuries are motor vehicle associated, whether the child is an occupant, pedestrian, or cyclist. The nonfatal injury patterns for different mechanisms are listed here:
   1. Pedestrian struck
      a. Low speed: lower extremity fractures
      b. High speed: multiple trauma, head and neck injuries, lower extremity fractures
   2. Automobile occupant
      a. Unrestrained: multiple trauma, head and neck injuries, scalp and facial lacerations
      b. Restrained: chest and abdominal injuries, lower spine fractures
   3. Fall from height
      a. Low: upper extremity fractures
      b. Medium: head and neck injuries, upper and lower extremity fractures
      c. High: multiple trauma head and neck injuries, upper and lower extremity fractures
   4. Fall from a bicycle
      a. Without helmet: head and neck injuries, scalp and facial lacerations, upper extremity fractures
      b. With helmet: upper extremity fractures
      c. Striking handlebar: internal abdominal injuries
      Other causes of death in descending incidence are:
   1. Drowning
   2. House fires
   3. Homicides
      a. Infants—most commonly due to maltreatment
      b. Children and adolescents—most commonly by firearm injuries
   4. Falls

3. How does one go about evaluating a child involved in a trauma?
   The initial evaluation of the pediatric trauma patient should follow the advanced trauma life support (ATLS) guidelines, beginning with the primary and secondary survey. A stable patient should have a normal primary survey with coherent vocalization, nonlabored breathing with good equal bilateral breath sounds, and hemodynamic stability with good perfusion. It should be noted that children are often anxious in an unfamiliar setting and are often tachycardic from nervousness and agitation. This can be differentiated from circulatory compromise if the heart rate normalizes when the child is comforted, especially by family members.

4. How does the size of the patient affect their injury pattern?

The smaller the child, the greater the force applied per unit of body area. Also, less fat, less connective tissue, and closer proximity of multiple organs translate to higher frequency of multiple injuries in pediatric patients. Younger children also have proportionally larger heads, leading to higher frequency of blunt brain injuries in this age group.

5. How else does their size affect their care?

The younger they are, the higher their body surface area to body volume ratio is. This means hypothermia will develop faster than their older counterparts. Removal of wet clothing and expedient covering with warm blankets should be performed.

6. If they have no obvious external signs of skeletal injury, does that mean the underlying organs are ok?

A child's skeleton is more pliable than adults. The younger they are, the less calcified the skeleton is, with multiple active growth centers. Therefore, internal organ damage is often present without overlying bone fracture such as rib fractures. In these cases, the mechanism of injury will better predict their potential injuries. Conversely, if obvious fractures are present, such as rib fractures or skull fractures, a significant amount of energy has impacted the patient and underlying organ injuries such as pulmonary contusion and brain injury should be suspected.

7. What equipment is essential for the initial assessment of pediatric trauma?

Care for pediatric patients is size and weight based. The best guide for the appropriately sized equipment is the Broselow Pediatric Emergency Tape, which allows for rapid determination of approximate weight based on length for the appropriate equipment size, drug doses, and fluid volumes. A complete list of required equipment for ambulances is in the July 2009 issue of *Pediatrics*.

KEY POINTS

- Blunt injury accounts for approximately 90% of all pediatric traumas.
- While falls account for the majority of all pediatric injuries, the most common causes of death from injuries are motor vehicle associated.
- The initial evaluation of the pediatric trauma patient should follow the ATLS guidelines.
- Internal organ damage in pediatric trauma victims is often present without overlying bone fracture such as rib fractures.
- The Broselow Pediatric Emergency Tape allows for rapid determination of appropriate equipment size, drug doses, and fluid volumes based on approximate weight, based on length of the child.

BIBLIOGRAPHY

Analas, inpress *ATLS—Advanced trauma life support.* Chicago, IL: American College of Surgeons, Committee on Trauma; 2012.
American College of Surgeons Committee on Trauma; American College of Emergency Physicians; National Association of EMS Physicians; Pediatric Equipment Guidelines Committee-Emergency Medical Services for Children (EMSC). Partnership for Children Stakeholder Group; American Academy of Pediatrics. Policy statement—equipment for ambulances. *Pediatrics.* 2009;124(1).
Management of Pediatric Trauma. Committee on Pediatric Emergency Medicine, Council on Injury, Violence, and Poison Prevention, Section on Critical Care, Section on Orthopedics, Section on Surgery, Section on Transport Medicine, Pediatric Trauma Society, and Society of Trauma Nurses Pediatric Committee. *Pediatrics.* Aug 2016;138(2).

CHAPTER 41

PEDIATRIC HEAD INJURIES AND FACIAL TRAUMA

Leah Kaye

QUESTIONS AND ANSWERS

1. A 12-year-old male steps too close to another golfer's backswing and is hit in the right eye by the club. How can you prevent further eye damage on the way to the emergency department (ED)?

   You should physically protect the eye as well as avoid an increase in intraocular pressure (IOP), which can cause secondary injury. Anchor the protective shield on bones around the eye. If no eye shield is available, you can use a styrofoam or plastic cup. To avoid an IOP increase:
   1. Elevate the head of the bed to 30 degrees if not otherwise contraindicated.
   2. Give analgesia to avoid pain—narcotics are preferred to nonsteroidal anti-inflammatory drugs (NSAIDs) due to bleeding risk.
   3. Give antiemetics to avoid Valsalva with vomiting, sedatives if needed to avoid agitation and hypertension.

2. This same patient has a piece of plastic from his sunglasses lodged in his eye. Should you remove it?

   Do not remove ocular foreign bodies in the prehospital setting. These foreign bodies can lodge deep in the eye, paranasal sinus, or intracranial space, and removing it can damage the surrounding structures. Wait until the patient is evaluated in the ED with imaging.

3. What are the important initial steps in care of chemical burns to the eye?

   Both acids and alkali burns can cause large corneal defects. Irrigate the eye immediately. You can use nasal cannula tubing to direct the flow of normal saline, lactated Ringer's solution (LR), or water away from the corner of the eye (away from the lacrimal punctum). It is also important to bring the container of the offending agent to the hospital, if available.

4. Which pediatric dental injuries require immediate medical attention?

   For *primary* teeth (kids under 5, and some teeth of kids 6–12 years): luxation (displacement of tooth) should be referred to a dentist to be seen within 1–2 days. Avulsion (completely displaced from socket) is urgent only if the tooth was not found, due to need for x-rays to evaluate for aspiration.

   For *permanent teeth* (some teeth age 6–12 years, all teeth over 13 years): luxation and avulsion. Avulsion is the **most serious** and the goal should be immediate replantation.

5. A 15-year-old male is hit by a baseball bat backswing. An incisor is avulsed, falling onto the field. How should you handle the avulsed tooth to maximize the chance of replantation of this permanent tooth?

   Handle the tooth only by the crown. If the tooth is dirty, wash for 10 seconds under cold water, do not wash for a long time with water. If the child will let you, reposition the tooth into the socket and have him bite down gently on a cloth to hold it in place. If he is in too much pain to do this, place the tooth in a tooth storage medium, cold milk, or the patient's own saliva. Do NOT place it in water or it will destroy the fibroblasts needed for reattachment!

6. A 19-month-old male was running in the living room with a pencil when he slipped and fell. The pencil jammed into his mouth. On your arrival, he is crying, and the pencil is on the ground. There is scant bleeding in his mouth. Does he need emergency care?

   Children with potentially penetrating trauma to the posterior pharynx should be evaluated emergently. Trauma to the lateral soft palate and tonsillar pillars places kids at risk of an injury to the carotid sheath; therefore, these children may require emergent computed tomography (CT).

7. A 14-year-old female jumps for a header at a soccer game and collides with another player's head. She falls to the ground but has no loss of consciousness (LOC), gets up, and keeps playing. Her coach notes she is playing in the wrong position and seems "spacy." Should she be removed from play?

   This athlete is showing signs of concussion. If an athlete has had any LOC, or has any concussion signs or symptoms, she should be removed from play. Signs include appearing dazed, staring/vacant facial expression, confusion or mistakes during play, disorientation to game/score, inappropriate/labile emotions, incoordination/

clumsiness, slow to answer questions, LOC, and behavior/personality changes. Symptoms include headache, nausea, vomiting, balance problems/dizziness, double or blurred vision, photo-/phonophobia, feeling foggy/hazy, changes in sleep patterns, impaired concentration or short-term memory, irritability, emotionality, and sadness.

8. The soccer player is stable for private transport to further medical care. Her mother asks if the child will need a head CT. Is there any way to predict this?

    The Pediatric Emergency Care Applied Research Network (PECARN) head trauma study identified which children are at low risk for a clinically important traumatic brain injury (TBI) and thus avoid a CT scan of the head, when presenting within 24 hours of head trauma. Clinically important TBI was defined as a TBI leading to death or requiring neurosurgical intervention, intubation longer than 24 hours, or hospitalization for 2 or more nights. Factors associated with low risk for a clinically important TBI can be found in Table 41.1.

9. A 9-month-old male was seated on the kitchen counter and leaned forward, falling and hitting his head on the kitchen floor. When you arrive, he is lethargic. The receiving hospital requests a Glasgow Coma Scale (GCS) score. How do you calculate GCS score in pediatric patients?

    GCS score ranges from 3 to 15 and depends on three groups of physical exam findings (Table 41.2). Head injuries can be classified as mild (GCS score 14–15), moderate (GCS score 9–13), and severe (GCS score $\leq$8).

10. You are called to the home of a 3-week-old infant with a head injury after rolling off a changing table. After completing your primary and secondary assessments, what other information should you collect?

    This scenario is suspicious for nonaccidental trauma (NAT) due to a mechanism inconsistent with the developmental age of the child. A 3-week-old is unlikely to be physically able to roll. It is important to include a clear description of the scene and communicate the reported story clearly on arrival to the hospital.

11. A 6-year-old female falls from 6 feet and loses consciousness. On arrival, her GCS score is 7 and she has sporadic spontaneous respirations. Do you need to perform endotracheal intubation (ETI) immediately?

    This child needs to be ventilated, but if you can successfully bag-mask ventilate (BMV), you do not need to intubate if the transport time is brief. In a study of two large, urban EMS systems looking at kids 12 years or younger needing airway management, there was no significant difference in survival between BMV and ETI. Ventilating in the least invasive way possible also minimizes elevations in intracranial pressure.

12. A 9-year-old boy is hit in the face by a basketball and develops epistaxis, bruising, and swelling. Should you transport him to an ED?

    Nasal injuries rarely need emergent management. After assessing ABCs, apply direct pressure for 5–15 minutes without interruption. Bend the head forward to avoid aspiration. Check for a septal hematoma: a boggy, bluish mass bulging from the nasal septum. If there is a hematoma, transport the child to the ED. Identify the location of the bleed; if it is a posterior bleed, this may be harder to control and require transport.

Table 41.1. Findings Associated with Very Low Risk of Clinically Important Traumatic Brain Injury in Children

AGE	CLINICAL CRITERIA FOR LOW RISK
<2 years	• Normal mental status (GCS score >14) • Normal behavior according to caregiver • LOC <5 seconds • No severe mechanism of injury (defined as fall >3 feet, struck by high-impact object, MVC with patient ejection/passenger death/rollover, car vs pedestrian or bicyclist) • No scalp hematoma other than frontal scalp • No evidence of skull fracture
>2 years	• Normal mental status (no agitation, somnolence, repetitive questioning, or slow responses, GCS score >14) • No LOC • No severe mechanism of injury (see earlier—all the same as for age <2 years, except that fall cannot be >5 feet) • No vomiting • No severe headache • No signs of basilar skull fracture (hemotympanum, CSF rhinorrhea, CSF otorrhea, Battle sign, raccoon eyes)

CSF, Cerebrospinal fluid; *GCS*, Glasgow Coma Scale; *LOC*, loss of consciousness; *MVC*, motor vehicle collision.

Table 41.2. Glasgow Coma Scale (GCS) Score and Pediatric GCS Score

SIGN	GCS	PEDIATRIC GCS	SCORE
Eye opening	Spontaneous	Spontaneous	4
	To command	To sound	3
	To pain	To pain	2
	None	None	1
Verbal response	Oriented	Age appropriate—smile, orientation to sound, interacts (coos or babbles), following objects	5
	Confused/disoriented	Cries, irritable	4
	Inappropriate words	Cries to pain	3
	Incomprehensible sounds	Moans to pain	2
	None	None	1
Motor response	Obeys commands	Spontaneous movements (to verbal command if age appropriate)	6
	Localizes pain	Withdraws to touch	5
	Withdraws	Withdraws to pain	4
	Abnormal flexion to pain	Abnormal flexion to pain	3
	Abnormal extension to pain	Abnormal extension to pain	2
	None	None	1
Best total score			15

13. A 13-year-old female was in the front seat without a seat belt when her car was involved in a motor vehicle collision (MVC). The windshield is spidered, and she is still in the car and conscious. After assessing ABCs, how can you assess for facial trauma?
Look for symmetry of facial structures; malocclusion of the jaw can be a sign of facial fracture; a sunken eye can be a sign of orbital fracture. Listen for gurgling, snoring, or stridor, which can be signs of obstruction from swelling, bleeding, or damaged airway structures. Listen to the tone and clarity of the child's voice. Slurring, hoarseness, or stridor can signal facial or neck trauma. Check for loose or missing teeth.

14. The earlier child has no signs of facial or orbital fracture and is maintaining her airway. You note copious bleeding from her tongue. What should you do next?
Position her in an upright or lateral recovery position and suction the blood. If she can cooperate, identify the site of bleeding and hold a gauze compress against the bleeding site. Many tongue lacerations will self-heal, but if this wound is actively hemorrhaging, she needs emergency medical care.

KEY POINTS

- To prevent further eye damage, take steps to prevent an increase in intraocular pressure en route to the ED.
- Do not remove ocular foreign bodies in the prehospital setting.
- Avulsion of permanent teeth is an emergency, with the goal of immediate preimplantation.
- Penetrating trauma to the posterior oropharynx in kids requires emergent evaluation for carotid sheath injury.
- PECARN head trauma criteria can help predict who needs a head CT after head injury.
- A clear description of the accident scene is important in evaluation of potential nonaccidental trauma.

BIBLIOGRAPHY

Collins M, Stemp J, Lovell MR. New developments in the management of sports concussion. *Curr Opin Orthop*. 2004;15:100-107.
Friese G. Facial trauma. EMS World Education/Training. April 2010. Available at: https://www.emsworld.com/article/10319711/facial-trauma.
Gausche M, Lewis RJ, Stratton SJ, et al. Effect of out-of-hospital pediatric endotracheal intubation on survival and neurological outcome. *JAMA*. 2000;283(6):783-790.

Keels MA. The section on oral health. *AAP clinical report: management of dental trauma in a primary care setting. Pediatrics.* 2014;133(2):e466-e476.

Kuppermann N, Holmes JF, Dayan PS, et al. Identification of children at very low risk of clinically-important brain injuries after head trauma: a prospective cohort study. *Lancet.* 2009;374:1160-1170.

Seiler M, Massaro SL, Staubli G, et al. Tongue lacerations in children: to suture or not?. *Swiss Med Weekly.* 2018;148:w14683.

Serrano F, Stack L, Thruman RJ, Phillips L, Self WH. Traumatic eye injury management principles for the prehospital setting. *J Emerg Med Serv.* 2013;38(12):56-62.

Stoner MJ, Dulaurier M. Pediatric ENT emergencies. *Emerg Med Clin N Am.* 2013;31(3):795-808.

PEDIATRIC CERVICAL SPINE AND SPINAL CORD INJURIES

James F. Parker

QUESTIONS AND ANSWERS

Case: *You respond to the scene of a motor vehicle collision to find a 5-year-old child complaining of neck pain. She does not report any other complaints.*

1. What challenges do children present in evaluation of neck injuries?

   Young children are not always able to reliably communicate the extent or even location of their injuries. You must rely on observation of their behaviors and response to your evaluation to guide interventions.

2. What special considerations are there in evaluation of neck injury in children?

   Children have relatively larger heads and shorter necks than their adult counterparts. This causes the fulcrum of the spine to be located higher in the neck. When cervical spine injuries occur in children, they are more likely to occur in the upper cervical spine (C1–C4).

   Additionally, the structures within children's necks are more mobile and their muscles are relatively weak, allowing for soft tissue and spinal cord injuries without fracture.

3. What is SCIWORA?

   SCIWORA is an acronym for Spinal Cord Injury WithOut Radiographic Abnormality. In addition to more mobile neck structures, the shape and development of the pediatric cervical spine make children more prone to these injuries. The facet joints of the cervical vertebrae in children are oriented horizontally, allowing for increased movement of the bones relative to each other. Their cervical vertebrae are also not fully ossified, making the bones themselves more flexible.

4. How common are cervical spine injuries and spinal cord injuries in children?

   The overall incidence of spinal cord injury in children is 2 cases per 100,000 children. Cervical spine is the most common level of pediatric spinal injury, accounting for 60%–80% of spinal injuries in this population. Cervical spine injury is reported to occur in 1%–2% of pediatric blunt trauma patients.

5. What mechanisms cause pediatric cervical spine and spinal cord injuries?

   The mechanisms that lead to spinal injuries in children vary greatly with the age of the patient. In young infants and toddlers, spinal injuries are most commonly the result of motor vehicle collisions and falls. In older (school-going) children, these injuries are frequently caused by motor vehicle collisions and sports-related injuries. Sports that are considered high risk include diving, football, hockey, gymnastics, cheering, and the use of trampolines.

   In the pediatric population, nonaccidental (inflicted) trauma must always be considered as a source of spinal injury.

6. What factors should cause suspicion for cervical spine injury?

   A combination of mechanism and physical assessment/exam should be considered when assessing for injury. High-risk motor vehicle crashes (death of a passenger in the same vehicle compartment, passenger space intrusion >12 inches, or ejection of the patient from the vehicle) and diving injuries/axial load injuries increase risk for spinal injury.

   Physical exam findings suspicious for spinal injury include neck pain or tenderness, neck muscle spasm, other associated high-risk injuries (head injury or multisystem trauma). A history of weakness or numbness (even if resolved) or children who are not actively moving their necks should raise concern for injury.

7. What symptoms may be found in patients with spinal cord injury?

   The most common finding in patients with spinal cord injury is an isolated sensory deficit. Focal changes in motor function or strength also suggest spinal cord injury.

   There are constellations of findings that suggest particular types of spinal cord injury.
   - Complete loss of motor, sensory, and autonomic function (with or without signs of shock) suggests a complete transection of the spinal cord. The level of the injury can be determined by the location of the symptoms.
   - Patients with paralysis and loss of pain sensation but preservation of light touch sensation and position sense likely have an injury to the anterior spinal cord. This injury usually occurs as the result of hyperflexion of the spine/neck.

- Patients who present with weakness that is more pronounced in the upper extremities as compared to the lower extremities likely have an injury to the central spinal cord. This injury is the result of hyperextension of the spine.
- Brown-Sequard syndrome results from a complete transection of only one side of the spinal cord, and patients present with loss of light touch sensation and position sense on the side of the injury along with loss of pain and temperature sensation to the opposite side of the body.

Case: *You have determined that you suspect an injury to your patient's neck/cervical spine and that he/she should be transported to the hospital for further evaluation.*

8. Are there any decision rules that can be used to determine the need for spinal motion restriction (SMR) in the pediatric population?
   There are studies that have shown high sensitivity in detecting spinal injury in adults (e.g., NEXUS). However, these data have not been demonstrated to have the same degree of sensitivity in pediatric patients.
   A clinical decision rule has been developed to help address this issue Pediatric Emergency Care Applied Research Network (PECARN). Children are considered to be at low risk for spine injury if all of the following are absent:
   - Altered mental status
   - Focal neurologic deficit
   - Complaint of neck pain
   - Torticollis
   - Significant injury to the torso
   - High-risk motor vehicle crash
   - Injury sustained from a diving mechanism
   - Factors predisposing the patient to spinal injury (Down syndrome, Klippel-Feil syndrome, osteogenesis imperfecta, etc.)
   Some of these factors require the patient to be a reliable reporter. If there is any uncertainty as to the presence of any of these symptoms, the provider should err on the side of caution and implement SMR.

9. What additional considerations are there for SMR in the pediatric population?
   There is great variability in neck size (both circumference and height) among pediatric patients. Particular attention must be paid to proper cervical collar sizing and position. Be aware that a young infant may not be fit into a cervical collar, so other methods of restriction may be necessary.
   Once you have determined to implement SMR in a pediatric patient, recall the anatomic factors that differ from their adult counterparts. In the setting of SMR, it is particularly important to recall the prominent occiput in young children. If the patient is placed in the supine position on a longboard or a stretcher, this results in a tendency to flex the neck. In order to maintain a neutral position of the neck and cervical spine, young children require additional padding/support under their shoulders. If a rigid longboard is to be used, specially designed pediatric longboards (with a cutout for the patient's occiput) or additional padding behind the patient's shoulders is needed.
   With or without a longboard, the patient needs to be secured to the transport stretcher with an age-/size-appropriate restraint. The standard seat belts on transport stretchers are often insufficient and may, in fact, be detrimental in this population.

10. How do I transport a young infant with a suspected spinal injury?
    If the infant was properly secured in a car seat at the time of the crash or if the injury occurred from a mechanism other than a motor vehicle crash, consider transporting the infant in their own car seat. Be sure to assess the car seat for damage and ensure that it can be properly secured to your transport stretcher. If the car seat is undamaged and sitting in a car seat will not interfere with the care you expect to provide to the patient, you may restrain the patient with their usual five-point harness and padding to limit head and spine movement.

11. Do car seats really reduce the likelihood of injury in the pediatric patient?
    Car seat use reduces the risk of injury in a crash by 71%–82%. Booster seat use reduces the risk for serious injury by 45% for children aged 4–8.

KEY POINTS

- The physiologic and anatomic differences of the pediatric spine must be taken into account when evaluating these patients for spine injury. Pediatric injury patterns differ significantly from those of their adult counterparts.
- Communication challenges with younger patients create a need for a thorough objective exam. Although spine injury is uncommon in the pediatric population, a high index of suspicion should be maintained in the proper injury setting.
- Proper SMR in the pediatric population requires an understanding of anatomic and developmental status of the patient.

BIBLIOGRAPHY

Babcock L, Olsen CS, Jaffe DM, et al. Cervical spine injuries in children associated with sports and recreational activities. *Pediatr Emerg Care*. 2018;34:677.

Gopinathan NR, Viswanathan VK, Crawford A. Cervical spine evaluation in pediatric trauma: a review and an update of current concepts. *Ind J Orthop*. 2018;52:5.

Leonard JR, Jaffe DM, Kuppermann N, et al. Cervical spine injury patterns in children. *Pediatrics*. 2014;133:e1179.

Mohensi S, Talving P, Branco BC, et al. Effect of age on cervical spine injury in pediatric population: a National Trauma Data Bank review. *J Pediatr Surg*. 2011;46:1771.

Slaar A, Fockens MM, Wang J, et al. Triage tools for detecting cervical spine injury in pediatric trauma patients. *Cochrane Database Syst Rev*. 2017;12:CD011686.

CHAPTER 43

CHEST, ABDOMINAL, AND PELVIC INJURIES

Dorothy Rocourt

QUESTIONS AND ANSWERS

Case: You are called to the scene of a moderate-speed (45 miles per hour) motor vehicle crash and find a 10-year-old female in the back seat, restrained with a seat belt. Her mother's vehicle was "T-boned" on the driver's side, causing the vehicle to rollover several times. She is awake and alert. Her vital signs are blood pressure 110/76, heart rate of 110 beats per minute, respiratory rate of 26 breaths per minute. Her Glasgow Coma Scale (GCS) score is 15. She denies any head injury, headache, loss of consciousness, or amnesia to the event. She denies any neck or back pain. She complains of mild chest pain associated with shortness of breath. She states that her "belly doesn't hurt," but when you transfer out of the vehicle, she has a seat belt sign noted just above her umbilicus. Her abdominal examination reveals mild tenderness on palpation without distention. Her chest, back, and extremities have no external evidence of trauma.

1. How common are chest and abdominal injuries in children?
   Trauma is the leading cause of death and disability in children, and torso trauma is the second most frequent cause of death among children, following head injury. Blunt abdominal trauma accounts for approximately 80% of all abdominal trauma in children. Unfortunately, blunt abdominal trauma also accounts for the most common unrecognized fatal injury. Therefore, the prompt recognition and initial management of children with intraabdominal injury (IAI) following blunt torso trauma is of upmost importance in order to reduce morbidity and mortality.

2. What is the mechanism associated with chest and abdominal injuries in children?
   Patterns of injury are usually related to age and stage of development. Falls predominantly occur between ages of 0 years to 9 years, with a peak incidence of 1 year to 4 years of age. Resultant injuries will range from soft tissue contusions and extremity fractures when heights are low. With heights >10 feet, polytrauma will result involving head, face, spine, abdomen, and extremities.
   Pedestrians versus auto injuries can range in severity based on rate of speed, which can be minor from soft tissue and extremity fractures to polytrauma involving the head, chest, abdomen, and extremities.
   Automobile accidents when unrestrained typically result in polytrauma involving the head, neck, abdomen and pelvis, and extremities. Restrained occupants are also at risk for polytrauma and have a risk of seat belt complex.
   Bicycle handlebar injury to the abdomen typically results in injuries to liver, spleen, pancreas, and duodenum.

3. Children are not just small adults, especially when discussing chest and abdominal trauma. What is unique about children?
   Patterns of injury in children are different from those sustained by adults. Pediatric patients have unique considerations for both body habitus and physiology. Hypotension is a late finding and heart rate is the most important early vital sign. The abdominal wall tends to be thinner and is less muscular, offering less cushion for intraabdominal structures. The anterior-to-posterior diameter in children is smaller, resulting in more energy being dissipated over a smaller surface area. Solid organs in children are larger. The spleen is the most commonly injured abdominal organ following blunt trauma. The pelvis is shallower, providing less protection to the bladder.
   The chest wall in children is also unique. It is broader than long, providing less protection to solid organs. Ribs are also more flexible and pliable, allowing for more dissipation of energy to the lungs and mediastinal structures without overt rib fractures. As a consequence, rib fractures in children require a tremendous amount of force and severe injury should be suspected when identified. Blunt trauma accounts for 85% thoracic injuries in the pediatric population and has a 5% mortality rate. Mortality increases to 20% with an associated abdominal injury and up to 35% when associated with a concomitant head injury. Penetrating trauma has a 15% mortality rate.

4. How should you assess a child with possible chest and abdominal trauma?
   Advanced trauma life support (ATLS) principles are applied to children with the same priorities:
   ABCDE: airway, breathing, circulation, disability, exposure/environment
   Some pitfalls associated with children include:
       Airway—obstructs easily
       Breathing—avoid barotrauma and tension pneumothorax

Circulation—vascular access may be difficult in children <6 years of age
Disability—pediatric GCS or AVPU (alert, verbal, pain, and unresponsive)
Environment—watch out for heat loss

When assessing the pediatric trauma patient, identify the unique anatomic and physiologic characteristics. Keep in mind the common patterns of injury and responses to the injury.

Additional information from the EMS team is crucial. The state of Pennsylvania has adopted a standard algorithm for transmission of information from the EMS team to the trauma team, also known as DMIST:

DMIST

    D—Demographics
    M— Mechanism of Injury
    I —Injuries Identified
    S—Vital Signs
    T—Treatments already completed

5. What physical exam findings are associated with intrathoracic injury?
Two single-center studies reported findings associated with intrathoracic injury. Homes et al. determined that low systolic blood pressure, elevated age-adjusted respiratory rate, abnormal results on thorax physical exam, abnormal chest auscultation findings, femur fracture, and GCS score <15 were associated with intrathoracic injury. McNamara et al. determined that predictors of intrathoracic injury included loss of consciousness; hypoxia; GCS score <15; abnormal cervical spine findings; thoracic, lumbar, and/or sacral spine findings; and abnormal pelvic findings.

6. What physical exam findings are associated with IAI?
In an effort to create a prediction rule to identify children at very low risk for clinically important IAI following blunt abdominal trauma, the Pediatric Emergency Care Applied Research Network (PECARN) conducted a large, multicenter study, using only history and physical exam findings. Children were included if they presented to the emergency department with blunt torso (thorax and abdomen) trauma within 24 hours of the injury and either one of the following: (1) decreased level of consciousness (GCS score <15) in association with blunt torso trauma (but not isolated head trauma); (2) blunt traumatic event with any of the following: paralysis or multiple nonadjacent long bone fractures; (3) blunt torso trauma due to any of the following mechanisms of injury: motor vehicle crash (high speed [>40 mph], ejection, or rollover), automobile vs. pedestrian/bicycle, falls ≥20 feet, crush injury to the torso, or physical assault involving the abdomen; and (4) physician concern for abdominal trauma resulting in any of the following diagnostic or screening tests: abdominal computed tomography (CT) or ultrasound (US), laboratory testing to screen for IAI, or chest or pelvic radiography. Clinically important IAIs were defined as injuries associated with an acute intervention, such as death caused by the IAI, a therapeutic intervention (laparotomy, angiographic embolization to treat bleeding), a blood transfusion for anemia as a result of hemorrhage, or administration of intravenous fluids for two or more nights in patients with pancreatic or gastrointestinal injury.

Seven variables were associated with a clinically important IAI: evidence of abdominal wall trauma or seat belt sign, GCS score <14, abdominal tenderness, evidence of thoracic wall trauma, complaints of abdominal pain, decreased breath sounds, and vomiting. Therefore, pediatric patients who sustain blunt abdominal trauma without any of these variables may be discharged from the emergency department without diagnostic imaging.

7. In addition to physical exam findings, what radiologic and diagnostic studies can be associated with intrathoracic and intraabdominal injuries?
Adjuncts used in evaluating the pediatric trauma patient consist of laboratory tests and x-rays (chest x-ray [CXR], pelvis, lateral c-spine). Additional imaging will include focused assessment with sonography for trauma (FAST) and CT of the abdomen and pelvis. CT is the gold standard for evaluating abdominal trauma, particularly for evaluating solid organ injury. CT scans are highly sensitive and specific. It allows for grading of injury and may be useful for follow-up. Other adjuncts such as US are operator dependent.

Laboratory values tend to be nonspecific. In pediatric blunt abdominal trauma (pBAT), the combination of US, laboratory tests including ALT/AST and urinalysis for hematuria, and physical exam is useful in identifying intra-abdominal injuries. Elevated transaminase (Aspartate Aminotransferase [AST] >200 IU/L and Alanine Aminotransferase [ALT] >125 IU/L) is sensitive in detecting hepatic injury, level II data. Urinalysis with gross hematuria >50 red blood cells (RBCs) per high-power field screens for renal injuries, level II data. The combination of FAST, clinical exam, and lab tests can be useful to guide the need for radiation exposure. Worrisome clinical exam findings consist of abdominal distention; tenderness, which can be focal or diffuse; vomiting; and a rigid abdomen.

8. How common are cardiac injuries associated with blunt torso trauma in children?
Children have a low incidence of cardiac and great vessel injury. CT of the chest is typically indicated when there is radiographic abnormality on the CXR and mechanism of injury involves a high-velocity acceleration/deceleration event. Clinical exam with respiratory distress, distended neck veins, and hypotension suggest severe chest injury with pericardial tamponade. Suspicious radiographic abnormalities include left apical cap, obscured aortic knob, wide mediastinum, large pneumothorax or hemothorax. First rib fractures should also raise red flags. FAST exam

with pericardial effusion will raise concern. Motor vehicle collision at a high rate of speed and falls from a height >10 feet are common mechanisms of chest injuries in children.

9. How often is abdominal injury associated with nonaccidental trauma?
Nonaccidental trauma (NAT) is the fifth leading cause of death in children <1 year. Up to 50% of deaths are secondary to abdominal trauma. Overall mortality rate from NAT surpasses death from accidental trauma. Prevalence is 2.33 cases per million children <5 years of age.

Children who are physically abused tend to be younger and have a delayed presentation when seeking medical attention. Conflicting or changing stories and stories not consistent with pattern of injury for age and stage of development should raise suspicion. Bruises in various stages of healing are concerning. However, less than 12% of children with abdominal injuries will have bruising. Abdominal injury is the second most common cause of death in physically abused children.

KEY POINTS

- Torso trauma is the second most frequent cause of death among children, following head injury.
- A standard algorithm for the transmission of information from the EMS team to the trauma team utilizes the mnemonic DMIST: demographics, mechanism of injury, injuries noted, signs (vital), and treatments given.
- Low systolic blood pressure, elevated age-adjusted respiratory rate, abnormal results on thorax physical exam, abnormal chest auscultation findings, femur fracture, and GCS score <15 are associated with intrathoracic injury.
- Seven variables associated with a clinically important IAI include evidence of abdominal wall trauma or seat belt sign, GCS score <14, abdominal tenderness, evidence of thoracic wall trauma, complaints of abdominal pain, decreased breath sounds, and vomiting.
- Children have a low incidence of cardiac and great vessel injury.

BIBLIOGRAPHY

Boleken ME, Cevik M, Yagiz B, et al. The characteristics and outcomes of penetrating thoracic and abdominal trauma among children. *Pediatr Surg Int.* 2013;29:795-800.

Chu FY, Lin HJ, Guo HR, et al. A reliable screening test to predict liver injury in pediatric blunt torso trauma. *Eur J Trauma Emerg Surg.* 2010;36:44-48.

Holmes JF, Lillis K, Monroe D, et al. Identifying children at very low risk of clinically important blunt abdominal injuries. *Ann Emerg Med.* 2013;62:107-116.

Holmes JF, Sokolove PE, Brant WE, et al. A Clinical Decision Rule for Identifying Children with Thoracic Injuries after Blunt Torso Trauma. *Ann Emerg Med.* 2002 May;39(5):492-499.

Maguire SA, Upadhyaya M, Evans A, et al. A systemic review of abusive visceral injuries in childhood—their range and recognition. *Child Abuse Negl.* 2013;37:430-445.

McNamara C, Mironova I, Lehman E, Olympia RP. Predictors of intrathoracic injury after blunt torso trauma in children presenting to an emergency department as trauma activations. *J Emerg Med.* 2017 Jun;52(6):793-800.

Perez-Brayfield MR, Gatti JM, Smith EA, et al. Blunt traumatic hematuria in children. Is a simple algorithm justified? *J Urol.* 2002;167:2543-2546.

Schacherer N, Miller J, Petronis K. Pediatric blunt abdominal trauma in the emergency department: evidence-based management techniques. *Pediatr Emerg Med Pract.* 2014;11:1-23.

CHAPTER 44

EXTREMITY INJURIES

Matthew Cully and Kaynan Doctor

QUESTIONS AND ANSWERS

1. You are en route to the local children's emergency department having picked up a 3-year-old male who fell off the monkey bars at a playground. The patient has a left elbow deformity (Fig. 44.1). What are key characteristic features of pediatric bones compared to adult bones that can affect presentation and management?
   - The presence of a growth plate or physis. The growth plate is the manufacturing center of long bone growth. It is also an area of weakness and is more susceptible to fracture.
   - Thicker, more vascular, and more elastic periosteum. The periosteum helps stabilize the bone when a fracture occurs. The periosteum allows many pediatric fractures to be managed through closed reduction rather than open surgery.
   - Remodeling. Pediatric bones will remodel extremely well compared to adults. Therefore, timely, appropriate reduction or splinting is paramount.

2. What fractures are unique to the pediatric population?
   Most pediatric fractures fall into five categories: plastic deformation/bowing, buckle/torus, greenstick, complete fracture, and physeal injury.

3. While preparing to transport a 9-year-old female patient who sustained a left ankle injury, you are told by the referring general emergency department that her x-rays show a Salter-Harris type IV growth plate injury. What is the Salter-Harris classification system? (See Fig. 44.2.)
   - Salter I—The fracture extends through the physis
   - Salter II—The fracture extends through the physis and metaphysis
   - Salter III—The fracture extends through the physis and epiphysis
   - Salter IV—The fracture extends through the physis and both the epiphysis and metaphysis
   - Salter V—Crush or compression of the physis

4. What is the most common Salter-Harris fracture?
   Salter-Harris II

5. Which Salter-Harris fracture has high risk for growth plate injury, which can affect bone growth?
   Salter-Harris V

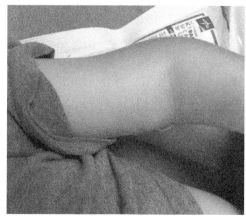

Fig. 44.1. Left elbow deformity. *(Courtesy of Kaynan Doctor, MD, MBBS, BSc.)*

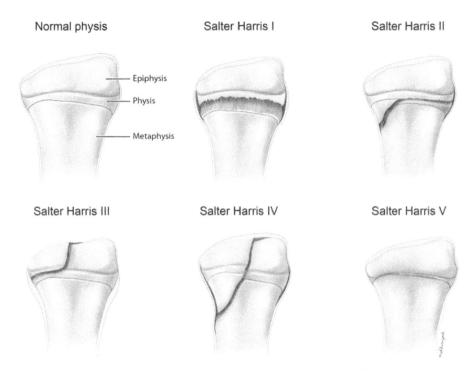

Normal physis — Epiphysis — Physis — Metaphysis

Salter Harris I

Salter Harris II

Salter Harris III

Salter Harris IV

Salter Harris V

Fig. 44.2. The Salter-Harris classification of physeal injuries. *(From Little JT, Klionsky NB, Chaturvedi A, Soral A, Chaturvedi A. Pediatric distal forearm and wrist injury: an imaging review.* Radiographics. *2014;34:472-490.)*

6. You have been called to assess and transport a 17-year-old football player. He is complaining of right shoulder and clavicular pain after being tackled. What questions should you ask regarding any pediatric extremity injury as part of your initial assessment?
   - Mechanism of injury
   - Location of the injury
   - Coexistent injuries
   - Prior injuries
   - Chronic medical conditions and medications
   - Allergies
   - Last meal (with consideration of the patient being kept nil by mouth)

7. How should pediatric extremity injuries be examined?
   General assessment includes palpating the area around the injury including at least one joint above and below, evaluating neurovascular function and looking for soft tissue damage or breaks in the skin.

8. What should the neurovascular examination include?
   Neurovascular examination includes palpating distal pulses, measuring capillary refill, and testing motor function and sensation.

9. Describe the motor and sensory function of the upper extremity.
   See Table 44.1.

10. Describe the motor and sensory function of the distal lower extremity.
    See Tables 44.2 and 44.3.

11. Should an extremity injury be immobilized prior to arrival to the emergency department?
    Yes. Immobilization prevents displacement of a potential fracture or loss of reduction. This protects the area from further injury and can reduce pain.

Table 44.1. Motor and Sensory Function of the Upper Extremity

NERVE	MOTOR	SENSORY
Median	Wrist flexion Pronation Thumb abduction	Palmer thumb and index finger
Ulnar	Finger spread Thumb adduction Flexion ring and little finger	Ulnar side of 4th and 5th digit
Radial	Wrist extension Supination Thumb extension	Dorsal web between web and index finger
Musculocutaneous	Elbow flexion	Lateral forearm

Table 44.2. Sensory Nerve Function of the Distal Lower Extremity

NERVE	SENSORY
Deep peroneal	Dorsal web 1st and 2nd toes
Superficial peroneal	Dorsum foot
Sural	Lateral foot and ankle
Saphenous	Medial ankle

Table 44.3. Motor Nerve Function of the Distal Lower Extremity

NERVE	MOTOR
Peroneal	Ankle dorsiflexion Big toe extension
Tibial	Ankle plantarflexion Toe flexion Big toe flexion

12. What is the preferred method of immobilization by EMS?
Splinting.

13. What are the basic techniques to apply for splinting?
   • Provide pain control, as needed, prior to splinting.
   • Assess full extent and exposure of injury.
   • Apply padding to boney protuberances.
   • Ensure adequate and comfortable splinting; make the splint long and wide enough to cover approximately one-half of the circumferences of the extremity.
   • Immobilize the joint above and below.
   • Splint in a position of function and comfort.
   • Evaluate neurovascular status before and after splint application.

14. What are the complications of poor splint placement?
Complications of poor splint placement include excessive swelling, skin breakdown, and poor immobilization. Abzug et al. showed that splints applied incorrectly or left on for too long could result in unintended injury. Special care and attention to detail and proper splinting technique with reevaluation are necessary.

15. In addition to immobilization and splinting, how else can prehospital analgesia be provided?
Prehospital analgesia should be based on local or state emergency service guideline protocols. Prehospital pain management may include ibuprofen, acetaminophen, and opioid administration. Intranasal fentanyl (1.5 μg/kg) has been shown to be safe and effective in prehospital management of acute pain administered by advanced paramedics (Murphy et al., 2017).

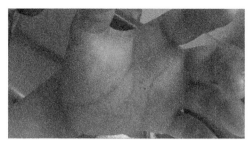

Fig. 44.3. View of the palm in a crush injury to the hand. *(Courtesy of Kaynan Doctor, MD, MBBS, BSc.)*

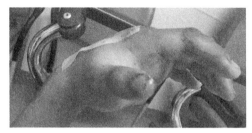

Fig. 44.4. Another view of a crush injury to the hand. *(Courtesy of Kaynan Doctor, MD, MBBS, BSc.)*

16. What fractures require immediate emergency and orthopedic attention?
    - Compartment syndrome with and without fracture
    - Open fracture
    - Fractures associated with significant deformity, vascular or nerve injuries
    - Irreducible joint dislocations

17. An 8-year-old male had his left hand run over by a vehicle in a skateboarding accident. You arrive at the scene. Despite splinting and analgesia, he is extremely anxious and is complaining of severe pain to his swollen left hand (Figs. 44.3 and 44.4). You are concerned that the patient has sustained a crush injury and is developing compartment syndrome. What are the symptoms and consequences of compartment syndrome?
    The pressure buildup in tissue compartments that occurs with compartment syndrome can result in irreversible damage to muscle, nerves, and surrounding tissue if not addressed in a timely manner by trained specialists.
    In older teenagers and adults, consider the P's of compartment syndrome as clinical indicators:
    - P—Pain (on passive stretching)
    - P—Pallor
    - P—Pulselessness
    - P—Paresthesias
    - P—Paralysis
    - P—Perishingly cold

    In children, however, consider the 3 A's of compartment syndrome to alert you:
    - A—Anxiety
    - A—Agitation
    - A—Analgesia (increased need)

18. A 13-year-old female patient was an unrestrained, front seat passenger involved in a motor vehicle collision. She has sustained this injury to her left knee (Fig. 44.5). How are open fractures managed in children?
    - Initial resuscitation and management should be guided by pediatric advanced life support and advanced trauma life support; stabilization of the airway, breathing, circulation should take priority.
    - All pediatric open fractures should be irrigated with sterile saline or water, once bleeding is controlled and adequate analgesia has been achieved. A saline- or betadine-moistened gauze should be applied and the extremity should be immobilized. Antibiotics should be given as soon as possible and tetanus prophylaxis should also be considered. The patient should be transferred to for evaluation by a pediatric-trained ortho- pedic team.

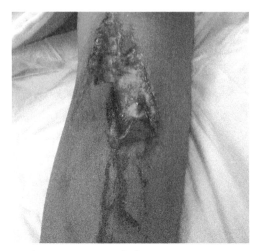

Fig. 44.5. Knee laceration. *(Courtesy of Kaynan Doctor, MD, MBBS, BSc.)*

19. Compared to adults, how do open fractures differ in children and adolescents?
    - Children experience more rapid and reliable healing due to their more vascular periosteum.
    - Children have more potential for periosteal bone formation.
    - Children have lower reported open fracture infection rates.

20. Name the two most common complications of open fractures in pediatrics.
    - Infection
    - Compartment syndrome

21. You have transferred a 7-year-old girl who has sustained a lower extremity injury and deformity after falling at a trampoline park. You are about to hand off care. List the key information that should be communicated to the emergency department.
    - Age and sex of the patient
    - Dominant extremity
    - Mechanism of injury (if known)
    - Location of bone or injury
    - Presence or absence of an open injury
    - Neurovascular status of the injury
    - Intervention (immobilization or splint)
    - Pain assessment (and intervention)

22. A 3-year-old male managed to get his left third finger caught in the hinged seat of a golf cart. The tip of his finger was amputated (Fig. 44.6). You arrive on scene and his father nervously hands you the amputated tip of the patient's thumb. What is your initial management?
    Amputations or partial amputations should be managed similar to open fractures (see earlier). Avulsed tissue should be wrapped in sterile saline moistened gauze and placed in a closed specimen bag. This specimen bag should then be placed in another specimen bag containing ice and water. The tissue should not be placed directly in water or ice to avoid further tissue damage. Rapid transport is key. Although avulsed tissue may often not be viable, it can serve as a biological dressing to promote wound healing.

23. The mother of a 4-month-old male reports that her son was crawling on their bed and fell off it. She subsequently reports that he was in his crib and fell from the crib. He is now crying whenever his right leg is moved. On closer examination, you note right thigh swelling and bruises in various stages of healing on the patient's extremities and torso. The mother reports that he is a "very active child." What should you be concerned about?
    It is highly unusual for a 4-month-old to be actively crawling. The description of the injury does not coincide with the developmental capabilities of this patient. This, along with the inconsistency of the story and physical examination findings, should raise suspicion of nonaccidental trauma and be reported by all mandated reporters.

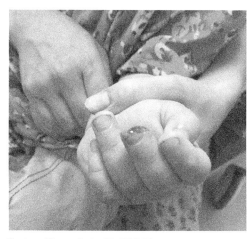

Fig. 44.6. Fingertip amputation. *(Courtesy of Kaynan Doctor, MD, MBBS, BSc.)*

KEY POINTS

- Unique characteristics of fractures in children:
  - The presence of the growth plate and physis
  - Thicker and more elastic periosteum
- Fractures or dislocations with neurovascular compromise, compartment syndrome, and open fractures require immediate emergency and orthopedic intervention.
- Immobilization with splinting should be immediately applied following examination to protect the area from further injury and reduce pain.
- Increased need for analgesia for pain out of proportion associated with pediatric fractures should raise the suspicion for developing compartment syndrome.

BIBLIOGRAPHY

Abzug JM, Schwartz BS, Johnson AJ. Assessment of splints applied for pediatric fractures in an emergency department/urgency care environment. *J Pediatr Orthop.* 2017;39:76-84.

Cepela DJ, Tartaglione JP, Dooley TP, Patel PN. Classifications in brief: Salter-Harris classification of pediatric physeal fractures. *Clin Orthop Relat Res.* 2016;474:2531-2537.

Little JT, Klionsky NB, Chaturvedi A, Soral A, Chaturvedi A. Pediatric distal forearm and wrist injury: an imaging review. *Radiographics.* 2014;34:472-490.

Murphy AP, Hughes M, Mccoy S, Crispino G, Wakai A, O'Sullivan R. Intranasal fentanyl for the prehospital management of acute pain in children. *Eur J Emerg Med.* 2017;24:450-454.

Noonan K, McCarthy JJ. Compartment syndromes in the pediatric patient. *J Pediatr Orthop.* 2010;30:S96-S101.

Okike K, Bhattacharyya T. Trends in the management of open fractures: a critical analysis. *J Bone Joint Surg Am.* 2006;88:2739-2748.

Shaw KN, Bachur RG, Chamberlain JM, Lavelle J, Nagler J, Shook JE. *Fleisher & Ludwig's Textbook of Pediatric Emergency Medicine.* 7th ed. Philadelphia, PA: Wolters Kluwer; 2016.

Shore BJ, Glotzbecker MP, Zurakowski D, Gelbard E, Hedequist DJ, Matheney TH. Acute compartment syndrome in children and teenagers with tibial shaft fractures: incidence and multivariable risk fractures. *J Orthop Trauma.* 2013;27:616-621.

Trionfo A, Cavanaugh PK, Herman MJ. Pediatric open fractures. *Orthop Clin North Am.* 2016;47:565-578.

CHAPTER 45

THERMAL BURNS AND INHALATION INJURIES

Ellen Beth Rodman

QUESTIONS AND ANSWERS

1. What is the prevalence of burn injuries in children in the United States?
   Over 250,000 children require medical attention for burns; of these, 200,000 are scald injuries. Males outnumber females 2:1. Approximately 15,000 kids per year require hospitalization for burn injuries. Burns and fires kill 1100 children aged 14 years and under in the United States each year. Children aged 5 years and under are more than twice as likely to die in a fire as any other age group. Most fire-related deaths are caused by smoke inhalation of toxic gases. Actual flames and burns account for 30%. The majority of children under 4 years who are hospitalized for burns suffer from scald injuries (65%).

2. How are children different from adults?
   - Larger body surface area-to-mass ratio.
   - Smaller airway diameter.
   - Shorter trachea.
   - Thinner skin, especially in infants and toddlers, leading to deeper burn injury.
   - Vascular access more challenging.
   - More susceptible to hypothermia
     (Fig. 45.1).

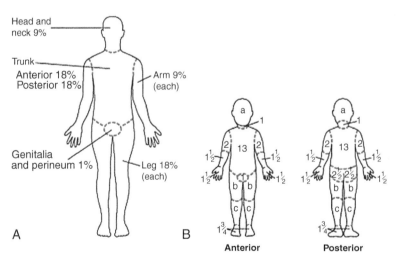

Relative percentage of body surface area (% BSA) affected by growth

Body Part	Age				
	0 yr	1 yr	5 yr	10 yr	15 yr
a = 1/2 of head	9 1/2	8 1/2	6 1/2	5 1/2	4 1/2
b = 1/2 of 1 thigh	2 3/4	3 1/4	4	4 1/4	4 1/2
c = 1/2 of 1 lower leg	2 1/2	2 1/2	2 3/4	3	3 1/4

Fig. 45.1. Total surface calculations: pediatrics versus adults. *BSA*, Body surface area. *(Redrawn from Artz CP, Moncrief JA. The Treatment of Burns. 2nd ed. Philadelphia: WB Saunders; 1969.)*

3. Name the different degrees of burn injury.
   - First degree—red, dry, and painful.
   - Second degree—wet and most painful.
   - Third degree—dry and insensate.
   - Fourth degree—injury to underlying muscle and bone.

4. What are the body's responses to burn injury?
   - Local: denatures and coagulates protein with irreversible tissue destruction. Surrounding area with decreased tissue percussion, which is potentially salvageable.
   - Systemic response: release of vasoactive mediators (cytokines, prostaglandins, and oxygen radicals). Increased capillary permeability leads to fluid extravasation in interstitial space. Destruction of red blood cells may also reduce oxygen carrying capacity. Metabolic response: hypermetabolic increase in energy use and protein metabolism.

5. Describe the initial treatment of burns and inhalation injuries.
   - ABC's:
     - Airway—early airway intubation for upper airway injury before the anatomy becomes distorted by edema.
     - Breathing—decreased level of consciousness, inhaled smoke or toxins, and associated injuries can interfere with ventilation and/or oxygenation. Chest wall compliance may be compromised by circumferential burns to the chest or abdomen.
     - Circulation—at initial presentation, signs of compromised circulation such as unexplained tachycardia, poor peripheral percussion, or hypotension suggest associated traumatic injuries.
   - Stop the burning process. Remove clothing and jewelry. Cool (not less than 8°C) water for 10–20 minutes for small scald burns. Dry clean sheets for flame burns.
   - Oxygen for any smoke inhalation.
   - Pain management.
   - Preserve core temperature (most house fires occur in winter, and children lose heat rapidly).
   - Rapid transfer to hospital.
   - Fluid administration not necessary in field with short (<1 hour) transport time or small burns.
   - Intravenous (IV) fluids for large burns or prolonged transport.
   - Chemical burns require immediate decontamination at scene. Brush off any dry powders, then copious irrigation with water. Avoid contaminating rescuers.

6. How do you determine how much fluid to give in burns?
   Fluid resuscitation is based on the Parkland formula:
   4 cc/kg/% total body surface area (TBSA) burn (disregarding first-degree burns). Generally only needed for burns of greater than 15% TBSA. Half of the volume calculated is given over the first 8 hours, and the remainder, over the next 16 hours. The initial burn fluid of choice is lactated Ringer's. This is a starting point only; actual volumes are titrated to patient response (goal is urine output of 0.5–1 cc/kg/hour).

7. What are the best places to obtain intravascular access?
   Preferably to the nonburned area. You can go through burned tissue if necessary including using interosseous access. Children with small (<15% TBSA) or superficial burns can generally take extra fluids by mouth and do not need an IV.

8. What are the methods of pain management for children with burns?
   For small superficial burns, cooling with cool water for 10–20 minutes. (No ice application; water should be no colder than 8°C [45°F] to prevent further tissue damage). Acetaminophen 15 mg/kg orally or rectally or ibuprofen 10 mg/kg orally can be given. Large or deep burns usually require narcotics or pain relief. Morphine can be given IV at 0.05–0.15 mg/kg. Where protocols allow, ketamine or fentanyl can be given IV or intranasally. No medications should be given intramuscularly as absorption is unpredictable.

9. Where is the best place to transport a pediatric patient with burn or inhalation injury: local emergency department, trauma center, or burn center?
   There are many factors to consider, including transport times, availability, and local protocols. Most emergency departments should be able to provide initial care and stabilization. If you are in an urban area and there is a choice within a reasonable transport time, the facility offering the highest level of care is preferred.
   The American Burn Association guidelines include:
   - Moderate partial thickness >10% TBSA <10 years old.
   - >20% TBSA >10 years old.
   - Any significant burn to the face, hands, feet, genitalia, perineum, or major joint.
   - Full-thickness burns (third degree) >5% TBSA.
   - High-voltage electrical burns, including lightning injury.

- Chemical burns.
- Inhalation injury.
- Burns in children with preexisting conditions that could complicate management, prolong recovery, or affect mortality.
- Any child with burn and traumatic injury in which burn poses greatest risk of mortality or morbidity.
- Children requiring social, emotional, or rehabilitative services, including suspected child abuse.
    Patients with both burns and trauma in which trauma poses the greatest risk of morbidity and mortality may be stabilized at a trauma center first.
    Small burns 5%–10% TBSA second degree and 2%–5% TBSA third degree, as well as most scald burns, can be treated at local hospitals that have pediatric surgical capabilities.

10. What are signs of burn injury being a result of nonaccidental trauma?
    Circumferential scald burns with well-demarcated boarders. Classically "stocking, glove, or donut" pattern (Fig. 45.2).
    - Patterned burns such as from cigarette, iron, and branding.
    - Contact burns to the dorsum of the hands or feet.
    - Inconsistent story or not fitting the child's developmental stage.

11. Name some indicators of significant inhalation injury and impending respiratory failure.
    Stridor, wheezing, drooling, hoarseness, facial burn, or edema. History of entrapment in closed space such as house fires.

12. How should endotracheal intubation be performed on a burn patient?
    Cuffed oral tracheal tube with ties to secure. Often, these patients will require high pressures to ventilate. Swelling and sloughing skin make tape difficult to secure tube.

13. What are signs and symptoms of carbon monoxide poisoning?
    - Headache
    - Dizziness
    - Nausea
    - Shortness of breath
    - Weakness
    - Confusion
    - Drowsiness
    - Blurred vision
    - Chest pain
    - Seizure
    - Altered level of consciousness

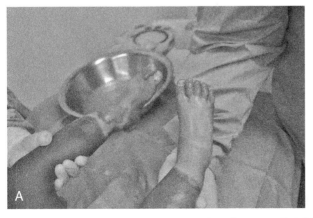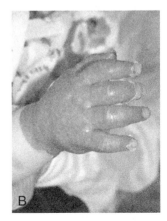

Fig. 45.2. Stocking (A) and glove (B) distribution of burns. *(From (A) Letson MM, Tscholl JJ. Bruises, burns, and other blemishes: diagnostic considerations of physical abuse.* Clin Pediatr Emerg Med. *2012;3(3):155-16; and (B) Jenny C.* Child Abuse and Neglect: Diagnosis, Treatment, and Evidence. *Philadelphia: Saunders; 2011.)*

14. Describe the causes of lung injury.

   A combination of direct and systemic toxicity. Gas constitutes of smoke include carbon monoxide, cyanide, acidic, and aldehyde gases. Inhalation leads to impaired ciliary function, increased bronchial vessel permeability, and alveolar destruction. Release of Tumor Necrosis Factor and neutrophil infiltration alter microvascular barrier function, which leads to pulmonary edema.

15. What scene characteristics should prehospital providers relay to the hospital to enhance patient care?
   - Where was the patient found?
   - Was the fire in an open or enclosed space?
   - What was burning?
   - How long was the patient exposed to smoke?
   - Are there other injuries suspected (explosion or falling debris)?
   - Loss of consciousness?
   - Length of transport?
   - Therapy prehospital?

KEY POINTS

Burns

- Airway, breathing, and circulation (ABC's) with basic life support (BLS) is first priority.
- Children with burns are susceptible to:
  - Hypoxia
  - Hypovolemia
- Infection
- The patient's palm equals 1% of their TBSA.
- Depth of burn injury on initial exam can be inaccurate; the full extent of tissue necrosis can take days to develop.

Inhalation

- Children's airways are more narrow and shorter than those of adult's, making them more likely to occlude.
- Pulse oximetry is unreliable with carbon monoxide poisoning.
- Oxygen by nonrebreather should be given to all patients exposed to flame or smoke.

BIBLIOGRAPHY

Burn statistics. http://www.burninuryguide.com.
Fire safety and burns—injury statistics and incidence rates. http://www.stanfordchildrens.org.
Fishe JN, Psoter KJ, Anders JF. Emergency medical services bypass of closest facility for pediatric patients. *Prehosp Emerg Care.* 2019;23(4.).
Herndon DN. *Total Burn Care.* 5th ed. Edinburgh, Elsevier; 2018.
Joffe MD. Moderate and severe thermal burns in children: emergency management. http://www.uptodate.com.
McCullah CJ, Nordin A, Tolbot L, et al. Accuracy of prehospital care providers in determining total body surface area burned in severe pediatric thermal injury. *J Burn Care Res.* 2018;39(4):491-496.
Mellion SA, Adelgais K. Prehospital pediatric pain management; continued barriers to care. *Clin Pediatr Emerg Med.* 2017;18(4): 261-267.
Shah AR, Liao LF. Pediatric burn care. Unique considerations in management. *Clin Plast Surg.* 2017;44(3):603-610.
Sheridan RL. Burn care for children. *Pediatr Rev.* 2018;39(6):273-286.

CHAPTER 46

GENERAL PRINCIPLES IN DISASTERS AND MASS CASUALTY INCIDENTS

Jessica Mann and Ryan Kelly

QUESTIONS AND ANSWERS

1. What is a disaster?

    A disaster is defined by the World Health Organization as a sudden ecologic phenomenon of sufficient magnitude to require external assistance. Essentially, it is any event that overwhelms the capabilities of a particular service. For example, a multicar accident on a highway can easily overwhelm the nearest trauma center if there are multiple serious injuries or a power outage in a hospital that is already operating at 110% capacity for patients. At any time during any day where the resources on hand cannot handle the task that needs to be done, a disaster can happen.

2. What are the different types of disasters?

    Natural disasters are probably the event that is thought of the most when the word *disaster* is mentioned. These are events like earthquakes, wildfires, floods, hurricanes, and tornados. Damage to infrastructure can occur at the same time that a large volume of patients may be presenting to the local hospital. Terrorist events, like the Boston Marathon bombing in April 2013, create a large number of seriously wounded patients that overwhelm the local EMS and hospital capabilities. Internal disasters happen when a hospital or facility has an event that only affects that facility, like a power outage or fire. In all of these cases, the potential for loss of life is high and exacerbated by the lack of normally available and prepared personnel, equipment, and resources. These types of disasters can lead to a mass casualty incident (MCI).

3. What is an MCI?

    The World Health Organization describes an MCI as a disaster and major incident characterized by a quantity, severity, and diversity of injuries in patients that can rapidly overwhelm the ability of local medical resources to deliver comprehensive and definitive medical care. Multiple resources, such as EMS, police, hospitals, and equipment, will likely be depleted/exhausted during an MCI.

4. How do you respond to an MCI?

    The response to an MCI needs to be organized and approached in a team effort. Decisions need to be made early, including assignment of roles. Communication is key to any MCI response. It is important to perform an assessment of the scene for both safety and scale of incident and request resources early. All of these points and the process for approaching an MCI are outlined by the National Incident Management System (NIMS).

5. What are the challenges with an MCI?

    An MCI can be a very chaotic and stressful scene at first. There are many challenges, including location of the incident, scene safety, ongoing disaster, available resources and equipment, available professionals, and untrained first responders. Depending on the MCI, crowd control, traffic control, and media can also be challenging.

6. What is the NIMS?

    According to the Department of Homeland Security, NIMS is a comprehensive, national approach to incident management that is applicable at all jurisdiction levels and across functional disciplines. NIMS provides a common standard for approach to an incident that can be used at any level, including federal, state, tribal, and local. It allows for efficient and effective responses to any incident that can vary from an individual structure fire to a natural disaster.

7. Name the components of NIMS.

    There are five main components to NIMS. They include preparedness, communications and information management, resource management, command and management, and ongoing management and maintenance.

8. Why do we use NIMS?

    An MCI begins locally and can include many organizations including police, fire, EMS, and private sectors. The incident may be large enough to require higher-level resources at the state or federal level. NIMS provides the structure and guidance for these entities to work together to respond to an incident. It allows multiple organizations to use a common language for communication. It encourages organizations to work together to prevent, protect against, mitigate, respond to, and recover from incidents.

KEY POINTS

- Disasters can be manmade, terrorist events, hospital specific, community wide, limited time frame, or have an unknown endpoint.
- Disasters all have similar characteristics in that they can easily overwhelm the normal community resources for any length of time and usually cause an MCI.
- MCIs can be stressful and require an organized approach with clear roles and communication.
- A comprehensive approach to an MCI is using the NIMS.

BIBLIOGRAPHY

Tintinalli JE, Cline D. *Tintinalli's Emergency Medicine Manual.* New York: McGraw-Hill Medical; 2012.

U.S. Department of Homeland Security. NIMS: Frequently Asked Questions. Available at: https://www.fema.gov/pdf/emergency/nims/nimsfaqs.pdf.

World Health Organization: Disasters and emergencies. Available at: https://www.who.int/surgery/challenges/esc_disasters_emergencies/en/.

CHAPTER 47

PREHOSPITAL TRIAGE FOR MASS CASUALTIES

Jessica Mann

QUESTIONS AND ANSWERS

1. What is a mass casualty incident (MCI)?
   The World Health Organization describes an MCI as a disaster and major incident characterized by a quantity, severity, and diversity of injuries in patients that can rapidly overwhelm the ability of local medical resources to deliver comprehensive and definitive medical care. Multiple resources, such as EMS, police, hospitals, and equipment, will likely be depleted/exhausted during an MCI.

2. How do we approach the multiple patients of an MCI?
   It is important that a rapid and effective triage system be performed to evaluate the number and severity of patients. During an MCI, resources are limited. The goal is to perform the greatest good for the largest number of people. Overall, patients should be rapidly organized into categories by using a triage system.

3. What triage system should be used for an MCI?
   There are numerous triage systems currently available that include START (simple triage and rapid treatment), SALT (sort, assess, lifesaving interventions, treatment/triage), SAVE (secondary assessment of victim endpoint), and STM (sacco triage method). No matter which system is used, the goal is to perform minimal care to determine which patients have the greatest survival chance. This can be difficult as training always encourages giving comprehensive care and saving lives, but in an MCI, there will be severely ill patients who are determined to have a poor survival chance and there should be no attempt to save their life. All triage systems organize patients using a universal color coding system.

4. What do the color of tags mean in a triage system?
   See Table 47.1.

5. What is the most widely used triage system in the United States?
   START, which was developed in 1983.
       See Fig. 47.1.

6. How do you triage using the SALT system?
   See Fig. 47.2.

7. Are there any pediatric triage systems that can be used?
   Yes, JumpSTART can be used for the pediatric population, which is similar to START for adults (Fig. 47.3).

8. Describe other concerns/issues that should be considered with triage of an MCI.
   There should always be consideration of scene safety before entering/engaging in any MCI. Large areas will need to be identified and marked for patients to be placed based on the color of the tag. Always notify the local hospital as early as possible so that preparation and resources can be allocated to help care for the multiple patients.

Table 47.1. Tag Color in the Triage System

COLOR	CATEGORY	MEANING
Black	Expectant	Unlikely to survive given injuries
Red	Immediate	Requires immediate medical attention for survival
Yellow	Delayed	Has serious injuries, but not immediately life threatening
Green	Minor	Minor injuries that patient could survive for days

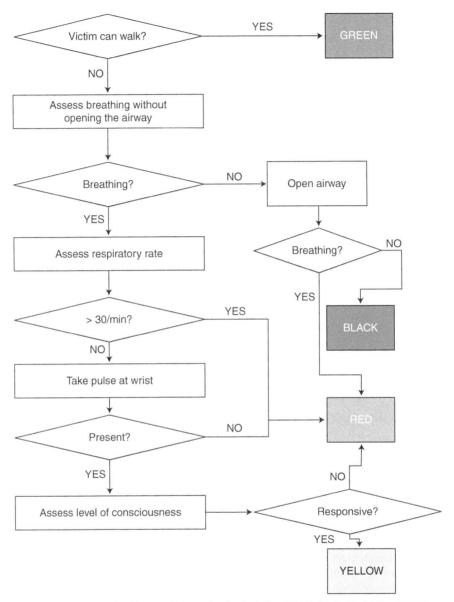

Fig. 47.1. START (simple triage and rapid treatment) triage system flowchart. *(From Kahn CA, Schultz CH, et al. Does START triage work? An outcomes assessment after a disaster. Ann Emerg Med. 2009;54(3):424-430.e1.)*

9. Once a patient is triaged with a color tag, is that patient's status permanent?
   No, the severity level of a patient can change. The triage system is fluid. It is important that patients are monitored once organized into a certain color tag zone. It is possible for any patient to become more ill or decompensate. If this happens, a patient's color tag may need to be upgraded to a more severe color. Frequent reevaluation of patients is imperative in any triage system.

10. You arrive to a mall shooting and police report that the scene has been cleared and is safe. You enter to find multiple victims. There is a 56-year-old male who is walking toward you with a hand that is bleeding. There is a 34-year-old female who is not breathing and when you reposition her airway, she still does not breathe.

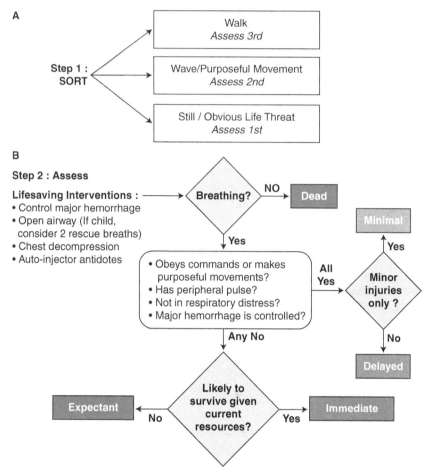

A

Step 1 :
SORT

Walk
Assess 3rd

Wave/Purposeful Movement
Assess 2nd

Still / Obvious Life Threat
Assess 1st

B

Step 2 : Assess

Lifesaving Interventions :
• Control major hemorrhage
• Open airway (If child, consider 2 rescue breaths)
• Chest decompression
• Auto-injector antidotes

Breathing? NO → Dead

Yes

• Obeys commands or makes purposeful movements?
• Has peripheral pulse?
• Not in respiratory distress?
• Major hemorrhage is controlled?

All Yes → Minor injuries only ? Yes → Minimal

No

Delayed

Any No

Likely to survive given current resources?

Expectant ← No

Yes → Immediate

Fig. 47.2. (A and B) SALT (sort, assess, lifesaving interventions, treatment) triage method. *(From Bhalla MC, Frey J, Rider C, et al. Simple triage algorithm and rapid treatment and sort, assess, lifesaving, interventions, treatment, and transportation mass casualty triage methods for sensitivity, specificity, and predictive values.* Am J Emerg Med. *2015;33(11);1687-1691.)*

There is a 12-year-old boy who is breathing and the respiratory rate is 12 breaths per minute. There is a 19-year-old female who is lying on the ground breathing with a respiratory rate of 20 breaths per minute with a radial pulse and is able to blink her eyes. How would you triage these patients using START and Jump-START?

56-year-old male—Green
34-year-old female—Black
12-year-old boy—Red
19-year-old female—Yellow

• There are multiple triage systems that are available to use for an MCI, with the most popular being START.
• No matter which triage system is used for an MCI, the color tags are the same and should be familiar to providers.
• The goal of triage in an MCI is to perform little care to determine which patients have the best survival chance.
• Triage is a fluid process that requires frequent reevaluation to determine if a patient's status becomes more critical/severe.

JumpSTART Pediatric MCI Triage ©

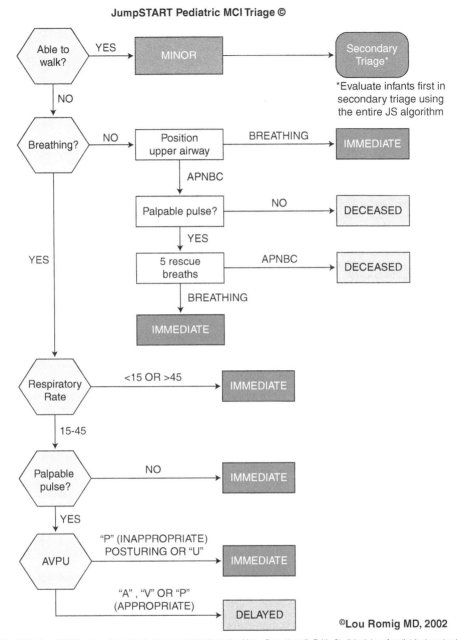

Fig. 47.3. JumpSTART prehospital pediatric mass casualty triage algorithm. *(From Heon D, Foltin GL. Principles of pediatric decontamination. Clin Pediatr Emerg Med. 2009;10(3):186-194.)*

BIBLIOGRAPHY

Clarkson L, Williams M. EMS, mass casualty triage. StatPearls [Internet]. Treasure Island, FL: StatPearlsPublising; 2020.
Edgerly D. The basics of mass casualty triage. *J Emerg Med Serv*. 2016;41(5.).
START Adult Triage. https://chemm.nlm.nih.gov/.
World Health Organization. Disasters and emergencies. https://www.who.int/surgery/challenges/esc_disasters_emergencies/en/.

CHAPTER 48

MASS CASUALTY EVACUATION AND PATIENT MOVEMENT

Jessica Mann

QUESTIONS AND ANSWERS

1. What are casualty collection points that are used during a mass casualty incident?

   These are areas that have been designated to move patients from the scene of the incident. They need to be in a safe area, usually a distance from the scene, and should not be accessible to the public. The collection points usually coincide with the levels of triage to help keep patients organized. Patients are moved to these areas by any means possible, including walking, wheelchairs, litters, or flexible stretchers.

2. What are the overall steps in casualty movement and evacuation during a mass casualty incident?
   - Evaluate the current situation.
     - This means identifying any threats at the scene, estimating the number of patients, and figuring out the resources available and the resources needed for transportation.
   - Develop a plan for evacuation.
     - Once the situation is evaluated, use that knowledge along with the availability of healthcare facilities to figure out a plan for patient evacuation.
   - Implement the plan and perform effective communication.
     - Execution of a plan will require flexibility and adaptability. There will need to be communication with the incident commander, 911 dispatch, and the emergency operations center.

3. How do we estimate the number of patients and the mode of transportation they will need?

   The estimate of patients present will be calculated as they are moved to the casualty collection points. At the casualty collection points, triage will determine the level of medical care needed using a triage system. The mode of transportation the patient will need will likely be determined by the triage level of care. This level of care can change and patients will have frequent reevaluations at these collection points. Minimal medical care is actually given at the casualty collection points.

4. Where will patients be evacuated to during a mass casualty incident?

   Patients can go to numerous places during a mass casualty incident. The obvious site is local hospitals. However, due to these resources getting overwhelmed quickly, patients can also be sent to hospitals that are further away. Patients can also be assigned to go to an alternate care facility that is established specifically for the mass casualty incident, for example, a firehouse that has been designated to provide care to the walking wounded.

5. List the modes of transportation that can be used for patient evacuation.
   - Ambulances—these will likely be used for the critical patients who may require acute medical care during transport and need to go to a hospital; it is possible that an ambulance could transport more than one patient at a time.
   - Buses (school or public)—these may transport a large group of walking wounded to an alternate care facility.
   - Private vehicles—some patients will escape the incident without being triaged and arrive at a hospital by their own means.
   - Police vehicles—police are usually one of the first services to arrive to any scene and have a tendency to perform basic first aid care and transport some patients immediately to a local hospital without waiting for the evacuation plan; this especially occurs with shootings.
   - Taxis and share rides—during the Las Vegas mass shooting of 2017, it was noted that more patients arrived to the emergency department by this mode of transportation than by ambulances.
   - US Department of Defense—has available resources to deploy to assist in patient evacuation.

6. How can these various modes of transportation hinder the evacuation process?

   If patients are taken by police, private vehicles, and ride shares without following the evacuation plan, this will lead to disorganization and lack of control of the transportation flow. This will also cause patients to arrive at local hospitals without notification. It also means that most of these patients were not triaged and receiving hospitals will need to perform mass casualty triage upon arrival.

7. When developing a plan for evacuation, how do we communicate with hospitals?
    There are numerous applications and software programs available to alert an area of a mass casualty incident. These same programs allow the hospitals in that region to communicate with the emergency operations center giving their available resources and amount of patients they can receive. This reinforces the importance of communication between the incident command, transport officer, dispatch centers, and emergency operations center.

8. What is an ambulance exchange point?
    This is a designated area where a patient may be transported from one mode of transportation to another. There are many reasons to utilize an exchange point. One is that if the distance to a specialty resource is far and a patient may need air services. Another is if the incident is so large and there may be multiple casualty collection points, patients may be transported from these multiple points to a central holding area before final transport to a facility.

9. What are some general considerations for evacuation as the plan is implemented?
    There will need to be designated traffic flow and likely local law enforcement to help implement. There will need to be evaluation and estimation of the need of medical professionals at each component of patient movement/evacuation. Landing zones for helicopters will need to be identified early and how patients will move to these areas (ambulance exchange point).

10. Can patients be tracked during a mass casualty incident?
    Yes. The same applications and software programs that are used to communicate with hospitals regarding available resources can also track patients. Most of the triage tags used today have a bar code on them that can be used to track patients. This tracking will begin at the scene and continue upon patient's arrival to a hospital. With that being said, there is still a large number of patients that independently arrive at an emergency department or do not seek medical attention, and these patients are sometimes lost to tracking.

11. What do local healthcare facilities need to consider with patient evacuation during a mass casualty incident?
    One of the most important considerations is the offloading process. The ideal scenario is a quick offload so the mode of transportation can quickly get back to the incident and offer continued services. Usually, this is achieved with a drive-through set-up where the drivers/caretakers of the transport unit may not even get out of the unit. Another consideration for the facility is how the mass influx of patients will be registered. It is also important for receiving facilities to reevaluate a patient upon arrival for appropriate triage level. This is why it is important that healthcare facilities also practice and perform drills on responding to a mass casualty incident.

KEY POINTS

- Evaluating, planning, and effective communication are key to patient movement and evacuation during a mass casualty incident.
- There are many modes of transportation that may be used during a mass casualty incident, not just ambulances.
- Organizing traffic flow, evaluating need of medical professionals, and identifying landing zones are all imperative to the implementation of patient evacuation during a mass casualty incident.
- It should be expected that not all patients will be easily tracked during a mass casualty incident and area hospitals should expect to receive a number of patients that arrive by their own mode of transportation.
- Receiving health care facilities will need to communicate with the emergency operations center and also have planned on how they will receive the influx of patients during an evacuation of a mass casualty incident.

BIBLIOGRAPHY

Cone DC, Brice JH, Delbridge TR, Myers JB, eds. *Emergency Medical Services: Clinical Practice and Systems Oversight.* Vol 2, 2nd ed. United Kingdom: John Wiley & Sons; 2015: 303-312.

Koser B, Suchenski M, EMS, casualty evacuation. In: StatPearls [Internet]. Treasure Island, FL: StatPearlsPublishing; 2020.

Zane RD, Rich T, Biddinger PD. Recommendations for a national mass patient and evacuee movement, regulating, and tracking system. Homeland Security Digital Library. 2009. Available at: https://www.hsdl.org.

CHAPTER 49

BIOLOGICAL AND CHEMICAL TERRORISM

Walker Foland

QUESTIONS AND ANSWERS

1. What is the importance of preplanning regarding chemical and biological terrorism?
   Without preplanning, the risk of injury or death to first responders is greatly increased. Each responding organization should develop standard operating procedures (SOPs) to implement personal protective equipment (PPE) use, decontamination of casualties, and technical decontamination of first responders. Individual SOPs should be part of the overall incident response plan. Frequent multiagency training is necessary to unify resources, decision-making, and information exchange.

2. List examples of PPE regarding chemical and biological terrorism.
   Organizations must identify potential threats and have appropriate PPE to address these threats. Gowns, gloves, air-purifying respirators (APRs), self-contained breathing apparatus (SCBA), or supplied air respirators (SARs) are all examples of PPE. Frequent training with all required PPE is necessary to surmount real-world limitations in delivering care.

3. What chemical agents are most likely to be used in a terrorist attack?
   Table 49.1 lists the chemical agents most likely to be used in a terrorist attack.

4. What steps can hospitals take to prepare for a biochemical attack?
   See Table 49.2.

5. What type of dissemination techniques are most likely to be used for chemical terrorism?
   Chemical agent release is most likely to occur using a recognized dissemination device precipitated by a fire or explosion, also known as point source dissemination. The chemical agent could also be aerosolized from a point of elevation, from an airplane or helicopter, also known as line source dissemination. Regardless of dissemination, such an event would be recognizable by a large group of casualties presenting simultaneously.

Table 49.1. Common Chemical Agents in Terrorist Attacks

CATEGORY	AGENT
Nerve	Tabun (GA), soman (GB), sarin (GD), and VX gases
Pulmonary	Phosgene and chlorine gases
Riot control	CS (tear gas), OC (oleoresin capsicum)
Vesicants	Mustard gas, Lewisite
Blood agents	Cyanide

Table 49.2. Planning Steps for Hospitals

Community-based hospital planning
Personnel trained in recognition, mass casualty triage, and treatment
Decontamination facility
Supplies and training of personal protective equipment
Immediate access to antidotes, cyanide kits, and anticonvulsants
Hospital incident management system in place
Quick access to experts

Table 49.3. Biological Agents

CATEGORY	AGENT
Bacterial	Anthrax, brucellosis, cholera, plague, tularemia
Viral	Viral hemorrhagic fever, smallpox
Toxin	Botulinum, ricin, staphylococcal enterotoxin B

Table 49.4. Signs of Biological Terrorism

SYNDROMES	EPIDEMIOLOGY
Pulmonary symptoms	Multiple simultaneous events
Rashes	Dead animals
Sepsis-like syndrome	Large patient influx with high death rate and toxicity
Flulike symptoms (fever, malaise, myalgias)	

6. What symptoms do nerve agents cause?
   Nerve agents cause DUMBELS—defecation, urination, myosis, bronchorrhea, emesis, lacrimation, and salivation. This could be better pictured as liquids pouring from every part of the body. Neurological manifestations include muscle twitching, seizures, and coma. Treatment includes atropine, pralidoxime, decontamination, and supportive care.

7. What symptoms do pulmonary agents cause?
   Pulmonary agents cause mucosal irritation (burning eyes, throat, mouth) in small doses but choking and dyspnea can occur in higher doses related to pulmonary edema. Phosgene has a pleasant odor at low concentrations, like corn or freshly cut hay. Chlorine gas smells like bleach and is very irritating. Treatment is decontamination and supportive care.

8. What symptoms do vesicants (mustard gas and lewisite) cause?
   The presenting signs and symptoms of vesicants are respiratory, dermal (partial thickness burns with blistering), gastrointestinal (vomiting), and ocular (conjunctivitis and corneal burns). Treatment is decontamination and supportive care.

9. What symptoms do blood agents (Cyanide) cause?
   The presenting signs and symptoms of cyanide exposure are skin flushing, respiratory distress, and shock. Cyanide is a highly volatile toxic asphyxiant that shuts down cellular oxygen use. This can cause rapid decompensation, multisystem organ failure, and death.

10. What biological agents are most likely to be used in a terrorist attack?
    Table 49.3 lists the biological agents most likely to be used in a terrorist attack.

11. What are the signs suggesting biological terrorism?
    See Table 49.4.

12. How does anthrax inoculation present in casualties?
    Anthrax presents in two primary varieties, cutaneous and pulmonary. Spores are inhaled, ingested, or inoculated. The spores germinate into bacilli inside macrophages releasing toxins that cause edema and cell death. Pulmonary anthrax presents with flulike symptoms (fever, cough, malaise) 2–10 days after exposure. Cutaneous anthrax presents in 1–5 days with a progression from papule, vesicle, to black eschar. Treatment includes one of the following antibiotics: doxycycline, ciprofloxacin, or amoxicillin.

13. How does plague present in casualties?
    Plague comes in three varieties: bubonic, pneumonic, and septicemic. Pneumonic plague is the most likely to present in a terrorist attack because it can be aerosolized and disseminated. Casualties will present with flulike symptoms and hemoptysis with pneumonic plague. Onset occurs in 2–3 days. The mortality rate is nearly 100%. The disease rapidly progresses to systemic organ failure and death. Septicemic and bubonic plague will present with terrorist attacks but will likely be secondary to primary pneumonic plague. Treatment is the same for all types of plague, which includes doxycycline or tetracycline.

Table 49.5. Criteria for Smallpox	
MAJOR CRITERIA	**MINOR CRITERIA**
Febrile prodrome	Centrifugal pustule distribution
Classic smallpox lesions	First pustules of mouth, face, and forearms
All lesions in same stage	Toxic appearance
	Slow evolution of lesions
	Pustules of palms and soles

14. How does smallpox present in casualties?

    Smallpox can present in many forms: variola major, variola minor, hemorrhagic, and malignant. Variola major and minor are the more common forms of smallpox, representing 90% of cases. Casualties present 8–12 days after exposure and present with fever, prostration, and headache. Pustules form around day 12–15. When making a diagnosis of smallpox, there are three major criteria and five minor criteria. If a casualty has all three major criteria, they require immediate isolation and reporting. Supportive care is the only available therapy (Table 49.5).

15. How does ricin poisoning present in casualties?

    Casualties present 4–12 hours after exposure (ingestion, inhalation, or injection). Ingestion and inhalation are most likely used in terrorism and present with flulike symptoms, nausea, vomiting, and shock. Inhalation of ricin is characterized by cough, respiratory distress, and bronchospasm. Treatment is supportive. Death occurs within 72 hours.

16. How does botulism present in casualties?

    Presentation of symptoms from botulism occurs anywhere from 6 hours to 10 days after exposure. Symptoms include facial paralysis, bulbar weakness, and descending muscle paralysis. The symptoms can progress to paralyze the diaphragm and lead to death. Treatment is supportive.

17. What are the red flags for identifying biological terrorism?

    Red flags for biological agents include off-season flu symptoms, unexpected antibiotic resistance, large numbers of patients presenting simultaneously with similar complaints, localization of outbreaks, infected animal populations, and excessive morbidity and mortality. Biological agents are difficult to identify and require observation of signs and symptoms along with progression of disease.

18. What type of dissemination techniques are likely to be used for biological terrorism?

    Biological agents can be dispersed by unrecognized methods such as food or water tampering. Line source exposure from a mobile aerosol sprayer via boat or airplane is the most effective dissemination technique used to disperse biological agents. A less effective dissemination technique is point source exposure, which can occur with use of stationary aerosol sprayers, explosives, or missiles.

19. What major factors determine the effectiveness and severity of a biochemical terrorist attack?

    The severity of presentation can depend on atmospheric conditions, agent stability, and particulate size of the agent. Airborne pathogens must be less than 5 microns in size to be effective inhalation agents.

20. What is the most common device used in terrorist attacks?

    Incendiary devices are more common than biological and chemical devices because they are easily produced, transported, and deployed. If an explosion has occurred, secondary explosions meant to injure or kill first responders should be considered. First responders must remain observant for suspicious people and activity.

21. What methods are commonly used to identify chemical agents after a terrorist attack?

    Nerve and blister agents can be identified with M8 and M9 chemical detector paper, which uses an enzyme method for detection. Other methods to identify chemical agents include flame spectrophotometry, acoustic infrared spectroscopy, filter-based infrared spectroscopy, and ion mobility spectroscopy.

22. Terrorist attacks can seem like typical HAZMAT exposures. What are red flags for terrorism?

    Red flags for terrorism include explosions or large numbers of ill patients arriving at the same time. All personnel must remain vigilant to the possibility of terrorism and know red flags.

23. At the sight of a terrorist attack, evidence collection is paramount and second to only one thing. What is always the primary objective?

    First responder safety and casualty care will always take priority, even over evidence collection.

24. Evidence collection for terrorist attacks is under what authority?

Evidence collection for terrorist attacks is under the authority of the FBI Hazmat Response Unit. Evidence collection includes hazard identification, evidence identification, determination of collection methods and containers, the necessary PPE, and maintaining the chain of custody.

KEY POINTS

- Biological agents most likely to be used in terrorist attacks include bacterial pathogens, viral pathogens, and toxins.
- Chemical agents most likely to be used in terrorist attacks include nerve agents, pulmonary agents, riot control gasses, vesicants, and blood agents.
- Red flags to identify biological terrorism include off-season flu symptoms, unexpected antibiotic resistance, large numbers of patients presenting simultaneously with similar complaints, localization of outbreaks, infected animal populations, and excessive morbidity and mortality.
- Red flags to identify chemical terrorism include explosions and/or large numbers of patients presenting simultaneously with similar complaints.
- Biological agents are most effectively released using line source dissemination from mobile aerosol devices attached to airplanes, vehicles, or boats.
- Chemical agents are most effectively released using point source dissemination precipitated by a fire or explosion.

BIBLIOGRAPHY

Centers for Disease Control and Prevention. Cyanogen chloride. 2019. Available at: https://www.cdc.gov/NIOSH/ershdb/EmergencyResponseCard_29750039.html.

Centers for Disease Control and Prevention. Phosgene. 2019. Available at: https://emergency.cdc.gov/agent/phosgene/basics/facts.asp.

Centers for Disease Control and Prevention. Ricin. 2019. Available at: https://emergency.cdc.gov/agent/ricin/clinicians/treatment.asp.

Centers for Disease Control and Prevention. Vesicants. 2019. Available at: https://emergency.cdc.gov/agent/vesicants/casedef.asp.

Hauda W, et al. Medical support for hazardous material response. In: *Special Operations Medical Support*. Dubuque, IA: Kendall Hunt Professional; 2009:186-201.

Schultz CH, Koenig KL. Chapter 194. Weapons of mass destruction. In: Marx JA, Hockberger RS, Walls RM, et al., eds. Rosen's Emergency Medicine Concepts and Clinical Practice. 8th ed. Elsevier Saunders; 2013:3021-3032.

CHAPTER 50

RADIATION AND RADIATION INJURY

Puneet Gupta

QUESTIONS AND ANSWERS

1. Is it safe to treat patients who have been exposed or contaminated during a radioactive disaster?

   This is the first question because it is the most important. Like any other situation in the field, *safe* is a relative term. There are three primary sources of danger: the origin of the radiation, the hazards of the disaster environment, and the patient. By maintaining vigilance about the environment and wearing the proper personal protective equipment (PPE), it is safe to treat patients during a radiation event. Well, as safe as one can be in the field during any disaster.

   Do not let the myths surrounding radiation prevent you from doing your job. We have seen this occur during mock disasters. In the words of the Greek poet Archilochus, "We don't rise to the level of our expectations, we fall to the level of our training."

2. What is the difference between exposure and contamination?

   There are three methods by which individuals will be affected by radiation:
   A. Irradiation (or exposure): radiation from the field passing through the body.
   B. External contamination: radioactive materials outside the body.
   C. Internal contamination: radioactive materials that have entered the body (usually from inhalation or ingestion).

   While it is important to understand the difference, it is not a focus for providers in the field retrieving patients; it is more of an academic point. Every patient should be approached as if they are contaminated until proven otherwise.

3. What is the concern about radiation?

   The radiation to be concerned about in a radiological event is ionizing radiation. Every person has constant exposure to background radiation, but it is usually nonionizing. Ionizing radiation causes more damage as it has the power to penetrate tissues and remove electrons from atoms or molecules, generating free radicals that are highly reactive. Although the body has cellular repair mechanisms, these are generally operating at capacity just dealing with background radiation.

   When human cells are exposed to ionizing radiation, three things can happen: they repair themselves, they die, or they mutate. Low levels of ionizing radiation do not have any immediate health effects but might cause a small increase in the possible risk of cancer. High doses can cause acute radiation syndrome (ARS), which can be fatal.

4. How can a provider be protected from irradiation in the event of a radiological event?

   There are two main ways to limit radiation exposure. Either block it or stay away from it. There are four types of radiation particles that can be encountered: alpha, beta, gamma, and neutrons. Alpha particles will not penetrate skin, clothing, or paper. Beta particles can and will penetrate through 1 cm of flesh. Standard turnouts will stop the first two but are useless against gamma rays and neutron particles.

   Gamma rays can only be stopped by a substantial amount of concrete, lead, or water. Neutrons require plastic and water. To limit exposure, in addition to wearing turnouts, a provider should attempt to keep concrete or water shielding between them and the source of radiation at all times. Concrete shielding is easy to find, but what about water shielding? At least 50% of your partner is water! If you do not need to expose yourself to carry out your duties, stand behind them to limit irradiation.

5. What can help prevent internal contamination?

   Internal contamination is one of the deadliest means of exposure. It will be necessary to protect against particles, so the minimum protection is an N-95, R-95, or an equivalent mask in the field. Understandably, in a disaster, these may be in scarce supply, but utilize what is available. Abstain from hand-to-mouth activities such as eating/drinking/smoking until you have been decontaminated and are in a cold zone.

6. How far away should a provider remain from the radiation source?

   The amount of radiation that rescuers in the field will expose themselves to will be dependent on the situation. How many volunteers are there? How many victims? How much radiation is acceptable? Moral questions that will need to be answered by the responding team. That being said, there are a few principles to use as a guide.

   First, as noted previously, do not run from a contaminated patient. Unless they are physically holding the radiation source, decontaminating the patients will be enough to make them safe to treat and can be done with minimal risk. Second, the radiation from a source increases linearly with time (i.e., 50 hours equals 50 times the radiation received in 1 hour). Lastly, the effects decrease exponentially the further you are from the source (known as the "inverse square

Table 50.1. EPA's Emergency Action Dose Guidelines	
DOSE LIMIT (WHOLE BODY)	**EMERGENCY ACTION DOSE GUIDELINES**
5 rem (.05 Sv)	All activities allowed (maximum whole body dose limit for occupational workers)
10 rem (.05 Sv)	Protecting major property
25 rem (.05 Sv)	Lifesaving or protection of large populations only
>25 rem (.05 Sv)	Lifesaving or protection of large populations ONLY on a volunteer basis knowing the risks involved

law"). Radiation detectors in the field should give a provider an idea of the radiation being faced. See Table 50.1 for the Environmental Protection Agency's (EPA's) Emergency Action Dose Guidelines.

7. Where is a radiation detector found during a nuclear disaster?
Radiation detectors can be found in different places in different systems. They can be portable or built into the infrastructure. It is recommended that every provider locate where a detector is in their system. If there is a radiation-based disaster and a detector cannot be located, do not panic! There are a few locations that are highly likely to have a radiation detector: hospitals (especially major trauma centers), fire apparatus may have them built-in, and the HAZMAT teams should have them. A disaster coordinator or their equivalent will likely be able to provide more specific information.

8. Where should patients be decontaminated?
It is essential to understand that there is a lack of research on this topic. Where to decontaminate patients is mostly based on expert opinion. Decontamination points should be set by incident command. There are a few principles to guide these choices. First, there should be decontamination at any point that may potentially release patients. This usually means decontamination will occur at the casualty collection point (CCP) in the warm zone. Second, never assume that a patient has been decontaminated. In this spirit, when patients arrive at the hospital, they will usually be decontaminated more thoroughly. This is known as secondary decontamination. Lastly, do not delay lifesaving care for decontamination care. A patient can be transported and treated while rescuers/medical personnel are wearing protective equipment.

9. How should a patient be decontaminated?
Removal of a patient's clothing will remove the vast majority of the material. Once the patient's clothing has been removed, wash the patient with water and soap. Now the patient should be safe to treat as necessary. When decontaminating the patient, ensure they do not ingest any radioactive material as that could be fatal. Be mindful of water runoff as it will be considered contaminated. As mentioned previously, if a patient has a life-threatening injury that cannot wait for decontamination, provide interventions to stabilize the patient while clad in protective equipment. If you require rapid decontamination of a large number of patients, remove their clothing and have them go through a water source such as a fire hose or sprinklers.

10. What can gauge the severity of a victim's radiation exposure?
While there are lab tests to evaluate for this, the classic one being the white blood cell count, in the field, there is no access to these resources. See Table 50.2 for reference to estimate how bad the severity of radiation is. As a general rule, if the patient is symptomatic within an hour of exposure, the prognosis is grim.

Table 50.2. Clinical Effects from Whole-Body Radiation						
	AMOUNT OF RADIATION (RAD)					
	0–100	100–200	200–600	600–800	600–3000	>3000
Nausea and vomiting	None	5%–50%	50%–100%	75%–100%	90%–100%	100%
Time of onset		3–6 hours	2–4 hours	1–2 hours	<1 hour	Minutes
CNS function	No impairment	No impairment	Routine task impairment 6–20 hours	Simple and routine task impairment for >24 hours	Rapid incapacitation may have lucid interval of several hours	Decreases within hours

CNS, Central nervous system.

Based on Table 50.2, it is suggested to observe patients for up to 4 hours in field hospital triage. If they develop symptoms during this time, they need to be transported to a higher level of care to manage the ARS. If they remain asymptomatic, radiation exposure is probably negligible; transport/release per local guidelines.

11. What communication difficulties should you expect in a mass casualty that are unique to nuclear disasters?
Communication will already be affected by multiple users overwhelming the wireless network. AT&T's FirstNet has promised priority communication to first responders. This is a potential resource if available to the system. Regardless, have backup ways to communicate (i.e., radio). If there is a nuclear explosion, an electromagnetic pulse (EMP) may be released after detonation (a dirty bomb will not release one). This will disrupt unshielded electronics and electrical systems. The distance of effect will vary based on the explosion and altitude. Experts have theorized that current weapons could affect the entirety of the country. Fear not, experts also theorize it is unlikely for terrorists to use such sophisticated technology. They are much more likely to use a dirty bomb as they are easier to obtain and create.

12. What preparation should be done for a radiation event?
Train. As noted in this chapter, radiation events are manageable, and patients are treatable with equipment that should be available. When people do not understand this, they panic, and care is affected. An example of this is in 2004 a major "dirty bomb" drill was held, and when hospitals realized patients were contaminated, many of them attempted to go on diversion. A quick decontamination was all that was needed. The fear of radiation slowed operations significantly and could have been critical in a real disaster. By holding regular drills, not only will radiation treatment knowledge disseminate but also the location of esoteric equipment will become known. With proper training and education, a team will be well prepared to handle a radiation event should one arise.

KEY POINTS

- You can retrieve patients, decontaminate them, and treat them with equipment and supplies that most systems should have readily available with minimal radiation exposure to the rescuer.
- Limit radiation exposure during a rescue by keeping objects between you and the source; this includes your partner.
- Becoming symptomatic within 1 hour of radiation exposure is a very bad sign and the person will likely die.
- Set up decontamination points at every place that you may discharge or receive patients.
- Prepare to lose communication capabilities and have backups prepared.
- The fear of radiation can paralyze a system; train to prevent this.

BIBLIOGRAPHY

Berger ME, Leonard RB, Ricks RC. *Hospital Triage in the First 24 Hours after a Nuclear or Radiological Disaster*. Oak Ridge, TN: Oak Ridge Institute for Science and Education (ORISE); 2010.
Department of Veteran Affairs. *Pocket Guide: Terrorism with Ionizing Radiation General Guidance*. Bethesda, MD: Armed Forces Radiobiology Research Institute; 2003.
Environmental Protection Agency. 2017 PAG manual. https://www.remm.nlm.gov/EPA_PAG_Manual_FINAL_01-26-2017.pdf.
Jisha R. *Texas Motor Speedway Exercise Summary*. Austin, TX: Incident Investigation and Environmental Program, Texas Department of State Health Service; 2004.
Prehospital radiation triage scheme. https://orise.orau.gov/resources/reacts/documents/prehospital-radiological-triage-poster.pdf.

CHAPTER 51

BLAST INJURIES

Chadd E. Nesbit

QUESTIONS AND ANSWERS

1. Why is this chapter important and what is the chance that an EMS provider will see injuries from a blast or explosion?
   The frequency of blast injuries due to military conflict and terrorist activities has increased dramatically in the last 15 years. Injury patterns that used to be seen only in military conflicts are now being seen outside of these areas of conflict due to terrorist activities. Industrial accidents also frequently produce blast injuries that are indistinguishable from those caused by military ordnance. Transportation accidents involving trucks and railcars carrying flammable liquids are also a source of potential blasts that may be seen on any roadway and set of railroad tracks running through EMS service areas.

2. How can an EMS service prepare to handle these kinds of injuries should an explosion happen?
   We tend to act in emergency situations in the manner that we have trained for them, and preparing for disasters such as an explosion in the communities we serve is something for which we should all train. Boston EMS was able to respond very effectively to the events of April 2013 due to timely training covering very similar scenarios. All prehospital providers should be familiar with their departmental triage scheme for use in mass casualty events. Providers should also be aware of the capabilities of local hospitals and if hospitals have specialized capabilities for adult/pediatric trauma and/or burns. In a bombing or explosion, basic triage principles apply as they would in any mass casualty situation. Every provider should be familiar with the role or roles that may be expected of them to fill in the triage process.

3. How do explosions cause injury to people and do all explosions cause the same types of injuries?
   Explosives are broadly categorized into high order (HE) and low order (LE) types. HEs can be thought of as being detonated. Examples of HE include military explosives and dynamites. HEs need not be large. A military hand grenade is an HE. HEs are unique in that they cause an overpressurization wave, which results in unique types of injuries that the rescuer will encounter. These waves travel faster than the speed of sound.
   In contrast, LEs are best thought of as deflagration or burning. Gunpowder and gasoline-based devices are LEs. LEs need not be small. Technically the 9/11 airplane attacks were LEs. These explosions are subsonic and generally cause burns, blunt trauma, and shrapnel/penetrating-type injuries.

4. What determines the patterns of injuries seen in explosives?
   There are three factors that determine the injury patterns seen after an explosion. These can broadly be thought of as the agent, the environment, and the host. The agent includes factors such as the size of the bomb and the type of explosive. The environment includes factors such distance from the source, any shielding between the victim and the source, and whether the explosion is in a confined or open space. Confined space explosions are much more lethal than open space explosions. Host factors include the age, sex, and health of the victim, as well as the access to care after the event.

5. HEs are unique in that they cause an overpressurization wave. Does this cause any unique patterns of injury?
   The pressure wave of an HE causes unique injuries, generally to the air-filled structures of the body. These are called primary blast injuries. The tympanic membranes (TMs), lungs, and gastrointestinal (GI) tract, in that order, are the most commonly injured. Pulmonary barotrauma is the most frequently seen critical injury and is the most common fatal injury among initial survivors. It may have a delayed presentation. GI injuries such as mesenteric tears, leading to ischemia, may be insidiously difficult to detect and may not become apparent for days. The TM ruptures at a much lower pressure than that needed to cause pulmonary and GI injuries. An intact TM makes the likelihood of other serious primary injuries less likely but does not exclude it completely, and a high index of suspicion must be maintained.

6. What are the other types of injuries caused by HEs?
   In addition to the primary injuries discussed earlier, there are secondary, tertiary, quaternary, and quinary patterns of injury. Secondary injury is caused by flying debris propelled by the blast and may be blunt or penetrating injuries. Tertiary injury results in the body being thrown by the blast into a solid object or the ground. Quaternary injuries consist of injuries such as chronic obstructive pulmonary disease (COPD) or asthma exacerbations, burns, inhalation injuries, or radiation sickness. Some texts include a quinary injury pattern that is thought to be a hyperinflammatory state caused by an adverse reaction to material aerosolized by the bomb and internalized by the body.

Table 51.1. Classes of Blast Injury and Associated Injury Patterns

CATEGORY	MECHANISM OF INJURY	TYPE OF INJURY
Primary	Overpressurization wave seen only in high-order explosions	Blast lung Bowel injury TM ruptures Traumatic brain injury
Secondary	Flying debris	Penetrating injury Traumatic amputations Soft tissue injuries
Tertiary	Patient thrown by blast	Blunt trauma Traumatic amputations Head injuries
Quaternary	Injuries not due to the first three categories. This includes exacerbation of existing health problems.	Burns Radiation illness Angina Exacerbation of asthma/COPD
Quinary	Hyperinflammatory state due to components of bomb	Fever Sepsis Exposure to biological contaminants

COPD, Chronic obstructive pulmonary disease; *TM*, tympanic membrane.

7. What kinds of injuries are seen in low order explosions?
   LEs are subsonic and lead to the secondary, tertiary, and quaternary injury patterns due to flying debris or being the victim thrown by the explosion. They do not cause blast lung, organ injuries, or TM rupture, due to the fact that they do not cause an overpressurization wave. These types of explosions produce patterns of injury more familiar to most prehospital providers such as orthopedic and soft tissue injuries. Blast injuries do not occur in isolation. It is infrequent that a patient has only one type of injury. Blunt force, penetrating, and traumatic amputation–type injuries may all be seen in the same patient. See Table 51.1 for a summary of categories of injuries caused by blasts and the types of injuries associated with each category.

8. What are the initial treatment concerns for victims of blast injuries and are any of these different from treatment of other traumatic injuries?
   In general, treatment of blast injuries should follow the same protocols that prehospital providers would follow in treating any traumatic injury such as a fall or motor vehicle accident. A patent airway must be secured and the patient must be ventilated if needed. Any visible external hemorrhage should be aggressively controlled using direct pressure or tourniquets. Obvious fractures should be splinted and impaled objects stabilized in place to prevent movement and possible additional injury to underlying structures. The patient should be fluid resuscitated to a systolic pressure of about 90 mm Hg, perhaps 100 mm Hg if there is a severe head injury. Transport of patients should be guided by local, regional, or state trauma transport protocols. If transport time to an appropriate facility is more than 30 minutes by ground, consider transport by air medical helicopter if available.

9. Are there any injury patterns that may alert prehospital personnel to the most severely injured patients?
   Patients found at triage to be dyspneic or have altered mental status may have serious injuries that are not immediately obvious. The triad of dyspnea/apnea, bradycardia, and hypotension ("blast triad") is indicative of blast lung, the most common fatal injury among initial survivors. Severe abdominal pain along with nausea and vomiting may indicate the presence of a serious intra-abdominal injury such as a perforated viscous. Traumatic amputations are associated with multisystem injury and it should be assumed these patients are critically injured.

10. Explosions may produce large numbers of patients at a scene requiring triage. Are there any particular triage schemes for blast events as opposed to other types of mass casualty event?
    Standard triage schemes (SALT [sort, assess, lifesaving interventions, treatment/triage], START [simple triage and rapid treatment]) should be applied to the presentation of patients at the initial event. Expect that many of the minor injuries and walking wounded will present directly to the local hospital, bypassing EMS triage. Your local hospital must have a plan in place to address this "upside down" triage where the least injured arrive to definitive care first. A rough estimate of total casualties expected at a facility can be obtained by doubling the number of casualties presenting in the first hour after the event. If the bombing has caused structural collapse, the presentation of victims will be delayed.

11. Do "dirty bombs" pose a threat to first responders?

Any blast scene has the potential to have been caused by a "dirty bomb" containing radioactive, biological, or chemical contaminants. Immediate lifesaving procedures and triage should not be delayed out of concern for the possibility of contamination by radioactive material. Personal protective equipment (PPE) in the form of masks, gloves, and gowns effectively protects against radiation and blood-borne pathogens such as hepatitis. Secondary explosions and chemical or biological contaminants are possible, and if there is significant concern, surveillance for these hazards should be carried out as soon as possible by appropriately trained personnel.

Provider safety at the scene of a blast is paramount. Do not become another victim. If there is danger of fire or structural collapse do not enter the area unless you have the necessary specialized training to operate in that environment safely.

12. Are there any special populations that should be of higher concern in these situations?

Any pregnant woman, no matter how seemingly minor the injury is, should be transported for further evaluation. The amniotic fluid surrounding the fetus offers some degree of protection. However, fluid transmits force much more effectively than air. Children who are injured in these types of incidents require more intensive care than adults with similar injuries. If possible, children who are suspected of having the possibility of significant injury should be cared for in a pediatric trauma center.

KEY POINTS

- Blast injuries are increasing due to military and civilian casualties of conflicts and as a result of terrorist acts worldwide.
- The type of explosive device, surroundings, and distance from the device will determine the pattern and severity of injuries.
- Response to any type of mass casualty event caused by a blast must be guided by a system of triage of the injured and rapid transport of the most severely injured to the closest appropriate facility. Systems of care should be prepared for an upside down triage as the least injured will bypass EMS and present to the nearest care facility by private vehicle.
- Every EMS agency should routinely drill for the eventuality of a mass casualty incident. This may or may not be a bombing, but the general principles of incident command and triage will be applicable to any scenario causing a large number of casualties.
- Most initial survivors of blasts will have injuries familiar to prehospital personnel. Some initial survivors may have injuries caused by primary blast injury. These may have delayed presentation and often require specialized care.

BIBLIOGRAPHY

Centers for Disease Control and Prevention. Explosions and blast injuries: a primer for clinicians. www.cdc.gov/masstrauma/preparedness/primer.pdf.
Centers for Disease Control and Prevention, American College of Emergency Physicians. Bombings: injury patterns and care. ACEP.org/blastinjury.
DePalma RG, Burris DG, Champion HR, Hodgson MJ. Blast Injuries. *N Engl J Med*. 2005;352:1335-1342.
Jorolemon MR, Krywko DM. Blast injuries. Stat Pearls. https://www.ncbi.nlm.nih.gov/books/NBK430914/.
Kapur GB, Pillow MT, Nemeth I. Prehospital care algorithm for blast injuries due to bombing incidents. *Prehosp Disaster Med*. 2010;25:595-600.
Matthews ZR, Koyfman A. Blast injuries. *J Emerg Med*. 2015;49:573-587.
Wolf SJ, Bebarta VS, Bonnett CJ, Pons PT, Cantrill SV. Blast injuries. *Lancet*. 2009;374:405-415.
Yeh DD, Schecter WP. Primary blast injuries—an updated concise review. *World J Surg*. 2012;36:966-972.

CHAPTER 52

HAZARDOUS MATERIALS RESPONSE

Philip S. Nawrocki and Brendan Mulcahy

QUESTIONS AND ANSWERS
INITIAL RESPONSE CONSIDERATIONS

1. What is the best way to plan for potential hazardous material (HAZMAT) incidents in a particular region or community?

   Management of HAZMAT incidents begin well before the alarm goes off. Every organization involved in HAZMAT response should perform a comprehensive vulnerability analysis to identify any and all potential threats for their particular community. This includes working with governmental organizations, businesses, and other community stakeholders to develop a comprehensive plan for any incident that may develop within the local region. This "all-hazards preparedness approach" is supported by the Homeland Security Presidential Directive, a Presidential Policy directive by President George W. Bush in 2003 in response to the September 11 terrorist attacks. Its goals are to strengthen preparedness capabilities at the federal, state, and local levels and to enhance the preparedness and response to terrorist incidents, major disasters, and other emergencies.

2. How should EMS agencies plan for HAZMAT incidents?

   The development of standard operating guidelines (SOGs) is an essential process that delineates the roles, responsibilities, and response procedures of all parties involved in the response. These guidelines address specific procedures such as personal protective equipment (PPE) use, medical decontamination, and decontamination for emergency personnel. Of particular importance to EMS is the need to identify which agency will be providing medical support throughout the various stages of the incident, and ensuring mutual aid is available as necessary. This ensures that the personnel responsible for providing medical care have the necessary protocols, resources, and training to successfully respond to an incident. Ongoing multiagency training and education are essential in maintaining peak response capabilities at the provider and operational level.

3. What are the initial considerations for first responders who are responding to a reported HAZMAT incident?

   The primary consideration following a HAZMAT incident should be to ensure scene safety. This includes protecting responders from exposure, isolation of the scene from additional persons, and limiting additional exposure of victims to the material. Attempts to identify the actual or suspected material may then be safely conducted. The scale of the incident should be assessed to determine the resources needed and the number of victims that require care. Establishment of incident command should be performed as soon as possible to provide structured response and unified command. Local evacuation may be considered if deemed necessary by the incident commander and often requires substantial EMS resources.

4. What are the three "zones" that should be established in the initial phase of a HAZMAT incident?

   Once a perimeter has been established, three zones must be designated with respect to contamination. The exclusion zone (hot zone) is the area of actual or potential contamination that poses the highest risk to responders and patients. The contamination-reduction zone (warm zone) is generally the transition point between hot and cold zones and is where most decontamination occurs. The support zone (cold zone) is free from contamination and is where planning, staging, medical care, and rehabilitation operations are performed. This zone should ideally be situated upwind and uphill from the incident.

5. What properties of the material should be known prior to entering the hot zone?

   The actual or suspected nature of the material should be assessed prior to entering the hot zone. Placard information may be available on vehicles or storage tanks and can be cross-referenced with the Emergency Response Guide (ERG). Safety Data Sheets (SDS), transportation manifests, and other documentation should be obtained and referenced. Oxygen concentration and the risk of airborne or vapor exposure should also be assessed. These factors govern the initial PPE necessary to safely respond to the incident. Decontamination corridors, including contingency plans for emergency decontamination, should be in place prior to providers entering the hot zone.

Disclosures: The authors, their immediate family, and any research foundation with which they are affiliated have not received any financial payments or other benefits from any commercial entity related to the subject of this article.
Funding/sources of support: Not applicable (no financial, pharmaceutical, or industry support received).

Table 52.1. Characteristics, Advantages, and Disadvantages of the Various Levels of PPE

PPE LEVEL	CHARACTERISTICS AND ADVANTAGES	DISADVANTAGES
Level A	– Fully encapsulated chemical resistant suit including self-contained breathing apparatus (SCBA), double layers of chemical-resistant gloves, and chemical-resistant boots – Highest level of protection against vapor and splash threats	– Expensive – Bulky; limited dexterity – Heat retention – Limited amount of time due to SCBA and heat
Level B	– Consists of an SCBA, chemical-resistant suit, chemical-resistant gloves, and boots – Provides full respiratory protection – Can be used in warm zone for decontamination	– Less vapor protection – Heat retention – Limited amount of time due to SCBA and heat
Level C	– Full-face air purification device, nonencapsulating chemical-resistant suit, chemical-resistant gloves, and boots – Can be used in warm zone for decontamination	– Less vapor and splash protection – Heat retention
Level D	– Standard work clothes with no respiratory protection (e.g., firefighter turnout gear) – Increased dexterity and mobility	– Minimal respiratory, vapor, splash protection

PPE, Personal protective equipment.

6. What are the different types of PPE that are used during an incident?
   There are four levels of PPE that may be utilized in HAZMAT response. Characteristics, advantages, and disadvantages are listed in Table 52.1.

MEDICAL CARE DURING A HAZMAT INCIDENT

1. What are the initial considerations for medical responders once incident command has been established?
   There are many features of an incident that impact medical care, including environmental features, agent characteristics, and necessary medical equipment and supplies. The number of casualties should be determined as early as possible. Supplemental resources may need to be activated as part of a mass casualty response. Additional decontamination lanes may be needed to ensure adequate patient flow. The type of agent is an important initial consideration as this dictates the immediate hazard to life and limb, as well as the level of decontamination required. Specific therapies and medications may also be required depending on the agent.

2. What barriers exist to patient care in the HAZMAT environment?
   Many barriers exist when providing medical care in the HAZMAT environment. The provider's PPE limits manual dexterity and makes a thorough physical examination extremely challenging. The bulky nature of the suit may also limit access to confined spaces or those with obstacles. It also limits the provider's ability to perform procedures such as intravenous access, airway management, and medication delivery.
   Other barriers that limit medical providers in this setting relate to environmental factors. These include heat stress due to PPE, cold exposure in specific environments, dehydration due to overexertion, limited oxygen when utilizing self-contained breathing apparatus (SCBA), decreased communication abilities while in PPE, and the potential for decreased visibility and hearing in specific situations.

3. What medical care should be provided in each of the three zones of a HAZMAT incident?
   The previous factors limit the ability of medical responders to spend significant time and deliver thorough medical care while in the hot or warm zones. Similar to the concepts developed in Tactical Combat Casualty Care, medical interventions in the hot and warm zones should be limited to patient extrication and immediate lifesaving measures including use of tourniquets, autoinjector antidotes, and basic airway maneuvers. Once appropriately decontaminated and in the cold zone, a thorough assessment of the patient can be performed with routine medical intervention and transportation as required.

4. How should patients be triaged in a mass casualty incident that involves HAZMAT?
   Existing triage algorithms, including SALT (sort, assess, lifesaving interventions, treatment/triage) and START(simple triage and rapid treatment), should be practiced and utilized. In terms of decontamination, patients exposed to vapors should be addressed first, followed by those exposed to liquids and then those with severe injuries.

Table 52.2. Standards and Guidelines for Provider Safety and Medical Monitoring During HAZMAT Incidents

REFERENCE	DESCRIPTION
OSHA 29 CFR 1910.120	Federal regulations that set requirements for hazardous waste operations and emergency response (HAZWOPER)
NFPA 472	Standard for Professional Competence of Responders to Hazardous Materials Incidents
NFPA 473	Standard for Competencies for EMS Personnel Responding to Hazardous Materials/Weapons of Mass Destruction Incidents
NFPA 1584	Standard on the Rehabilitation Process for Members During Emergency Operations and Training Exercises
NFPA 1992	Standard on Liquid Splash-Protective Ensembles and Clothing for Hazardous Materials Emergencies. Establishes PPE requirements for responders in the hot and warm zones.

NFPA, National Fire Protection Association; *OSHA*, Occupational Safety and Health Administration; *PPE*, personal protective equipment.

5. How should decontamination of patients be conducted?
Gross decontamination may begin in the hot zone or warm zone and includes removal of clothing, removal of obvious contamination, and briefly rinsing the patient from head to toe using warm water. Removal of clothing may remove up to 80% of contamination. Secondary decontamination is the more thorough process of making the patient as clean as possible prior to transfer to the cold zone. Emergency decontamination occurs when responders sustain injury or are inadvertently exposed to a contaminated material. For injured or exposed patients, attention should be directed to contaminated mucous membranes as well as wounds. Specific decontamination products or agents may be required with certain chemical agents. The ERG and other resources should be referenced in these instances.

MEDICAL OVERSIGHT OF RESPONDERS DURING A HAZMAT INCIDENT

1. What are the standards that guide the medical monitoring and safety of HAZMAT responders?
The National Fire Protection Association (NFPA), Occupational Safety and Health Administration (OSHA), and National Institute of Occupational Safety and Health (NIOSH) set requirements and guidelines for provider safety and medical monitoring during HAZMAT incidents. A selection of these guidelines is provided in Table 52.2.

2. What are the primary responsibilities of medical providers attached to HAZMAT teams?
One of the most critical roles for EMS on the scene of a HAZMAT incident is the monitoring and medical care of response personnel. Medical providers should perform an assessment of each team member prior to their entry into the hazardous environment. This should include evaluation of vital signs, underlying medical conditions (both acute and chronic), hydration status, and overall physical and mental condition. Upon exiting the hazardous environment, responders should again be assessed for vital signs, hydration status, and symptoms that developed during the response. Medical providers should ensure adequate access to hydration, nutrition, and rest for responders. Following an incident, providers should perform short- and long-term surveillance for health problems or symptoms related to possible exposure during an incident.

ADDITIONAL RESOURCES

1. I am interested in becoming a medical provider for a HAZMAT response team. What additional training or education is needed?
Additional training is required by OSHA for EMS providers responding to HAZMAT incidents and is based on the duties and functions the provider will be performing. Various levels of Hazardous Waste Operations and Emergency Respond (HAZWOPER) training are available online at https://www.osha.com. Specific guidelines for your state, local area, and EMS agency should also be reviewed.

2. What additional resources exist to help guide responders during HAZMAT incidents?
   - **Emergency Response Guide (ERG)**—A common reference book that provides information on chemical agents and their associated health risks, PPE requirements, and decontamination information.
   - **Wireless Information System for Emergency Responders (WISER)**—Mobile application to assist first responders in HAZMAT incidents by providing information regarding hazardous substances, emergency resources available, and surrounding environmental conditions.

- **Federal Emergency Management Agency (FEMA)**—Provides online and live courses regarding HAZMAT response and disaster preparedness. Learn more at https://training.fema.gov.
- **Toxicology Data Network (TOXNET)**—A resource for searching databases on toxicology, hazardous chemicals, environmental health, and toxic releases.
- **CHEMTREC**—A 24/7 service that provides immediate critical response information for emergency incidents involving chemicals, HAZMATs, and dangerous goods.

KEY POINTS

- Ensuring scene and provider safety is of the utmost importance and should be conducted on an ongoing basis throughout a HAZMAT incident.
- Be aware of the significant constraints to patient care that exist outside of the "cold zone."
- Adequate preparation using an "all hazards preparedness approach" in conjunction with multiagency training is essential in ensuring a successful response to a HAZMAT incident.
- Use the ERG and other available resources to help identify hazardous substances, guide incident response, and optimize patient management.

BIBLIOGRAPY

Federation of American Scientists. Homeland Security Presidential Directive/HSPD-8. Subject: national preparedness. Available at: https://fas.org/irp/offdocs/nspd/hspd-8.html.

National Fire Codes. NFPA 472: Standard for Competence of Responders to Hazardous Materials/Weapons of Mass Destruction Incidents, 2018 Edition. In NFPA National Fire Codes Online. Available at: http://codesonline.nfpa.org.

National Fire Codes. NFPA 473: Standard for Competencies for EMS Personnel Responding to Hazardous Materials/Weapons of Mass Destruction Incidents, 2018 Edition. In NFPA National Fire Codes Online. Available at: http://codesonline.nfpa.org.

National Fire Codes. NFPA 1584: Standard on the Rehabilitation Process for Members During Emergency Operations and Training Exercises, 2015 Edition. In NFPA National Fire Codes Online. Available at: http://codesonline.nfpa.org.

National Fire Codes. NFPA 1992: Standard on Liquid Splash-Protective Ensembles and Clothing for Hazardous Materials Emergencies, 2018 Edition. In NFPA National Fire Codes Online. Available at: http://codesonline.nfpa.org.

United States Department of Labor. Occupational Safety and Health Administration. 1910.120—Hazardous waste operations and emergency response. Available at: https://www.osha.gov/laws-regs/regulations/standardnumber/1910/1910.120.

CHAPTER 53

TACTICAL EMERGENCY MEDICAL SERVICES

Walker Foland

QUESTIONS AND ANSWERS

1. Describe the origin of Tactical Emergency Medical Services (TEMS).
   The concept of TEMS was born at a series of national conferences in 1989 and 1990 with representatives from EMS, law enforcement, and emergency medicine. The National Tactical Officers Association endorsed that TEMS should be on every tactical team in 1994 and again in 2007.

2. What is the injury rate among SWAT team officers?
   An injury occurs in 33 of every 1000 missions. Suspects are injured nearly 19 (18.9) of every 1000 missions, while bystanders are injured at a rate of 3 in every 1000 missions.

3. How much is casualty survival increased by having TEMS on tactical teams?
   Survivability is increased by 44%.

4. What are the unique attributes that TEMS provides?
   TEMS provides many unique attributes that include care under fire, weapons safety, hazardous material expertise, forensics, unconventional patient situations, preventative medicine, primary care, special equipment and training, medical threat assessment (MTA), remote assessment methodology, sensory deprived physical assessment, sensory overload physical assessment, medicine across a barricade, and hasty decontamination (Fig. 53.1).

5. What are the principle guidelines for TEMS?
   The Tactical Emergency Casualty Care (TECC) Guidelines are the predominant source for protocols in TEMS. TECC is written and controlled by the Council for Tactical Emergency Casualty Care (C-TECC). TECC covers such a broad level of topics that not all content applies to all TEMS units. TECC allows for TEMS units to customize the content of its education per the needs of each individual unit.

6. What is the Tactical Primary Survey?
   A tactical primary survey is a medical survey that considers the dynamic and austere circumstances that occur on tactical teams. It can be remembered by two different mnemonics: SMARCH or XABCDE: SMARCH = Security/Safety, Massive hemorrhage, Airway, Respirations, Circulation, Head trauma/Hypothermia and XABCDE = eXsanguinating hemorrhage control/eXtrication, Airway, Breathing, Circulation, Disability, Evacuation. Regardless of the mnemonic used, security is the first priority.

7. What are the zones of care regarding TEMS?
   The zones of care include the hot zone, warm zone, and cold zone.

8. What is a hot zone?
   A hot zone is where a direct threat exists. Casualty extrication is paramount, but the X portion of the tactical primary survey can be addressed in the hot zone. This includes eXtrication of the casualty and controlling eXsanguinating hemorrhage. When it comes to extrication, the casualty should attempt self-extrication if possible. If the casualty cannot self-extricate, the team must extricate the casualty. Control of exsanguinating hemorrhage should be addressed with limb or junctional tourniquets.

9. What is a warm zone?
   A warm zone is where an indirect threat exists. Care is delivered based on risk/benefit ratio. Airway, breathing, and circulation are addressed in the warm zone, unless otherwise deferred due to risk.

10. What is a cold zone?
    A cold zone is where no threat exists. Care is delivered based on the tactical primary survey and secondary survey.

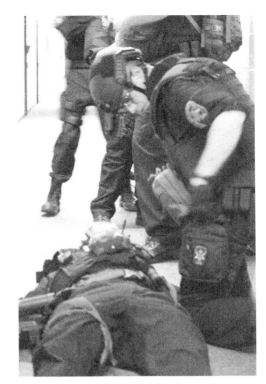

Fig. 53.1. Tactical emergency medical service physician Dr. Alec Weir applies a tourniquet during training exercise.

11. What is an MTA?

TEMS must provide an MTA during every operation. This assessment acts as a way of communicating environmental and operational health hazards to the team commander to optimize operational effectiveness.

12. What entails personal protective equipment regarding TEMS providers?

TEMS personal protective equipment (PPE) includes medical gloves, protective ballistic eyewear, body armor, and a Kevlar helmet (Fig. 53.2).

13. What are the less lethal weapons (LLWs) typical of tactical teams?

It is important that TEMS providers know how to handle all weapons on the tactical team, including LLWs, chemical irritants (oleoresin capsicum [OC] and ortho-chlorobenzylidene [CS]), kinetic impact weapons, conducted energy weapons (CEWs), and noise-flash diversionary weapons (NFDDs).

14. What are the two types of chemical irritants used on tactical teams?

There are two types of chemical irritants, OC and CS gas. Both irritate mucosal membranes, causing tearing and blephorospasm. They incapacitate most; however, some individuals are minimally affected and can "fight through" the symptoms.

15. What complication can occur from CS gas?

In rare cases, CS gas can cause laryngospasm. Typical delivery occurs via incendiary devices. Laryngospasm is temporary and generally lasts less than 1 minute, depending on length of exposure. Patients may require supportive care such as nasal cannula oxygen, venti mask, or nonrebreather.

16. How is OC delivered?

OC is typically delivered by spray, stream, or paintball.

17. How do kinetic impact weapons work?

Kinetic impact weapons function by incapacitating subjects with nonpenetrating blunt force trauma. Kinetic impact projectiles are larger than usual munitions. They travel much slower to expand the affected surface area and avoid penetration of skin; however, skeletal fractures are possible.

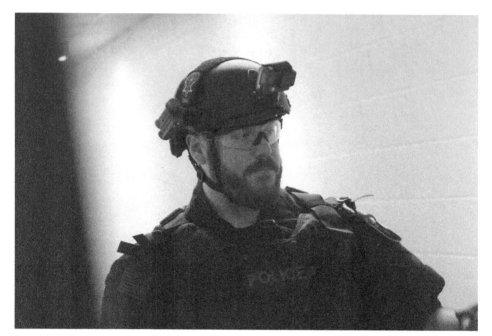

Fig. 53.2. Tactical personal protective equipment on tactical emergency medical service physician Dr. Walker Foland.

18. How do NFDDs work?
NFDDs are devices designed to saturate the subject with overwhelming sensory overload. This will temporarily stun anyone who is the target of these devices. An NFDD's blast pressure can burst the eardrums. The incendiary portion of the NFDD can burn furniture and subjects if detonated too closely. No fragmentation comes from these devices; they do not explode but instead release a bright flash and bang from the device in a controlled fashion.

19. How does a CEW work?
A CEW delivers low-current, high-voltage shocks by direct contact or by insulated wires capped with sharp metal probes. These cause involuntary muscle contraction. Another name for a CEW is a TASER. TASER is an acronym for Thomas A. Swift's Electric Rifle, named after a children's book of the 1950s. It delivers 19 pulses per second up to 50,000 volts at 0.36 Joules. Only 0.3% of real-world subjects had significant injury from CEWs. These injuries include ocular puncture, bone fracture, and other injuries sustained from loss of protective reflexes. Cardiac arrhythmias from CEWs are very low risk.

20. What is the most common injury pattern seen in law enforcement officers?
Limb injury is the most common. Body armor protects injuries occurring to the chest.

21. What is the most common injury pattern seen in civilians?
Civilians most often suffer injuries to the chest and abdomen.

22. How many in-custody deaths occur in the United States due to excited delirium?
Excited delirium results in 50–125 in-custody deaths per year in the United States. Positional asphyxia can result from physical restraint, which can be mitigated by the presence of TEMS. TEMS providers have a unique skill set to approach patients with excited delirium in the field. This knowledge allows for safer de-escalation and restraint techniques to be implemented by the tactical team. Interventions like removal of restraints after chemical sedation, as well as cooling, volume resuscitation, ventilation, and hospitalization, can save the lives of those in excited delirium.

CLINICAL CASE 1

Case: There is a barricaded gunman in a domestic structure. Your tactical team makes entry and shots are fired. You are the team medic and you are called in to treat a teammate who has been shot. You find a teammate lying on the floor unconscious with a large gunshot wound to the left leg. Shots are being fired and the gunman is still an active threat.

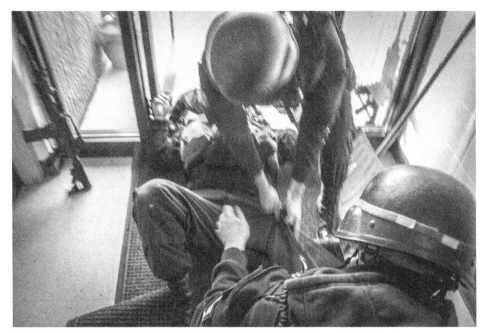

Fig. 53.3. Tactical emergency medical services paramedics respond to a casualty in the hot zone.

1. When you enter the structure, what zone do you assume you are entering?
   Always assume you are entering a hot zone (Fig. 53.3).

2. When you approach the casualty what is the first thing you should do?
   You should always make sure the casualty is safe. If there is a direct threat and you are in the hot zone, you must address the threat first.

3. After the threat is contained or eliminated, what steps should be taken to address the casualty?
   Hemorrhage control is paramount. Remember the tactical primary survey (XABCDE). Quick application of a tourniquet is essential in preventing exsanguination.

CLINICAL CASE 2

Case: During a high-risk warrant, your tactical team enters a domestic structure. Shots are fired and one of your teammates is down in a separate room from you.

1. In this scenario, what is the first thing you should do?
   In this case, the first thing you should do is call for the casualty to self-extricate. If the casualty cannot self-extricate, the team must secure the room and extricate the casualty.

2. Once the casualty is in your care, you perform the tactical primary survey. You quickly assess your teammate finding a chest wound on the right, just lateral to the body armor. Shots are no longer being fired and the suspect is no longer a threat. What is the first thing you do?
   In this scenario, the direct threat has been eliminated. It is presumed that you are now in a warm zone, because surrounding areas have not been cleared of threats. Being in a warm zone, you must address exsanguination, airway, and breathing (XAB). This casualty requires a chest seal and a needle decompression on the side of the injury. Circulation, decontamination, and disability (CD) on the tactical primary survey should be addressed once in the cold zone.

3. You have now extricated your casualty to the cold zone and you are transporting to the nearest trauma center. You expose the casualty to perform your secondary survey. The casualty's vital signs reveal tachycardia and a systolic blood pressure (BP) of 90. You determine there is no tension pneumothorax. What is the preferred intravenous (IV) resuscitation therapy?
   Blood products are preferred. Other IV fluids will thin the blood and can lead to dangerous coagulopathies. IV fluids can also contribute to hypothermia and increase mortality rates.

KEY POINTS

- TEMS increase survivability by 44%.
- The first step of the Tactical Primary Survey is always security.
- The zones of care in TEMS are the Hot Zone, Warm Zone, and Cold Zone.
- At a minimum, PPE in TEMS includes medical gloves, protective ballistic eyewear, body armor, and a Kevlar helmet.
- The most common injuries in law enforcement occur in the extremities, whereas civilians are more frequently injured in the chest, head, and abdomen.

BIBLIOGRAPHY

Fitzgerald D, Llewellyn C, Fisk B, et al. *CONTOMS Tactical Medic Handbook*. 2013:22-62.

Hauda WE, Collins D. Tactical emergency medical support. *Special Operations Medical Support*. Kendall Hunt Professional; 2009:203-213.

Heiskell LE, Carmona RH. Tactical emergency medical services: an emerging subspecialty of emergency medicine. *Ann Emerg Med*. 1994;23:778.

Swartz R. Tactical emergency medical support and urban search and rescue. In: Foland J, Weir A, eds. *Rosen's Emergency Medicine Concepts and Clinical Practice*. Philadelphia: Mosby Elsevier; 2010:3000-3009.

Wipfler JE. *Tactical Medicine Essentials*. Sudbury, MA: Jones & Bartlett Learning; 2010:4-15. 30-36, 42-49.

CHAPTER 54

SEARCH AND RESCUE

Ryan Kelly

QUESTIONS AND ANSWERS

1. What is search and rescue (SAR)?

   SAR is comprised of search functions and rescue functions. This is an important point not only because of differences in the skills and resources involved between these two types of operations, but sometimes due to differences in responsibilities, jurisdictions, and legal aspects. Search is an operation that uses available personnel and facilities to locate persons in distress. Rescue is an operation to retrieve persons in distress, provide for their initial medical or other needs, and deliver them to a place of safety.

2. Who performs SAR operations?

   Ideally, a SAR team would have the skills, knowledge, equipment, and training in the setting where the SAR is needed. At the local level, this task may fall on the shoulders of local police, fire, and EMS personnel. This is likely to be the first response when it is determined that someone is missing or lost. Once it is determined by the local responders that a specialized search team is needed, a call goes out for help. Most municipalities in the United States will have a process in place to handle this type of request, so it is important to find out what your local policy is for this type of situation. The vast majority of SAR teams are volunteer based and may not always be immediately available, so it is important to identify the need for a specialized SAR team as soon as possible.

3. What government organizations are responsible for SAR?

   The Air Force Rescue Coordination Center (AFRCC) based at Tyndall Air Force Base, Florida, is the primary Federal Government agency that is responsible for the coordination of inland SAR in the continental United States. AFRCC also offers assistance with SAR to Canada and Mexico. When a distress call is verified by the AFRCC, the staff determines the level of response and resources that are available in the area and notifies the appropriate personnel. This includes agencies like the Civil Air Patrol (CAP), US Coast Guard (USCG), and National Park Service (NPS).

4. What kind of special training do SAR teams have that police, fire, and EMS do not have?

   SAR teams are trained specifically to operate in areas where normal EMS operations are not able to go or involves special equipment that EMS teams do not have. This includes wilderness and remote locations, urban locations that are affected by natural disaster, and high angle rescues that require special equipment. Some SAR teams also have dogs that assist in tracking and locating lost and missing persons. Another emerging area of SAR is the use of cell phone forensics to locate the last known position (LKP) of a missing person. Initially used as a last resort option, due to the current prevalence of smart phones and positive results overtime, cell phone forensics is now a primary asset that is requested from the AFRCC.

5. If I am the first responder on a scene and determine that SAR is needed, what do I do next?

   As with any expanding EMS incident, an incident command system must be established so additional responders will know where to go and the search effort can be effectively coordinated. Next, personnel on the scene and early arriving personnel should be assigned to cover the hazards in the area, such as approaches to cliff areas, swift water, deep water, major roadways, etc. After that, gather as much information about the lost person as possible. This includes information about what they were wearing, any known medical problems, current medications, events in the hours and days before they were missing, and any other information that is relevant to the current situation. The next step is to begin an investigation and protect the LKP or place last seen (PLS). Assigning a staging area manager, setting up a staging area, and establishing check-in procedures are also necessary. Finally, analyze the mission and prioritize tasks.

6. List factors that may cause someone to be in a situation where they need to be rescued.
   - Inadequate planning
   - Inadequate clothing or footwear for the weather conditions
   - Inadequate physical conditioning
   - Unexpected illness including dehydration, hypo- or hyperthermia, orthopedic injuries, or exacerbation of chronic medical conditions
   - Lack of navigational proficiency
   - Inability to recognize or plan for sudden changes in the environmental conditions

7. What kind of specialized gear do SAR teams carry?

SAR teams will generally be self-sufficient in the field for up to 72 hours depending on the conditions of the search. This means that they may be carrying their own food, water, shelter, and appropriate clothing for the climate. This does not mean that they will remain in the field the whole time, but they can return to base and not need additional support from the local agencies for a period of time. SAR teams will also generally have a way to communicate with each other, but because expanding operations may involve several agencies, communication equipment may need to be standardized by a specific communications cell to ensure adequate communication from teams in the field to the mission base.

8. What type of SAR resources are available to assist in a search?

Resources vary depending on the area. Aviation resources are widely used and these include reviewing aircraft, which are great for low level searching over priority search areas, inserting or extracting rescue personnel and victims, and movement or transport of equipment and personnel. Local military and police resources are the most common to have rotary wing aircraft available for use in SAR missions. Fixed wing aircraft are also used for SAR and are able to search larger areas quickly, but usually from higher altitudes, making detection of smaller objects more difficult. Many ground SAR teams will also have access to search dogs that are specialized in the air scenting and/or tracking and trailing. Human trackers, aka "man-trackers," are specially trained team members who are highly efficient in determining a subject's initial direction of travel if an LKP is established. Other specialized SAR responders include rough terrain responders, swift water and underwater responders, winter environment responders, special vehicle responders, confined space responders, collapsed structure responders, and horse or mounted responders.

9. What happens if the person that is being searched for does not want to be found?

This can happen in a variety of situations. For example, lost children have a tendency to hide from strangers or from fear of being in trouble for getting lost. This can make detection exponentially more difficult. It is important in this case to involve the family to establish a way to identify likely places that the child may hide or items that may coax the child from hiding. Other situations may include persons that are purposefully evading detection for criminal reasons or because they have the intent to harm themselves. In this case, law enforcement must be involved and will likely be the lead organization on the search. When there is threat of physical harm to the searchers, most volunteer organizations will not be participating in that search. Those evading detection purposefully may also be armed and should not be approached by anyone other than trained law enforcement officers.

10. What happens when the missing subject is found?

It depends on the capabilities of your SAR team. The first thing to do is to determine if the person that you found is in need of any immediate medical interventions to preserve life, limb, or eyesight. Most SAR teams have at least one member that has basic or advanced first aid training. While the subject is being assessed, it is reasonable to simultaneously communicate with the mission base to notify them of the status of the team and give updates. Mission base will want to verify if the subject that has been found is the subject of the original search operation. Once the identity of the missing person is verified, the mission will transition to the rescue phase, which includes extraction from the area where the person was found. If the person is uninjured and otherwise medically stable, they may be able to walk out with the search team. Need for additional assistance to return to safety will depend on the capabilities of the search team, the terrain, the condition of the missing person, and the availability of specialized rescue vehicles or helicopters.

11. What should be done if the subject is found but they are deceased?

The first thing to be performed if one suspects that the person is deceased is to check for signs of life. Check responsiveness, check for breathing, and check for a pulse. If these are absent or there are obvious signs of death like dependent lividity, obvious decomposition, or mortal damage, then the scene should be secured and the mission base should be called for additional actions. Most likely, law enforcement will want to gather evidence if needed and the local coroner will be called to remove the decedent. Upon finding the subject, it is important to keep a log of actions and limit disturbing the scene until cleared by law enforcement in the event that foul play is suspected. While evidence preservation should not take precedence over saving human life, appropriate measures to preserve the scene should be taken when possible.

KEY POINTS

- SAR is a specialized function that requires special training, equipment, and personnel to perform.
- Most SAR teams are not 911 responders, but the earlier they are activated, the better the outcome can be.
- Different types of teams have different capabilities such as canines, helicopters, fixed wing aircraft, and waterborne vehicles.
- If the subject of the search is known to be violent, involved in criminal activity, or otherwise a danger to the search team, most volunteer search teams will be excluded from the search for safety reasons.
- Rescue operations are largely dependent on the capabilities of the team, terrain, weather, and the condition of the subject.

BIBLIOGRAPHY

Civil Air Patrol. *Capabilities Handbooks, Brochures & Briefings.* 2013. https://www.gocivilairpatrol.com/media/cms/Capabilities_ Handbook_HighRes_046ADDF6591BC.pdf.

National Search and Rescue Committee. Land Search and Rescue Addendum to the National Search and Rescue Supplement to the International Aeronautical and Maritime Search and Rescue Manual, Version 1.0. 2011. https://www.hsdl.org/?view&did=715465.

US Air Force. CONR-1AF (AFNORTH). 2014. https://www.1af.acc.af.mil/Library/Fact-Sheets/Display/Article/289622/air-force-rescue-coordination-center/.

CHAPTER 55

COMMUNITY DISASTER PREPAREDNESS

Melissa D. Kohn

QUESTIONS AND ANSWERS

1. How has emergency medical services been involved in disasters in the past?

   Emergency medical services (EMS) has been involved with disaster response as part of their routine responses. During a disaster, EMS will typically be called on through 911. EMS is likely to be the first to respond on a scene for an unexpected incident. EMS providers have acted as Incident Command to initiate response efforts until the rest of the system has been established. Simultaneously, EMS is expected to treat the injured and coordinate transport to definitive medical care as needed. As for predicted incidents, EMS has usually been involved in the planning and preparedness efforts in order to react and respond in the most effective and efficient ways possible.

2. During an epidemic, what are some ways that EMS is involved?

   Epidemics are described as the widespread manifestation of an infectious disease in a population during a particular time frame. Some epidemics can be expected, such as the potential for pandemic influenza during the winter months in the United States. The concept of an infectious disease that could easily be spread is a subject that EMS can prepare for, and in some ways can directly prepare the community. EMS providers can be prophylactically vaccinated against easily communicable diseases including influenza, but also measles or hepatitis A. Agencies can work together to determine the required level of isolation needed and potentially coordinate specific units to respond to calls that are suspected of an infectious disease. Working with the hospital system, specific sites can be predesignated to receive the potentially infected patients.

3. Who are members of the community that EMS should work with for emergency preparedness?

   EMS interacts with various organizations of the community in addition to their typical 911 response calls. EMS should participate in planning with hospitals for disaster response such as notification systems and distribution of patients. A fairly regular user of EMS is nursing homes. EMS could meet with nursing homes in the area to create plans for the response to an incident that could result in multiple victims, such as a fire. It is also possible that EMS could help the nursing homes develop an evacuation plan, which would end up being helpful for when EMS would have to respond. Another community area that has potential for a disastrous event would be a school. Community outreach to schools can help get students comfortable and educated about emergency response and preparedness.

   If the local community has an airport, there needs to be a plan developed with airport staff and security on how the EMS agencies would respond to an incident, whether it involves an event in a terminal or on an airplane. Most EMS agencies have an established relationship with the fire departments in their area and should work with them to create plans on how to manage disaster situations. Along the same vein, a relationship needs to be fostered with the local police since their response will undoubtedly be part of a disaster event.

4. Why types of training should EMS provide to the community?

   EMS should be providing education about their services at community outreach events. They should also help to provide education and training about topics related to possible epidemics and disasters that could affect their local areas. Certain parts of the country will benefit from education about hurricanes, such as having a box ready at all times that contains items like nonperishable food and water. Other areas will need training on what type of notifications will be provided should there be an approaching tornado and how to shelter from an imminent storm. If there are established shelters in the area for either a hurricane or a tornado, people should know where the shelters are and how to access them. EMS may even be called upon to staff the shelters, providing medical care to the chronically ill or acutely injured. Evacuation plans and routes should be distributed, and people need to be encouraged to follow these plans. EMS agencies would benefit from teaching this information since the emergency routes would then be more accessible for their needs.

   During infectious epidemics, EMS can distribute information regarding the disease, how it is spread, and the precautions that people can take in order to reduce the possibility of becoming infected and decreasing the spread of the disease. Again, EMS benefits as there would be less likelihood of an infected patient. If someone is infected, awareness of symptoms by the person might allow EMS to arrive more prepared to treat the patient with appropriate precautions.

5. Name examples of existing national programs for community emergency preparedness.

EMS providers can participate in programs developed for national community preparedness. EMS can partner with the local Department of Public Health to gather more resources and help circulate information. The American Public Health Association (APHA) has a "Get Ready" campaign that offers materials to share with the public on various topics such as heat waves and potential home disasters. One of the longest standing and beneficial programs is the teaching of cardiopulmonary resuscitation (CPR). The American Heart Association (AHA) has been traveling the United States since 2012 trying to demonstrate proper CPR techniques to the public. EMS agencies can pair up with the AHA and host events to teach the current recommended hands-only CPR method. Many EMS providers become instructors for CPR and other AHA classes to teach first aid to the public.

The Federal Emergency Management Agency (FEMA) developed a program called "Until Help Arrives." The program is aimed at showing the public what they can do in a disaster situation until emergency responders can get to them. As part of their program, FEMA encourages citizens to stop the bleeding. Another national program is specifically called "Stop the Bleed," which was developed by the Department of Homeland Security. The initiative is designed at teaching the public how to stop hemorrhagic bleeding with methods such as direct pressure and proper tourniquet use. Stop the Bleed education materials and training materials can be obtained by EMS agencies. By providing education and supplies, EMS could ultimately benefit since a patient may be more stable upon their arrival having not lost excessive amounts of blood.

6. What are some other ways that EMS providers could be involved in community disaster preparedness?

EMS providers will typically be responsible for responses during a disaster in their local area. Aside from responding with their agency, providers may wish to participate with other associations that help during the time of a disaster. The American Red Cross is a large and well-established organization that provides disaster relief throughout the country. A member of the Red Cross may be asked to serve in another area of the country if a disaster were to strike. More locally, there may be teams that EMS providers can join to provide assistance to their local area. The Medical Reserve Corps (MRC) are local teams with members who have a variety of skill sets. Many of the MRC teams are supported by local government funding. Another local team could be the Community Emergency Response Team (CERT), which is often supported through some form of federal funding via FEMA. Both MRC and CERT members could be asked to use their skills as part of an extended response to a disaster, which would typically not be asked of an EMS provider in the initial response phase.

7. What are mutual aid agreements?

Mutual aid agreements are agreements among agencies, organizations, and sometimes jurisdictions to provide assistance in an emergency. The arrangements are typically made beforehand but could be made emergently should the need arise. Agreements are made for personnel, materials, equipment, or services. The concept behind mutual aid agreements is to establish a relationship and construct a deal between agencies to facilitate the exchange of resources during a disaster situation. Some agreements occur on a regular basis when there is a system overload. For example, a neighboring ambulance service will respond to a call for another agency when the initial EMS agency has utilized all units for other calls. Such an agreement is a locally agreed-upon decision. For bigger incidents, a response may require resources from the region or from across the state. Agreements involving state-to-state exchange of resources may be developed with government agency involvement as certain declarations may need to be enacted to trigger the release of the resources. EMS agencies may be asked to respond as part of one of these agreements, although it was not initiated through the EMS agency directly.

8. What are the challenges to EMS and community emergency preparedness?

As with most subjects, funding will always be a challenge. Due to some of the recent epidemics and disaster incidents, some funding has been provided to EMS agencies to help them prepare themselves and subsequently their communities. This funding has come by way of national government agencies, primarily the Department of Homeland Security and the Department of Health and Human Services. Most agencies were able to purchase supplies and even vehicles that would aid in the response to disasters. Some supplies were aimed at isolation precautions during disease epidemics. There are funding resources available through the Emergency Preparedness Grant Coordination program and various federal agencies.

EMS also faces challenges when dealing with special populations. These populations can include patients with special needs, including those who are hearing or visually impaired, as these citizens may not be able to take advantage of typical notification systems during a disaster. The homeless population presents difficulties with disaster notification as well, but the same population can be a nidus for the spread of an infection during a disease epidemic. Similar issues could arise with an immigrant population, especially with a potential for a language barrier.

KEY POINTS

- EMS agencies have been participating in responses to disasters and epidemics for many years in various roles, including disease surveillance and direct patient treatment.
- Education to the community by EMS can involve instructing people on what resources are available, but also how they can personally prepare for a disaster.
- National campaigns like the AHA's CPR program and Department of Homeland Security's Stop the Bleed initiative can involve EMS agencies and providers.
- Working with other community organizations like hospitals, schools, and nursing homes, EMS can develop disaster plans in advance to provide better responses during an incident.

BIBLIOGRAPHY

American Public Health Association. Get the facts: ready-to-use materials from APHA's Get Ready campaign. Available at: http://aphagetready.org/new_pg_facts.htm.

McIntosh BA, Hinds P, Giordano LM. The role of EMS systems in public health emergencies. *Prehosp Disaster Med.* 1997;12(1):30-35.

National Highway Traffic Safety Administration. Preparedness. Available at: https://www.ems.gov/preparedness.html.

National survey on EMS preparedness for disaster and MCI response. Available at: http://www.naemt.org/docs/default-source/ems-agencies/EMS-Preparedness/2017-naemt-ems-preparedness-report.pdf?sfvrsn=0.

US Department of Health & Human Services. Public Health Preparedness and Response 2018 National Snapshot. Available at: https://www.cdc.gov/cpr/pubs-links/2018/index.htm.

US Department of Health & Human Services. What does coordinated emergency health preparedness look like? Available at: http://www.phe.gov/Preparedness/planning/hpp/Documents/em-prep-grant-coord-infographic.pdf.

US Department of Homeland Security. Mutual aid agreements and assistance agreements. Available at: https://emilms.fema.gov/IS703A/RES0102130text.htm.

US Department of Homeland Security. You are the help until help arrives. Available at: https://www.fema.gov/sites/default/files/2020-07/fema_nims_mutual_aid_guideline_20171105.pdf.

Williams T. Preplanned EMS role in emergency management. *J Emerg Med Serv.* 2018;. https://www.jems.com/2018/08/09/preplanned-ems-role-in-emergency-management/.

GENERAL PRINCIPLES IN WILDERNESS MEDICINE

CHAPTER 56

Christopher Davis and Stephanie Lareau

QUESTIONS AND ANSWERS

1. What is wilderness medicine?

   Wilderness medicine is, in general, as defined by Hawkins in *Wilderness EMS*, "medical care and problem-solving in circumstances where the surrounding environment, has more power over our well-being than does the infrastructure of our civilization." Many texts have defined wilderness medicine with various verbiage over the years, but as the field has matured, the definition has evolved. Historically, definitions have centered on time from "definitive care," often referring to a hospital or emergency department. Many organizations still use the definition of 1 or 2 hours from definitive care to activate "wilderness" protocols. This is based off of the increasingly questioned, historical concept of the "golden hour" for trauma, presuming that patients should arrive at a hospital within an hour of a traumatic injury. *Auerbach's Wilderness Medicine* defines wilderness medicine as "medical care delivered in those areas where fixed or transient geographic challenges reduce availability of, or alter requirements for, medical or patient movement resources." Practically speaking, this refers to any medical care provided in austere conditions, which may be anywhere from a remote Alaskan mountain, to a battlefield, in space or at sea, in an urban area on the side of a steep cliff, or during a natural disaster.

2. What is the relationship between wilderness medicine and wilderness EMS?

   Wilderness EMS (WEMS) is increasingly being recognized as its own distinct subspecialty. WEMS is truly a specific *subtype* of wilderness medicine. Traditionally, there has been a divide in wilderness medicine between "professional rescuers" and recreationalists. This has evolved over time, but the two primary contexts remain: recreationalists who are providing ad hoc care without a duty to act and organized teams of credentialed providers who do have duty to act. Wilderness medicine traditionally has had the connotation that it is ad hoc medical care provided in an unplanned manner. It is largely improvisational, and presupposes rescue. WEMS, on the other hand, as defined by Hawkins is "The systematic and preplanned delivery of wilderness medicine by formal healthcare providers." This includes special operations teams in both civilian EMS and the military, ski patrols, search and rescue (SAR) teams, or conventional EMS who have been unexpectedly placed in a "wilderness context." In the context of the definition discussed earlier, this could be a vehicle rescue over a cliff, an injury on a trail in a suburban park, or routine EMS care during a natural disaster. Although the resources available to a WEMS team are different than in conventional EMS, the public expectation for high-quality care does not change. While, traditionally, wilderness medicine has been referred to as "austere" or "resource-limited" medicine, within a WEMS system, there may be highly advanced resources such as helicopters, blood products, or antivenin that is not available in an urban context. This is the premise upon which the concept for preplanning and development of a WEMS system is built. Systems should be developed locally and designed to meet the anticipated needs based on the patient population and geographic areas served.

3. What training and certification are available in wilderness medicine?

   Unlike traditional EMS education, which grew from a system of government directives, oversight, and policy, wilderness medicine training grew out of private organizations and schools who offer training on a for-profit basis. There are currently no nationally recognized certifications and no governmental oversight for the common wilderness medicine certifications. Many private educational organizations offer training and certifications in wilderness medicine and WEMS. Some of the most common levels of training are Wilderness First Aid, Wilderness Advanced First Aid, Wilderness First Responder, and Wilderness EMT. These courses range in length from 1 or 2 days to 30 days or more for Wilderness EMT. While the Wilderness Medical Society (WMS) has published consensus recommendations for curriculum of Wilderness First Aid and Wilderness First Responder courses, they specifically do not approve or disapprove of any courses. Many of these courses are geared toward recreationalists or outdoor guides who may or may not have a duty to act. Without universal acceptance of these certifications, how individuals are integrated into an existing EMS system varies greatly among jurisdictions. More recently, NAEMSP (National Association of EMS Physicians) has published an expert opinion, consensus document outlining recommended educational core content, scopes of practice, and medical oversight for WEMS providers. They recommend four levels of WEMS provider: Wilderness Emergency Medical Responder (WEMR), Wilderness Emergency Medical

Technician (WEMT), Wilderness Advanced Emergency Medical Technician (WAEMT), and Wilderness Paramedic (WParamedic). The nomenclature used was chosen to align with the current recommendations for prehospital providers as outlined in the National EMS Scope of Practice Model and National EMS Education Standards. They also affirmed that WEMS providers are, in fact, providing healthcare and therefore should function within a defined scope of practice and physician medical oversight.

4. Is it appropriate to have an expanded scope of practice in the wilderness?
Most EMS protocols and national guidelines on scope of practice are written from the urban EMS context. There are numerous time-sensitive conditions that are typically deferred to hospital care that do warrant early intervention in a prolonged-care context. Some common examples of this are reduction of dislocated joints, insertion of Foley catheters, and antibiotic or blood product administration.

In 2010, the NAEMSP and NAEMSO (National Association of State EMS Officials) issued a joint position statement that stated operational EMS programs should function within and not outside the mainstream healthcare system and function within their defined scope of practice. It is appropriate, and critical, to have an expanded scope of practice in the wilderness; however, this should be defined locally in a systematic manner. Protocols for reduction of dislocated joints, prolonged pain management, management of infectious diseases, and nutrition/hydration, for example, should be developed in advance. Providers should not perform procedures for which they are not trained or credentialed within a WEMS system.

5. How are scene safety concerns addressed?
WEMS providers face many of the same scene safety concerns as urban EMS providers do. Violent, altered patients pose a threat, and there is the constant threat of exposure to potentially infectious body substances. There are unique scene safety concerns often faced by WEMS providers that are not generally of primary concern to the urban provider. Weather plays a big role in wilderness operations, and WEMS providers often spend a prolonged time in the elements. Extremes of heat and cold, lighting, and avalanche terrain are common scene safety concerns that must be mitigated. WEMS often takes place in inherently dangerous environments, which has spurred a movement to reexamine the concept of a safe scene, and some WEMS programs are now teaching a "risk mitigation" approach, rather than "scene safety." In general, risk and hazard mitigation in WEMS begins with training in situational awareness, survival skills, and risk assessment, as well as technical skills in rescue, backcountry travel, and hazard mitigation techniques specific to each operational environment (wilderness search, rock/snow/ice travel, high altitude, etc.).

6. What are common modes of patient transport in the wilderness?
Often, patients are able to be transported from the wilderness under their own power. This is usually the fastest method and requires the least external resources. When considering whether to have a patient evacuate under their own power, consider the risk of further injury or suffering to the patient, versus the risk to other rescuers, the resources required to evacuate the patient by other means, and the time required to perform a rescue. If the patient must be carried, stokes litters are often used. These are baskets that afford some rigid protection beneath and around the sides of the patient and allow for them to be secured for transport over uneven or technical terrain. Stokes litters are also typically used by technical rescue teams to move patients through vertical and technical terrain.

Arguably one of the most powerful assets for WEMS operations is helicopters. They allow for insertion of rescuers and patient evacuation in a fraction of the time that ground-based teams require. Often, a rescue that may take hours or even days can be completed in a few hours or less when helicopters are employed. While helicopters are used extensively in Europe, access to helicopter-based rescue and WEMS is limited in the United States. With some notable exceptions, most helicopter EMS (HEMS) systems in the United States are private, for-profit, or hospital based and do not perform SAR or WEMS activities. Some locales have access to helicopters via arrangements with law enforcement agencies or federal agencies who provide rescue services on a contractual basis. The National Park Service has a robust helicopter WEMS system in place in some parks providing hoist and short-haul (human external cargo) operations. This allows rescuers and patients to be inserted or extracted by either a hoist cable or a fixed line (short haul) without the helicopter having to land on the scene. This is particularly useful if the terrain is too steep or loose or significant ground obstacles do not allow for an acceptable helicopter landing zone, which typically must be at least 100 ft by 100 ft.

7. What equipment is commonly required?
WEMS providers must be prepared to care for their own needs and those of their patient for 24–72 hours, depending on the operational environment. This typically includes food and water, fire starting supplies, appropriate outerwear for anticipated weather, and some form of shelter. Medical equipment varies greatly depending on the operation and preferences of the teams or providers on the mission. Kits are often modular and allow for them to be customized prior to deploying based on the anticipated patient care needs. The weight and size of the equipment are primary considerations, as the kits usually have to be carried into the field by the provider. Some basic equipment is commonly carried regardless of the mission, such as basic wound care and hemorrhage control supplies, as massive hemorrhage is the most common cause of preventable death after trauma. Airway

management is also of primary concern, but due to the complexity of the procedure, and the size and weight of the supplies for endotracheal intubation, supraglottic devices are preferred. Oxygen is typically used very liberally in urban EMS, but the size and weight of oxygen tanks make them impractical for many missions. Typical type D portable oxygen cylinders will last approximately 3.5 hours at 2 liters per minute (LPM), 1.5 hours at 6 LPM, and only 30 minutes at 10 LPM.

8. Are there evidence-based guidelines for patient care in wilderness medicine?

Many concepts used within wilderness medicine arise from Tactical Combat Casualty Care (TCCC), which is evidence-based prehospital care guidelines used by the military on the battlefield. One of the concepts commonly used in patient assessment is MARCH, where M is massive hemorrhage, A is airway, R is respiration, C is circulation, and H is hypothermia (hyperthermia/hike/helicopter). This shifts from the typical A, B, C approach to patient care, with evidence showing in trauma in austere environments that uncontrolled hemorrhage is one of the leading causes of death, and in austere environments, blood volume cannot be readily replaced. This encourages the early use of tourniquets, which have fallen back into favor. This approach also reminds rescuers of the importance of protection from the environment by protecting patients from hypothermia and considering evacuation requirements (hike or helicopter). Additionally, the WMS has published a series of evidence-based guidelines for the treatment of conditions both related to wilderness exposures and for the care of patients in the wilderness. These guidelines cover such topics as hypothermia, drowning, altitude illness, and avalanche burial.

KEY POINTS

- Wilderness medicine, in general, is "medical care delivered in those areas where fixed or transient geographic challenges reduce availability of, or alter requirements for, medical or patient movement resources" and can apply to many locations and circumstances.
- While there are currently no nationally recognized certifications in wilderness medicine, there are many courses available to train both laypeople in advanced medical techniques, such as reduction of dislocated shoulders, while in the wilderness and for medical professionals to apply their medical skills in an austere environment.
- Patient transport is often one of the largest challenges facing wilderness clinicians.
- Wilderness medical kits should be individually tailored considering the training of the clinician, expected injuries and illnesses, length of trip, distance and time to definitive care, and size/weight constraints limiting the ability to bring the kit along.

BIBLIOGRAPHY

Bowman WD. The development and current status of wilderness prehospital emergency care in the United States. *J Wilderness Med.* 1990;1:93-102.

Butler FK, Bennett B, Wedmore CI. Tactical Combat Casualty Care and wilderness medicine: advancing trauma care in austere environments. *Emerg Med Clin North Am.* 2017 May;35(2):391-407.

Davis C, Abo B, McClure S, Hawkins S. Safety is third, not first, and we all know it should be. *J Emerg Med Serv.* November 2018;*http://bit.ly/34fneYr.*

Hawkins S. WEMS systems. *Wilderness EMS.* In: Hawkins S, ed. New York, NY: Wolters Kluwer; 2018:21.

Hawkins SC, Millin MG, Smith W. Wilderness emergency medical services and response systems. In: Auerbach PS, ed. *Auerbach's Wilderness Medicine.* 7th ed. Philadelphia, PA: Elsevier; 2017:1200-1213.

Millin MG, et al. Medical oversight, educational core content, and proposed scopes of practice of wilderness EMS providers: a joint project developed by wilderness EMS educators.

National Association of EMS Physicians and the National Association of State EMS Officials: medical direction for operational emergency medical services programs. *Prehosp Emerg Care.* 2010;14(4):544.

Otten E, Bowman W, Hackett P, Spadafora M, Tauber D. Wilderness prehospital emergency care curriculum. *J Wilderness Med.* 1991;2(2):80-87.

CHAPTER 57

BITES, STINGS, AND ENVENOMATIONS

Emily Hegamyer and Kaynan Doctor

QUESTIONS AND ANSWERS

1. A 60-year-old man was sweeping the floor of his garden shed when he was bitten by a large spider. He has managed to trap the spider under a glass jar. On arrival to his Houston, Texas, residence, you find him sitting on a chair anxiously holding his wounded left hand. You are unsure if the trapped spider is a black widow or brown recluse. How do these spider bites differ in presentation and management?
   See Table 57.1.

2. A 6-year-old girl was playing in her yard when she felt a sharp sting on her right arm and looked down to see a scorpion scurry away. You are called for further management given the severity of pain. What do you know about scorpion envenomation that you could share with the parents?
   In the United States, the vast majority of scorpions reside in the Southwest (Arizona, California, Nevada, New Mexico, and Texas). Venom is contained in the tail and has neurotoxic and cytotoxic properties. Fatality is rare from

Table 57.1. Differentiating Between Brown Recluse and Black Widow Spider Bites

	BROWN RECLUSE	BLACK WIDOW
Source	• South, Central, Midwest United States • Prefer dark, warm, protected areas (closets and garages)	• Throughout North America (except for Maine and Alaska) • Most commonly in South, Ohio Valley, Southwest, and West Coast • Attics, barns, trash piles
Description	Violin-shaped mark on the dorsal cephalothorax	Red hourglass-shaped marking on underside of the abdomen
Mechanism of action	• Cytotoxic • Usually only bite when threatened	• Affects neurotransmitters
Clinical manifestation	• Stinging sensation • Increased pain and pruritus within hours • Mild local irritation leading to large necrotic lesions • *Loxoscelism:* systemic reaction (40% of envenomations most common in young children): fever, nausea/vomiting, headache, arthralgias, morbilliform eruption with petechiae, hematuria, and renal failure	• Local reaction • *Latrodectism:* widespread, sustained muscle spasms/pain; tachycardia, diaphoresis, flushing, hypotension, "pavor mortis" (fear of death), grimaced face, conjunctivitis/rhinitis, periorbital edema • *Myopathic syndrome:* muscle cramps at the site of the bite, progression to muscle rigidity of large skeletal muscles (chest, abdomen, face); may mimic an acute abdomen
Treatment	• Supportive (pain control, local wound care, elevation) • AVOID early excision • Antibiotics if secondary wound infection • Tetanus	• Stabilize ABCDEs • Pain/muscle spasm management: benzodiazepine, opioids • AVOID beta-blockers • Severe envenomation may require antivenin (rare)

All images © iStock.

scorpion stings, but symptoms can be severe. The smaller sized scorpions can be the most venomous. Scorpion stings are most commonly seen in young children.

3. Describe the clinical manifestations of scorpion stings and how they are classified.
Clinical manifestations of envenomation vary widely:
Grade I: Local pain, burning, and paresthesia at the sting site
Grade II: Local AND remote pain with paresthesia
Grade III: Either neuromuscular hyperactivity or cranial nerve dysfunction
Grade IV: Both neuromuscular hyperactivity and cranial nerve dysfunction
Neuromuscular/systemic symptoms may include:
- Shaking/jerking of extremities, fasciculations, restlessness
- Roving eye movements, slurred speech, tongue fasciculations, hypersalivation, upper airway dysfunction
- Difficulty swallowing, tachycardia, hypertension, vomiting, stridor, hypoxia, respiratory distress, fever and/or anaphylaxis, development of pancreatitis

4. What are your next steps in the management of this patient?
Stabilize the ABCDEs
Grade I + II envenomations can be managed with ibuprofen and acetaminophen.
Grade III + IV envenomations require hospital care.
- Secure the airway and ensure appropriate oxygenation.
- Focus on pain control and excessive motor activity.
  - Oral/intravenous (IV) narcotics, benzodiazepines
- Vomiting
  - Usually transient and self-limited
  - Consider antiemetics such as ondansetron
- Hypersalivation
  - Atropine
- Antivenin
  - Consider use for Grade III + IV envenomation.

5. A 35-year-old man was cleaning his yard when he accidentally stepped on a large anthill. He sustained several ant bite wounds to his legs, which have become very painful and erythematous with associated swelling. You happen to see multiple ants in the patient's yard (Fig. 57.1). What are next steps in evaluation and management?
Fire ants reside primarily in the Southeastern United States. Symptoms of envenomation may include cytotoxic, hemolytic, and potentially cardiotoxic effects. Clinical manifestations include pain with localized wheals and erythema, the development of pustules within 24 hours, and possible systemic symptoms, including heart failure or anaphylaxis with multiple stings. Treatment is usually supportive care with topical steroid ointments, local

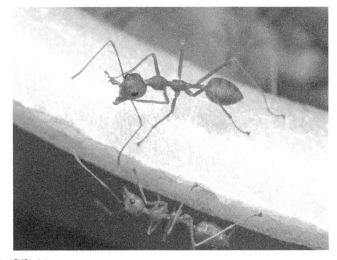

Fig. 57.1. Fire ants. *(© iStock.)*

anesthetic cream, oral antihistamines, and local wound care. Intramuscular epinephrine should be available to manage the rare occurrence of anaphylaxis.

6. You receive a phone call about an 8-year-old female who stepped on a beehive while playing soccer. She has sustained several bee stings over her body. What should you be prepared for prior to arrival?
   Envenomation from bee stings can affect histamine, serotonin, acetylcholine, and dopamine production. Patients may experience nausea, vomiting, diarrhea, hypotension, or tachycardia. Delayed symptoms may include rhabdomyolysis, hemolysis, acute kidney injury, pancreatitis, and shock. More than one sting/kg in children is associated with risk of systemic toxicity. Anaphylaxis may also occur with just one sting.

7. What are your first steps in evaluation and treatment of this patient?
   Evaluate and stabilize the ABCs. Rapid immediate removal of stingers is *not* necessary. Remove dead (or alive) bees from the nares, ears, and oropharynx. Initiate supportive care, including intramuscular epinephrine and IV fluids if there are concerns for anaphylactic shock. Securing an airway may be necessary with impending airway edema. Antihistamines and steroids may also help mitigate symptoms. Monitor for decreasing urine output, which may be an indicator for impending renal failure.

8. A 25-year-old man, while on vacation in Arizona, came across a large brightly colored lizard. In his attempts to take a "selfie" with the hissing lizard, he was bitten on his right arm. The patient described on the 911 call that the lizard would initially not let go and that he needed the help of his girlfriend to get the animal off him. His girlfriend reports that she thinks he might be having some difficulty breathing. As you travel to his location, you wonder what type of lizard may have bitten the patient.
   The Gila monster (Fig. 57.2) is one of the few venomous lizards on the planet. It is found in the deserts of the Southwestern United States and northern Mexico. Gila monsters are known to be tenacious in terms of their bite grip (especially when lifted off the ground); their teeth may break off if the animal is forced off. Removing a Gila monster may involve placing it on the ground, in cold water, or using nonlethal adjuncts to pry the jaws. Their bite venom consists of proteases that can cause pain, local edema, weakness, dizziness, nausea, and hypotension. Edema of the airway is also a rare but known complication. Initial management is supportive and consists of stabilizing the ABCs; letting the wound bleed; removing lodged teeth, watches, and rings; avoiding tourniquets; washing the wound; and providing analgesia, antihistamines, and possibly antibiotics.

9. A 40-year-old woman who was hiking in the Carolina Sandhills calls 911 after being bitten by a "multicolored snake" on her right ankle. On arrival, you ensure it is safe to approach the patient. You find her frantically looking up on her phone if the bite could be from a Coral snake. As you prepare to transport her to the nearest emergency department 40 minutes away, how should you stabilize the patient, what signs and symptoms should you be on the lookout for, and how would this presentation differ from a rattlesnake bite?
   See Table 57.2.

10. You have been called to assess a 22-year-old surfer who was stung by "something" while surfing off the coast of New Jersey. She is developing a generalized painful rash. On arrival, her friends recommend urinating on the rash. How would you best manage this patient?
    See Table 57.3.

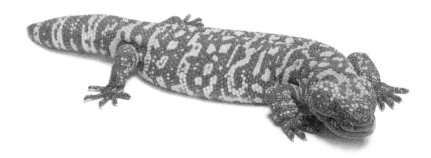

Fig. 57.2. Gila monster. *(© iStock.)*

Table 57.2. Pit Vipers vs. Coral Snakes

	CROTALIDAE FAMILY (PIT VIPERS)	ELAPIDAE FAMILY (CORAL SNAKES) *"RED ON YELLOW KILLS A FELLOW"*
Examples	Rattlesnakes, copperheads, water moccasins	Eastern Coral, Texas Coral, Sonoran Coral, cobras
Description	• Two pits on either side of head • Pupils are elliptical and vertically oriented • Triangular head • Two curved fangs that are widely spaced	• Black snout • May latch on and/or chew to deliver venom
	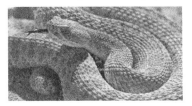	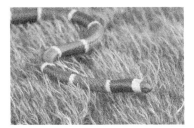
Source	Majority of US venomous snake bites	Less than 1% of poisonous snake bites
Mechanism of action	• Myotoxic (muscle involvement) • Hemotoxic (procoagulant + anticoagulant effects) • Neurotoxic (acts at neuromuscular junction)	• Venom contains α- neurotoxins • Postsynaptic neuromuscular junction blockade
Clinical manifes- tation	• Local tissue injury: severe pain, swelling, ecchymosis, hemorrhagic bullae • Increased risk of prolonged bleeding • Systemic effects: nausea/vomiting/ diarrhea, hypotension, airway edema (looks like anaphylaxis) • Muscle fasciculation: increased risk of respiratory compromise if involving upper extremities/torso • Weakness/respiratory failure	• Minimal local symptoms • CNS symptoms: paresthesia, dysarthria, ptosis, dysphagia, stridor, diplopia, fasciculation, muscle weakness, paralysis
Treatment	• ABCDE stabilization • Antivenin as indicated • Epinephrine + IV fluids if there are systemic symptoms • Elevate/immobilize affected extremity • Mark edges of swelling and tenderness every 15–30 minutes • Pain control • Basic labs, including coagulation studies	• ABCDE stabilization • Respiratory support • Antivenin (for systemic toxicity) • Admit all patients to the hospital for frequent neurologic monitoring (may occur up to 13 hours after initial bite)

CNS, Central nervous system; *IV*, intravenous.
All images © iStock.

11. You receive a 911 call reporting concern for allergic reaction. A 55-year-old woman was eating a tuna-containing sushi roll. She subsequently developed acute onset of flushing, vomiting, headaches, itching, and wheezing. What are your initial steps in management?
    While this presentation may mimic an allergic reaction, keep in mind the possibility of Scombroid poisoning, which occurs after eating improperly stored fish (tuna, mackerel, sardines, mahi-mahi). The patient may report that the fish tasted peppery and that the flesh had a honeycomb appearance. Symptoms may occur within 1 hour of in-gestion with resolution in 8–12 hours and may include flushing of the face and upper trunk with nausea, vomiting, or diarrhea. Patients may also develop tachycardia, headache, pruritus, and bronchospasm. Initial management includes ABC stabilization, antihistamines, and consideration of epinephrine with albuterol.

Table 57.3. Marine Animal Envenomation

	SOURCE	CLINICAL MANIFESTATION	TREATMENT
Jellyfish 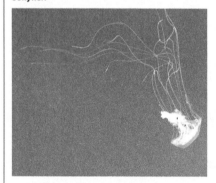	Most coastal waters	Local: Mild stinging with dermatitis and erythema. Systemic: generalized symptoms are extremely rare. Resolution is within hours.	• Sea water rinse • Removal of tentacles • Hot water for 60–90 minutes • Consider topical lidocaine, antihistamines, corticosteroid cream, and analgesics
Portuguese man of war 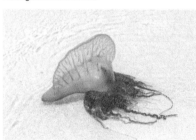	Atlantic, Pacific, and Indian oceans	Local: immediate localized pain, linear dermatitis, progression to vesicles, bullae, necrosis. Systemic: muscle spasm, nausea, vomiting, malaise, local numbness or paralysis. Rarely, hemolysis and acute kidney injury can occur. Symptoms usually resolve within 72 hours.	• Seawater rinse • Removal of tentacles • Hot water for 60–90 minutes • **AVOID** use of vinegar, which may activate nematocysts
Scorpion fish, lionfish, and stone fish 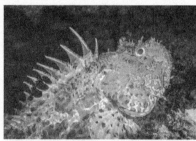 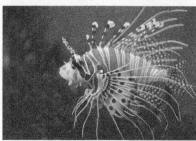	Tropical and temperate waters	Envenomation from bony spines along the fins that pierce the skin. Local: severely painful puncture wound with local edema and cyanosis. May develop blistering and necrosis. Systemic: stonefish are the most toxic; patients may develop systemic symptoms: altered mental status, fever, nausea, seizures, paralysis, pulmonary edema, heart failure.	• Irrigate with sterile saline • Hot water soak for 60–90 minutes and repeat as necessary • Pain control • Consider antibiotics for marine bacteria • Surgical debridement of wound if extensive • May consider stonefish antivenin if severe • Monitor for cardiotoxic effects and respiratory depression

(Continued)

Table 57.3. Marine Animal Envenomation (*Cont.*)

	SOURCE	CLINICAL MANIFESTATION	TREATMENT
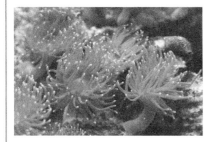			
Sea anemone 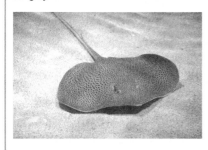	Reefs and tidal pools	Local: erythema, pruritus, blisters, ulceration. Systemic: fever, chills, weakness, nausea, syncope, cellulitis, lymphangitis.	• Seawater rinse • Topical 5% acetic acid • Pain control • Wound care
Stingray	Atlantic, Pacific, and Gulf coasts	Local: localized puncture laceration, edema, and cyanosis, which can develop into hemorrhage and necrosis. There can be moderate to severe pain. Systemic symptoms (rare): nausea/vomiting, cramps, dysrhythmias. Death from direct trauma. Secondary wound infection from retained foreign body.	• Direct pressure to control bleeding • Seawater rinse • Hot water immersion for 60–90 minutes • Pain control • Consider antibiotics • Surgical management (depending on site and extent of wound)

Jellyfish image courtesy of Kayan Doctor, MD. Other images © iStock.

12. How does Ciguatoxin poisoning typically present?
Poisoning occurs after eating barracuda, sea bass, parrotfish, red snapper, grouper, or sturgeon. Clinical signs occur within 2–6 hours of ingestion. Persistent central nervous system (CNS) symptoms, including a reversal of hot-cold temperature sensation, paresthesias, painful/loose-feeling teeth, a metallic taste, tongue numbness, paralysis, or seizures, are seen. Patients may also develop nausea, vomiting, diarrhea, cramps, bradycardia, or hypotension.

13. What are initial steps in the management of Ciguatoxin poisoning?
Key areas of management include supportive care for gastrointestinal symptoms and atropine for persistent bradycardia.

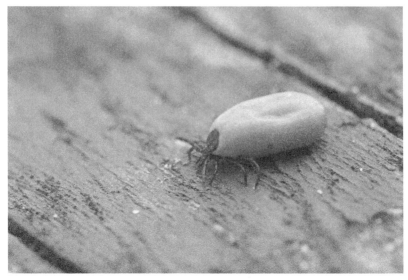

Fig. 57.3. American dog tick image. *(© iStock.)*

14. A patient contacted EMS with concern for worsening weakness and inability to move his lower extremities. On examination, you notice this large tick on the patient's left upper extremity (Fig. 57.3). What is the etiology of symptoms?

    This patient may be presenting with tick paralysis. There is often a latent period of between 4 and 7 days after tick attachment, after which patients can develop restlessness, irritability, and ascending flaccid paralysis. Respiratory paralysis and death may follow if the tick is not detected and removed.

15. What is the best technique for tick removal?

    In order to remove a tick, use a blunt forceps or tweezers. Grasp as close to skin as possible and pull upward with steady even pressure. Avoid twisting or a jerking motion and squeezing or crushing the tick's body. Ensure that all body parts are removed from the wound. Tick paralysis is reversible after removal of the tick.

KEY POINTS

- With any bite wound or sting, ensure that it is safe to approach the patient, evaluate the ABCs, perform a thorough full-body examination, and remove any watches, rings or other objects that could cause a tourniquet effect ahead of time.
- Many bites or stings can result in or mimic allergic reactions or anaphylaxis. Prioritize stabilizing the airway, breathing and circulation with oxygen, an artificial airway (if needed), IV fluids, epinephrine, diphenhydramine, and analgesia.
- Black widow envenomation may affect neurotransmitters, causing diffuse muscle spasm/pain, and ultimately lead to diffuse muscle rigidity.
- Pit viper envenomation causes localized tissue damage versus coral snake envenomation, which primarily affects the nervous system. Both may require antivenin.
- After stabilizing the ABCs, most marine animal intoxications can be initially managed with a seawater rinse, removal of foreign bodies, and a hot water immersion for 60–90 minutes.

BIBLIOGRAPHY

Abo B. Management of animal bites and envenomations. In: Hawkins SC, ed. *Wilderness EMS*. Philadelphia, PA: Wolters Kluwer; 2018.

Fenner P. Marine envenomation: an update—a presentation on the current status of marine envenomation first aid and medical treatments. *Emerg Med Australasia*. 2000;12(4):295-302.

Lachance L, Veillon D, Cotelingam J, et al. The black widow spider bite: differential diagnosis, clinical manifestations, and treatment options. *J La State Med Soc.* 2015;167:74-78.

Rahmani F, Banan Khojasteh SM, Ebrahimi Bakhtavar H, Rahmani F, Shahsavari Nia K, Faridaalaee G. Poisonous spiders: bites, symptoms, and treatment; an educational review. *Emerg (Tehran).* 2014;2(2):54-58.

Rodrigo C, Gnanathasan A. Management of scorpion envenoming: a systematic review and meta-analysis of controlled clinical trials. *Syst Rev.* 2017;6:74.

Seeyave DM, Brown KM. Environmental emergencies, radiological emergencies, bites and stings. In: Shaw KN, Bachur RG, eds. *Fleischer and Ludwig's The Textbook of Emergency Medicine.* Philadelphia, PA: Wolters/Kluwer/Lippincott Williams & Wilkins; 2016:744-758.

Tortorella V, Masciari P, Pezzi M, et al. Histamine poisoning from ingestion of fish orscombroid syndrome. *Case Rep Emerg Med.* 2014;2014:482-531.

Ward NT, Darracq MA, Tomaszewski C, Clark RF. Evidence-based treatment of jellyfish stings in North America and Hawaii. *Ann Emerg Med.* 2012;60(4):399-414.

CHAPTER 58

DYSBARISMS

Erica M. Simon

QUESTIONS AND ANSWERS

DYSBARISMS

1. What are dysbarisms?

   A collection of illnesses resulting from changes in ambient air pressure, to which an individual cannot readily adapt. Dysbarisms include barotrauma, decompression sickness (DCS), arterial gas embolism (AGE), nitrogen narcosis, and oxygen toxicity.

2. Who is at risk of developing dysbarisms?

   Astronauts, aviators, compressed air workers (e.g., caisson workers, tunnel workers, hyperbaric chamber observers), and scuba divers.

3. What is barotrauma?

   Trauma due to a failure to equalize pressure between an air-containing space and the environment. Barotrauma that occurs during descent is known as a "squeeze." A "reverse squeeze" or "reverse block" is experienced upon ascent. Anatomic structures frequently involved include the ear, sinuses, teeth (barodontalgia; air in dental caries or beneath fillings), lungs, and intestines. Facial injury (mask squeeze) results from a faulty mask seal, which does not allow for pressure equalization between the mask and the surrounding environment during exhalation. Although rare, cutaneous injury (suit squeeze) may appear if folds develop in a diver's wet/dry suit. During descent, these folds create pressure against the skin, which cannot be mitigated.

4. What is DCS?

   A clinical illness resulting from the formation of nitrogen bubbles in the blood and tissues. Upon rapid ascent from a depth, dissolved nitrogen comes out of solution (serum) and forms bubbles. Based upon the location and degree of bubble formation, symptoms manifest. Traditionally, DCS is classified into Type 1 (DCS I) and Type 2 (DCS II). DCS I affects the musculoskeletal system, the lymphatics, or the skin. DCS II involves any other organ system, often the central nervous system (CNS), inner ear, and lungs. Look for DCS following a prolonged dive given the duration of exposure to a high partial pressure of nitrogen.

5. What is an arterial gas embolism?

   A complication of pulmonary barotrauma in which damage to the lung parenchyma results in air bubbles entering the pulmonary venous circulation and, subsequently, the systemic circulation. AGEs are most deadly when they travel to the coronary and cerebral circulation, mechanically obstructing blood flow. Divers who panic and rapidly ascend without exhaling may experience an AGE.

6. What is nitrogen narcosis?

   Impaired cognition and motor skills resulting from an increased nitrogen concentration in the bloodstream. Nitrogen narcosis or "rapture of the deep" occurs when compressed air is utilized below 100 ft of seawater (fsw). For this reason, mixed gases with a lower concentration of nitrogen are recommended for sport diving to greater depths.

Disclaimer: The views expressed in this chapter are those of the author and do not necessarily reflect the official policy or position of the Department of the Army, Department of the Navy, Department of the Air Force, Department of Defense, or the US Government. "I am a military Servicemember. This work was prepared as part of my official duties. Title 17, USC § 105 provides that 'Copyright protection under this title is not available for any work of the U.S. Government.' Title 17, USC § 101 defines a U.S. Government work prepared by a military service member or employee of the U.S. Government as part of that person's official duties."

Disclosures: The author has nothing to disclose.

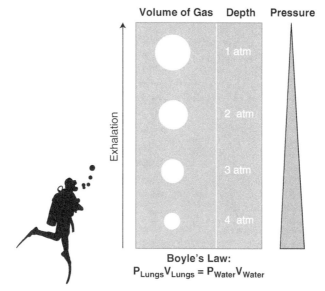

Fig. 58.1. Boyle's Law as applied to dysbarisms. Upon ascent, water pressure decreases ($\downarrow P_{water}$) and the volume of gas in the diver's lungs increases ($\uparrow V_{Lungs}$). In order to maintain the constant pressure-volume relationship, the diver must exhale to reduce lung pressure (P_{Lungs}), as the volume of the gas in the surrounding water (V_{Water}) cannot be controlled. *atm*, Atmosphere(s).

7. What is oxygen toxicity?

   Direct tissue injury from oxygen-free radicals. Exposure to oxygen, at elevated partial pressures for a prolonged duration, may result in neurologic or pulmonary symptoms. Oxygen toxicity is exceedingly rare as experienced divers utilize dive tables detailing safe dive depths and durations.

8. How can the pathophysiology of dysbarisms be explained?

   Through an understanding of the Gas laws. Barotrauma is a manifestation of Boyle's law. Boyle's law states that at a constant temperature, the volume of a quantity of gas varies inversely with the pressure on that gas. An illustration of this is a diver's requirement to exhale while ascending from a depth, in order to avoid pulmonary barotrauma and AGE (Fig. 58.1). According to Henry's law, the amount of gas that will dissolve in a liquid at a given temperature is directly proportional to the partial pressure of that gas. Partial pressures increase at depth; therefore, as compared to sea level (ambient pressure of 1 atmosphere [atm]), additional nitrogen will be taken into the bloodstream. This may result in nitrogen narcosis or, in the setting of a rapid ascent, DCS. Dalton's law further elucidates the pathophysiology of nitrogen narcosis and explains oxygen toxicity. The total pressure of the gases that a diver breathes is the sum of the partial pressures of each gas. Divers swimming with tanks of compressed air are exposed to higher partial pressures of nitrogen and oxygen at depths.

9. How can classifying the onset of symptoms aid in the diagnosis of a specific dysbarisms?

   Certain conditions occur during descent, at depth, during ascent, following ascent, and within 24 hours of resurfacing (Table 58.1).

10. What are the signs and symptoms of dysbarisms?

    See Table 58.2 and Fig. 58.2.

11. You suspect dysbarism. What should your prehospital assessment include?

    A history of present illness focusing on the dive profile:
    - Type of dive (commercial, rescue, etc.), gas used (compressed air, nitrox, heliox, other), body of water (fresh versus salt), water temperature, number of dives within 72 hours of symptom onset, dive profiles (maximum depth, time at depth, surface interval, decompression stops), time of onset of symptoms (descent, at depth, etc.).
      An assessment for DCS risk factors:
    - Patient obesity or advanced age, alcohol consumption, prolonged dive time, deep dives, repeated dives in a single day, dives in cold water, strenuous activity at depths, or exposure to decreased ambient pressure following dives (flying or driving over mountainous regions).
      A thorough previous medical history:

Table 58.1. Diving Injuries and Onset of Symptoms

SYMPTOM ONSET	INJURY
Descent	Ear, sinus, or facial barotrauma
At depth	Nitrogen narcosis
	Oxygen toxicity
Ascent	AGE
	DCS
	Pulmonary barotrauma
	Ear barotrauma
	Gastrointestinal barotrauma
	Barodontalgia
Following ascent	AGE
Within 24 hours of resurfacing	DCS

AGE, Arterial gas embolism; *DCS*, decompression sickness.
Data from Christiani D. Physical and chemical injuries of the lung. In: Goldman L, Schafer A, eds. *Goldman-Cecil Medicine*. 26th ed. Philadelphia: Elsevier; 2020:577-585; Byyny R, Shockley L. Scuba diving and dysbarism. In: Tintinalli J., Ma J., Yealy D, Meckler G, Stapczynski J, Cline D, Thomas S, eds. *Rosen's Emergency Medicine: Concepts and Clinical Practice*. 9th ed. Philadelphia: Elsevier; 2018:1773-1786; and Murphy-Lavoie H, LeGros T. Dysbarisms, dive injuries, and decompression illness. In: Adams J, Barton E, Collings J, DeBlieux P, Gisondi M, Nadel E, eds. *Emergency Medicine Clinical Essentials*. 2nd ed. Philadelphia: Saunders; 2008:1153-1161.

- Question specifically regarding patent foramen ovale (PFO), atrial septal defect (ASD), and arteriovenous malformation (AVM). In these conditions, gas bubbles may readily enter the arterial system (paradoxical emboli). The larger the PFO or ASD, the greater the risk of cerebral AGE.
- Pulmonary diseases. Work of breathing increases during dives, and the temperature of inhaled gas decreases at depths. Individuals with exercise- or cold-induced asthma may experience respiratory compromise. Persons with chronic obstructive pulmonary disease are frequently advised against diving, given their underlying pulmonary pathology, which may predispose to barotrauma.
  Vital signs and a focused physical examination:
- Obtain a temperature to evaluate for hypothermia.
- Perform a neurologic exam prior to securing the patient on a stretcher to avoid concealing motor weakness or a focal deficit.
- Evaluate for external signs of trauma. Trauma and dysbarisms may coexist.
- Look for signs detailed in Table 58.2.
  Perform an electrocardiogram in patients with chest pain:
- Ischemia, infarct, or dysrhythmias may suggest coronary AGE.
  Identify an on-scene legal authority to collect the patient's gear for testing:
- Compressed air inlets exposed to combustion sources may become contaminated with carbon monoxide (CO), ultimately resulting in tank contamination. As symptoms of CO poisoning—headache, nausea, and dizziness —are nonspecific and easily confused with DCS, assess for hypercapnia. If possible, utilize a co-oximeter to determine carboxyhemoglobin levels.

Table 58.2. Signs and Symptoms of Dysbarisms

INJURY	SIGNS AND SYMPTOMS
Ear barotrauma	Inner ear: ear pain on descent, hearing loss, vertigo, nausea. Romberg sign, ataxia, nystagmus, tympanic membrane (TM) injury, neuronal hearing loss.
	Middle ear (barotitis or ear squeeze): ear pain on descent, tinnitus, transient vertigo. Conductive hearing loss, TM injury, unilateral facial paralysis (elevated middle ear pressure presses against the facial nerve causing ischemic neurapraxia).
	External ear: ear pain on descent. Hemorrhages in the wall of the external auditory canal.
Sinus barotrauma (barosinusitis)	Facial pain on descent or ascent. Epistaxis.
Facial barotrauma (mask squeeze)	Facial pain or pressure on descent, vision changes (rare). Facial edema and conjunctival edema, petechial hemorrhages, subconjunctival hemorrhages, gross visual deficit (damage to the optic nerve).

(Continued)

Table 58.2. Signs and Symptoms of Dysbarisms (*Cont.*)

INJURY	SIGNS AND SYMPTOMS
Nitrogen narcosis	Confusion, disorientation, euphoria, numbness, and tingling of the lips and extremities. Symptoms resolve at shallower depths. Death may result due to drowning.
Oxygen toxicity	CNS: headache, irritability, dizziness, vision changes, nausea. Tremor, altered mental status, tonic-clonic seizure.
	Pulmonary: coughing, shortness of breath, chest burning on inhalation. Fever, hemoptysis, rales.
AGE	CNS: stroke-like symptoms, confusion, agitation, headache upon ascent. Altered mental status, hemiplegia, focal neurologic deficit, seizure, loss of consciousness.
	Cardiac: chest pain, palpitations, shortness of breath, nausea upon ascent. Diaphoresis, dysrhythmia, hypotension, death.
	Pulmonary: pleuritic chest pain, shortness of breath, coughing. Tachypnea, hemoptysis.
DCS	Type I
	Musculoskeletal pain (the bends) that is dull, aching, constant, and frequently localized to the joints upon ascent or within 24 hours of surfacing. Examination of the joints absent erythema and edema.
	Cutaneous DCS (skin bends): skin rash, itching, "insects crawling on skin." Mottled skin (cutis marmorata). Swelling in the axilla or groin. Lymphedema and tender lymph nodes.
	Type II
	Neurologic DCS: memory loss, difficulty speaking, vision changes, low back pain or abdominal pain, progressive limb numbness and tingling, loss of motor function, loss of bowel/bladder control within hours of ascent. Altered mental status, aphasia, ascending motor weakness, bowel or bladder incontinence.
	Vestibular DCS (the staggers): dizziness, nausea, vomiting, tinnitus upon ascent. Possible ataxia, hearing loss.
	Pulmonary DCS (the chokes): dry cough, chest pain. Rales/crackles (pulmonary edema), hypotension, death.
Pulmonary barotrauma	Pulmonary barotrauma includes diagnoses such as pneumomediastinum, mediastinal emphysema, subcutaneous emphysema, pneumothorax. Look for chest pain, chest fullness, coughing, or shortness of breath upon ascent.
	Pneumomediastinum and mediastinal emphysema: tachypnea, crepitus with cardiac auscultation (Hamman sign).
	Subcutaneous emphysema: hoarseness, difficulty swallowing. Crepitus of the chest, axilla, or neck.
	Pneumothorax: symptoms vary according to baseline pulmonary function and volume of air accumulating in the pleural space. Decreased or absent breath sounds. Possible hypotension and cardiovascular collapse if tension physiology develops.
Gastrointestinal barotrauma	Abdominal pain, nausea, belching, passing gas. Resolve upon resurfacing through eructation and flatus.
Barodontalgia	Dental pain upon ascent. Although rare, dental fractures may occur.

AGE, Arterial gas embolism; *CNS*, central nervous system; *DCS*, decompression sickness.
Data from Christiani D, Physical and chemical injuries of the lung. In: Goldman L, Schafer A, eds. *Goldman-Cecil Medicine*. 26th ed. Philadelphia: Elsevier; 2020:577-585; Murphy-Lavoie H, LeGros T. Dysbarisms, dive injuries, and decompression illness. In: *Emergency Medicine Clinical Essentials*. 2nd ed. Philadelphia: Saunders; 2008:1153-1161; Van Hoesen K, Lang M. Diving medicine. In: Auerbach P, ed. *Auerbach's Wildness Medicine*. 7th ed. Philadelphia: Elsevier; 2017:1583-1618; Smart D. Dysbarism. In: Cameron P, Little M, Biswadev M, Desey C, eds. *Textbook of Adult Emergency Medicine*. 5th ed. Philadelphia: Elsevier; 2020:706-713; and Bove AA. Diving medicine. *Am J Respir Crit Care Med*. 2014;189(12):1479-1486.

12. **How are dysbarisms treated in the prehospital setting?**
    Initial resuscitation should be in accordance with basic life support and advanced cardiac life support guidelines. Provide supplemental oxygen (100%). Triage the patient according to organizational protocols. Do not hesitate to consult a dive medicine expert who can assist with disposition and care (Divers' Alert Network (DAN) telephone numbers previously listed).

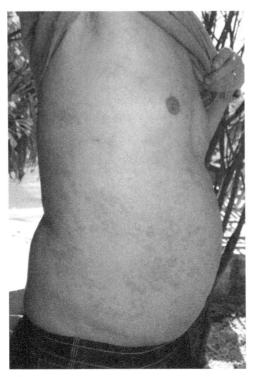

Fig. 58.2. Cutis marmorata. *(From Germonpre P, Balestra C, Obeid G, et al. Cutis marmorata skin decompression sickness is a manifestation of brainstem bubble embolization, not of local skin bubbles.* Med Hypothesis. *2015;85(6):863-869.)*

If DCS is suspected:
- Place the patient in the supine position (recovery position if unconscious) to avoid air embolization to the cerebral circulation.
- Administer oral or intravenous fluids, an action that may be lifesaving in severe DCS as hydration reduces venous gas emboli.
- Consider nonsteroidal anti-inflammatories (NSAIDs) if there are no contraindications. NSAIDs used as an adjuvant to hyperbaric oxygen therapy shorten recovery time for patients with DCS.
- Avoid hyperthermia, particularly in patients with neurologic symptoms.

If the patient has a pneumothorax, monitor for tension physiology requiring needle decompression or tube thoracostomy. Definitive treatment for DCS and AGE is hyperbaric oxygen therapy.

13. What are the considerations for air evacuation following a dive injury?
Exposure to low ambient air pressure may worsen DCS or AGE. If air evacuation is utilized, the aircraft should be pressurized to 1 atm or fly at low altitudes (≤150 m above the pickup location). In the patient with a pneumothorax, if you are licensed and credentialed, consider placing a chest tube prior to evacuation (Boyle's law: As altitude increases, air pressure decreases; therefore, the volume of gas in a confined space will increase. The pneumothorax will expand at altitude). For the same reason, weigh the risks and benefits of transporting a patient with subcutaneous emphysema. Airway compromise during flight may be a concern.

KEY POINTS

- Pilots, astronauts, compressed air workers, and scuba divers are at risk for dysbarisms.
- Middle ear barotrauma, also known as barotitis or ear squeeze, is the most common injury.
- AGE is a frequent cause of death among inexperienced scuba divers.
- DCS and AGE require recompression therapy.
- The prehospital treatment of dysbarisms is 100% supplemental oxygen and transport.

BIBLIOGRAPHY

Bove AA. Diving medicine. *Am J Respir Crit Care Med*. 2014;189(12):1479-1486.

Byyny R, Shockley L, Scuba diving dysbarism. In: Walls R, Hockberger R, Gausche-Hill M, eds. *Rosen's Emergency Medicine: Concepts and Clinical Practice*. Philadelphia: Elsevier; 2018:1773-1786.

Christiani D. Physical and chemical injuries of the lung. In: Goldman L, Schafer A, eds. *Goldman-Cecil Medicine*. Philadelphia: Elsevier; 2020:577-585.

Godden D, Currie G, Denison D, et al. British Thoracic Society Fitness to Dive Group: British Thoracic Society guidelines on respiratory aspects of fitness for diving. *Thorax*. 2003;58(1):3-13.

Mitchell SJ, Bennett MH, Bryson P, et al. Pre-hospital management of decompression illness: expert review of key principles and controversies. *Diving Hyperb Med*. 2018;48(1):25-55.

Murphy-Lavoie H, LeGros T. Dysbarisms, dive injuries, and decompression illness. In: Adams J, Barton E, Collings J, DeBlieux P, Gisondi M, Nadel E, eds. *Emergency Medicine Clinical Essentials*. Philadelphia: Saunders; 2008:1153-1161.

Smart D. Dysbarism. In: Cameron P, Little M, Biswadev M, Desey C, eds. *Textbook of Adult Emergency Medicine*. Philadelphia: Elsevier; 2020:706-713.

Van Hoesen K, Lang M. Diving medicine. In: Auerbach P, ed. *Auerbach's Wilderness Medicine*. Philadelphia: Elsevier; 2017:1583-1618.

CHAPTER 59

HEAT- AND COLD-RELATED ILLNESS

Erica M. Simon

QUESTIONS AND ANSWERS
HEAT-RELATED ILLNESS

1. What is the definition of a heat-related illness?

   An illness resulting from inadequate acclimatization, impaired heat dissipation, increased heat production, and/or an elevated wet bulb globe temperature.

2. How does the human body respond to heat and humidity?

   Sensors from the periphery alert the hypothalamus to an elevation in temperature. Signals are then sent to the sweat glands to begin producing sweat and to the vasculature to induce peripheral vasodilatation. In response to this vasodilation, the heart rate (HR) increases to maintain cardiac output (CO) (CO = HR × stroke volume [SV]).

3. What happens when physiologic cooling mechanisms fail?

   Increases in core temperature trigger the release of inflammatory mediators, causing cell damage. As blood is directed to the peripheral circulation, tissue hypoperfusion leads to organ ischemia. Ultimately, coagulopathy and organ failure result in death.

4. What is acclimatization?

   Acclimatization is the process of developing physiologic adaptations to environmental stress. After 7–14 days in heat and/or humidity, individuals experience an earlier onset of sweating (at lower core temperatures), increased sweat volume, and decreased sweat sodium concentration. During this time, aldosterone levels increase, expanding the plasma volume (increasing SV).

5. What are the risk factors for developing a heat-related illness?

   See Table 59.1.

6. What are the heat-related illnesses, and how do they present clinically?

   See Table 59.2 and Fig. 59.1.

7. Which conditions may masquerade as heat-related illnesses?

   See Table 59.3.

8. Which heat-related illnesses are commonly evaluated and treated in the prehospital setting?

   See Table 59.4.

9. What is classic heat stroke and how does it differ from exertional heat stroke?

   Classic heat stroke develops over days in older adults with chronic illnesses. Exertional heat stroke is sudden in onset; experienced by young athletes following periods of strenuous exercise.

Table 59.1. Risk Factors for Heat-Related Illness

INDIVIDUAL FACTORS	MECHANISM
Young age	As compared to adults: time to heat acclimatization is greater. Rate of sweat production is slower. Higher body surface area-to-mass ratio results in an increased rate of environmental heat absorption.
Advanced age	Decreased sweat gland function with age. Reduced ability to regulate vascular tone. Increased likelihood of comorbid medical conditions, which limit the body's ability to respond to heat stress.
Obesity	Adipose tissue produces more heat than lean muscle. Subcutaneous adipose restricts conductive heat transfer. An obese person has a smaller body surface area-to-mass ratio, reducing the efficacy of sweat evaporation.
Dehydration	Impairs the body's response to an elevated core temperature: Hypovolemia reduces SV. CO must therefore be maintained through an increase in HR; a compensatory response with limited sustainability.
Ethanol consumption	Predisposes to dehydration in the absence of water and electrolyte replacement.
Strenuous exercise	Increases heat production and raises the core temperature.
Heavy clothing	Hinders evaporative cooling through sweating.
Socioeconomic status	Limited access to transportation. Housing absent cooling mechanisms.
MEDICAL CONDITIONS	**MECHANISM**
Cardiovascular disease	Reduced ability to maintain CO when core temperature is elevated.
Pulmonary disease	Increased mortality in patients with asthma, chronic obstructive pulmonary disease (COPD), lung cancer, pneumonia, bronchitis, tuberculosis, and cystic fibrosis. Little evidence regarding the underlying mechanism. Reduced air quality accompanying heat waves is a leading hypothesis.
Hypertension	Hypertrophy of vascular smooth muscle and impaired response to neurohormonal mediators limit peripheral vasodilation.
Diabetes mellitus	Impaired thermoregulatory mechanisms secondary to hyperglycemia and/or neuropathy result in delayed responses to vasodilatory stimuli and decreased sweating.
Spinal cord injury	Thermoregulatory sensors from the periphery may be unable to alert the hypothalamus to alterations in temperature. Neurohormonal signaling to the sweat glands and peripheral vasculature is impaired.
Gastroenteritis	Profuse vomiting and diarrhea contribute to dehydration.
MEDICATIONS	**MECHANISM**
Anticholinergics	Decrease sweat production. Examples include ipratropium or tiotropium (asthma or COPD), oxybutynin (overactive bladder), benztropine mesylate (parkinsonism or dystonia), diphenhydramine (allergies), etc.
Antiepileptics	Topiramate and zonisamide inhibit sweating.
Atypical antipsychotics	Anticholinergic side effects. Patients may be taking olanzapine, risperidone, ziprasidone, aripiprazole, etc.
Stimulants or sympathomimetics	Increase bodily heat production and alter thermoregulatory mechanisms. Sweating and peripheral vasodilation begin at higher core temperatures. Cocaine, methamphetamine (Adderall or Ritalin for attention deficit disorder), ephedrine, (weight loss supplement), and pseudoephedrine (decongestant) are common examples.
Diuretics or laxatives	Reduce SV. Predispose to dehydration.
Beta-blockers or calcium channel blockers	Limit the cardiac response to increased core temperatures.

HR, Heart rate; *CO,* cardiac output; *SV,* stroke volume.

Data from Lipman GS, Gaudio FG, Eifling KP, et al. Wilderness Medical Society practice guidelines for the prevention and treatment of head illness: 2019 update. *Wilderness Environ Med.* 2019;S1080-6032(18)30199-6; and Cleland P. Heat-related illness. In: Kellerman R, Rakel D, eds. *Conn's Current Therapy.* Philadelphia: Elsevier; 2020:1259-1262.

Table 59.2. Heat-Related Illnesses

CONDITION	PRESENTATION
Heat rash	Pruritic vesicles on an erythematous base, confined to clothed areas. Heat rash results from blockage of sweat gland pores.
Heat edema	Self-limited swelling of the feet and ankles. The result of peripheral vasodilation and dependent positions (prolonged sitting or standing).
Heat cramps	Brief, severe cramps after exercise in muscles that have been fatigued. History of hypotonic fluid replacement and profuse sweating during activity. Frequently related to electrolyte derangement (hyponatremia and hypochloremia).
Heat syncope	Loss of consciousness secondary to dehydration and peripheral blood pooling.
Heat exhaustion	Alert and oriented patient with malaise, fatigue, and headache. Look for tachycardia and clinical signs of dehydration. Core temperature is often normal (if elevated, <40°C [104°F]).
Heat stroke	Sudden onset alteration of mental status (e.g., delirium, seizure, coma). Elevated core temperature (frequently >40°C [104°F]). Flushed and hot skin. Tachycardia. Tachypnea. Possible hypotension.

Data from Lipman GS, Gaudio, FG, Eifling KP, et al. Wilderness Medical Society practice guidelines for the prevention and treatment of head illness: 2019 update. *Wilderness Environ Med.* 2019;S1080-6032(18)30199-6; and Cleland P. Heat-related illness. In: Kellerman R, Rakel D, eds. *Conn's Current Therapy.* Philadelphia: Elsevier; 2019:1259-1262.

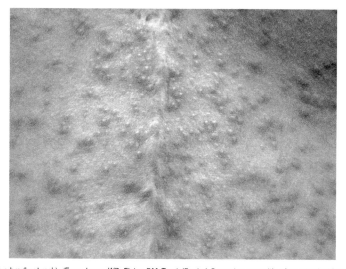

Fig. 59.1. Miliaria rubra (heat rash). *(From James WD, Elston DM, Treat JR, et al. Dermatoses resulting from physical factors. In: James WD, Berger T, Elston D, eds.* Andrews' Diseases of the Skin. *13th ed. Philadelphia: Elsevier; 2020.)*

COLD-RELATED ILLNESS

1. What is a cold-related illness?
   An illness resulting from environmental exposure or underlying medical conditions that alter thermoregulation. Cold-related illnesses include hypothermia, nonfreezing tissue injuries (frostnip, pernio, trench foot), and frostbite.

2. How does the human body lose heat, and what is the body's response to heat loss?
   Heat is lost primarily through transfer to the environment via electromagnetic radiation. Sweating and evaporation from the respiratory tract represent insensible losses. In response to heat loss, the hypothalamus sends signals to the thyroid to increase the basal metabolic rate. Simultaneously, the sympathetic nervous system stimulates constriction of peripheral arteries and veins, directing blood flow to the core. If the body is depleted of energy reserves, or if underlying medical conditions impair heat generation, the core temperature falls and cerebral

Table 59.3. Clinical Mimics of Heat-Related Illnesses

CONDITION	CLINICAL CLUES
Meningitis, encephalitis, or sepsis	History of recent illness or sick contacts. Meningismus.
Thyroid storm	History of Graves' disease. Agitated or altered patient with tachycardia or tachyarrhythmia and elevated core temperature. Lid lag and enlarged nodular goiter serve as clinical clues.
Neuroleptic malignant syndrome (NMS)	Patients prescribed dopamine receptor antagonists (haloperidol, droperidol, promethazine, chlorpromazine, etc.). NMS presents with altered mental status, fever, tachycardia, and diaphoresis. Look for "lead pipe" muscle rigidity.
Serotonin syndrome	Patients prescribed selective serotonin reuptake inhibitors (fluoxetine, escitalopram, etc.), tricyclic antidepressants (amitriptyline, doxepin, imipramine, etc.), or monoamine oxidase inhibitors (selegiline, phenelzine, tranylcypromine, etc.). Presents with fever, tachycardia, possible altered mental status. Differentiated by the presence of myoclonus.

Data from Lipman GS, Gaudio, FG, Eifling KP, et al. Wilderness Medical Society practice guidelines for the prevention and treatment of head illness: 2019 Update. *Wilderness Environ Med* 2019;S1080-6032(18)30199-6. and Cleland P. Heat-related illness. In: *Conn's Current Therapy.* Philadelphia: Elsevier; 2019:1259-1262.

Table 59.4. Heat-Related Illnesses and Prehospital Treatment

CONDITION	EVALUATION PEARLS	TREATMENT
Heat cramps	If limb pain is reported, history and physical exam should include an assessment for cellulitis and deep venous thrombosis.	Oral rehydration with an electrolyte solution. If severe, intravascular (IV) normal saline (0.9% NaCl). Caution in volume-sensitive patients: history of congestive heart failure. Local protocols dictate procedures; transport is rarely required.
Heat syncope	Auscultate for murmurs (aortic stenosis or regurgitation). Obtain a point-of-care (POC) blood glucose level; hypoglycemia may cause syncope. Perform an electrocardiogram. Assess for ischemia and arrhythmias.	Heat syncope is a diagnosis of exclusion. Patients frequently require transport to evaluate cardiac, neurocardiogenic, and metabolic etiologies of syncope.
Heat exhaustion	Obtain a core temperature. Perform a rapid neurologic exam. Patients with heat exhaustion are alert and oriented.	Place the patient in a cool, shaded area. Begin providing rapid hydration and salt replacement. Transport.
Heat stroke	Obtain a core temperature. Perform a rapid neurologic exam. If heat stroke is suspected, begin cooling measures immediately.	Perform initial resuscitation in accordance with basic life support (BLS) and advanced cardiac life support (ACLS) guidelines. Move the patient to a cool, shaded area. Remove all clothing. If possible, immerse the patient in cold water. If cold water immersion is unavailable, begin evaporative cooling with large circulating fans and skin misting. Ice packs may be placed in the axillae and groin as adjuncts. Obtain two large-bore IVs and initiate fluid resuscitation. If shivering occurs, consider benzodiazepines per protocol. Monitor core temperature once every 5 minutes. Discontinue cooling at 39°C (102.2°F) to prevent iatrogenic hypothermia. In a hypotense patient who does not respond to fluid resuscitation, avoid agents with alpha-adrenergic activity (e.g., norepinephrine), which cause peripheral vasoconstriction and limit cooling. Transport.

Data from Lipman GS, Gaudio FG, Eifling KP, et al. Wilderness Medical Society practice guidelines for the prevention and treatment of head illness: 2019 update. *Wilderness Environ Med.* 2019;S1080-6032(18)30199-6; and Cleland P. Heat-related illness. In: Kellerman R, Rakel D, eds. *Conn's Current Therapy.* Philadelphia: Elsevier; 2019:1259-1262.

perfusion suffers. Insufficient blood supply to respiratory centers of the brain results in reduced minute ventilation. Cold diuresis ensues as the release of antidiuretic hormone from the pituitary gland is inhibited. At 28°C–30°C (82.4°F–86°F), the majority of patients are unconscious. Bradycardia, arrhythmias, and hypotension predominate. Near 25°C (77°F), asystole is common.

3. What are the risk factors for cold-related illnesses?
   See Table 59.5.

Table 59.5. Risk Factors for Cold-Related Illnesses

INDIVIDUAL FACTORS	MECHANISM
Young age	As compared to adults: higher body surface area-to-mass ratio results in an increased rate of heat loss to the environment.
Advanced age	Reduced ability to regulate vascular tone. Increased likelihood of comorbid medical conditions that limit the body's ability to respond to cold stress.
Malnutrition	Shortage of energy reserves to generate heat.
Dehydration	Impairs the body's response to reduced core temperature: Hypovolemia reduces SV. Dehydration becomes particularly dangerous in the setting of cold diuresis.
Ethanol consumption	Predisposes to dehydration.
Strenuous activity	Increased heat loss through evaporative cooling.
Constricting or wet clothing/boots	Loss of heat through convection (e.g., transfer of heat to a fluid or gas).
Socioeconomic status	Homelessness. Inadequate clothing.
MEDICAL CONDITIONS	**MECHANISM**
Cardiovascular disease	Reduced ability to maintain CO when core temperature is decreased. In a healthy subject, CO is reduced to 45% at 25°C (77°F).
Diabetes mellitus	Impaired thermoregulatory mechanisms secondary to hyperglycemia and/or neuropathy result in delayed responses to vasoconstricting stimuli.
Spinal cord injury	Sensors from the periphery may be unable to alert the hypothalamus to alterations in temperature. Signaling to the peripheral vasculature may also be impaired.
Dermal disease	Burns, severe psoriasis, and exfoliative dermatitis: increase evaporative heat loss.
Acute trauma	Hypovolemia causes hypoperfusion. In the setting of hypoperfusion (depletion of cellular ATP), spontaneous hypothermia occurs.
Peripheral vascular disease	Insufficient peripheral circulation increases the risk for tissue injury.
MEDICATIONS	**MECHANISM**
Phenothiazines (typical antipsychotics)	Deplete catecholamine stores in the hypothalamus, reducing the body's ability to respond to hypothermia. Examples include thioridazine, prochlorperazine, chlorpromazine, fluphenazine, etc.
Sedative-hypnotics	Limit heat generation by inhibiting shivering. Impair cognition: inappropriate or absent response to environmental exposure. Clonazepam, lorazepam, diazepam, phenobarbital, and pentobarbital are sedative hypnotics.

ATP, Adenosine triphosphate; *CO*, cardiac output; *SV*, stroke volume.
Data from Stephen R. Hypothermia and frostbite. In: Adams J, Barton E, Collings J, DeBlieux P, Gisondi M, Nadel E, eds. *Emergency Medicine: Clinical Essentials*. 2nd ed. Philadelphia: Saunders; 2010:1142-1147.e1; Leikin J, Leikin S, Korley F, et al. Disturbances due to cold. In: Kellerman R, Rakel D, eds. *Conn's Current Therapy*. Philadelphia: Elsevier; 2019:1253-1259; and Zafren K, Danzl D. Accidental hypothermia. In: Tintinalli J, Ma J, Yealy D, Meckler G, Stapczynski J, Cline D, Thomas S, eds. *Rosen's Emergency Medicine: Concepts and Clinical Practice*. 9th ed. Philadelphia: Elsevier; 2018:1743-1754.e3.

4. How does a patient with hypothermia present, and what steps are taken in the prehospital setting to treat this condition?
See Table 59.6 and Fig. 59.2.

Table 59.6. Presentation and Treatment of Hypothermia

CONDITION	PRESENTATION	TREATMENT
Mild hypothermia 32.2°C–35°C (90°F–95°F)	Patient drowsy, shivering. Tachycardia. Tachypnea.	Passive external rewarming: Move the patient to a warm environment. Remove wet clothing. Wrap in blankets. Place warm packs in the axillae and groin. Provide oral hydration and food (energy for heat generation). Transport.
Moderate hypothermia 28°C–32.2°C (82.4°F–90°F)	Patient confused, lethargic, dysarthric. Possible shivering (ceases at < 30°C–32.2°C [86°F–90°F]). Bradycardia, hypotension, bradypnea. POC blood glucose: hyperglycemia (insulin ineffective outside of normal physiologic temperature range). Electrocardiogram (ECG): possible Osborn wave.	Modification to BLS guidelines: Assess breathing and pulse for 30–40 seconds. If the patient is not breathing, begin rescue breathing (utilize warmed [40°C–45°C], humidified oxygen through the bag valve mask). Remove wet clothing gently due to the irritable myocardium. Do not apply external warming devices in the field. For hypothermic patients in cardiac arrest with pulseless ventricular tachycardia or ventricular fibrillation: Deliver up to three shocks to determine responsiveness. If the rhythm is refractory, begin cardiopulmonary resuscitation and active internal warming (warm, humidified oxygen and warmed IV saline [40°C–42°C] if available). Contact medical control for disposition: extracorporeal membrane oxygenation may be considered. Transport in the horizontal position to avoid worsening hypotension.
Severe hypothermia <28°C (82.4°F)	Patient unresponsive. Pupils fixed and dilated. Muscular rigidity present. Bradycardia. Hypotension. Bradypnea or apnea. POC blood glucose as above. ECG: atrial fibrillation, ventricular fibrillation, or asystole.	Modification to ALS guidelines: If the patient has not developed cardiac arrest, focus on support of the airway, breathing, and circulation. Intubate patients who cannot protect their airway. External pacing may be worth trying in profound bradycardia (follow local protocols). In the setting of cardiac arrest, the hypothermic heart may be unresponsive to cardioactive drugs, pacemaker stimulation, and defibrillation. Begin active internal warming with warm, humidified, oxygen and warmed IV saline. If the patient fails to respond to initial drug therapy and/or three defibrillation attempts, additional medication boluses and defibrillations should be held until the patient's core temperature is >30°C (86°F). Contact medical control for disposition: extracorporeal membrane oxygenation may be considered. Transport in the horizontal position to avoid worsening hypotension.

ALS, Advanced life support; *BLS*, basic life support; *IV*, intravenous; *POC*, point of care.
Data from Stephen R. Hypothermia and frostbite. In: Adams J, Barton E, Collings J, DeBlieux P, Gisondi M, Nadel E, eds. *Emergency Medicine: Clinical Essentials.* 2nd ed. Philadelphia: Saunders; 2010:1142-1147.e1; Leikin J, Leikin S, Korley F, et al. Disturbances due to cold. In: Kellerman R, Rakel D, eds. *Conn's Current Therapy.* Philadelphia: Elsevier; 2019:1253-1259; and Zafren K, Danzl D. Accidental hypothermia. In: Tintinalli J, Ma J, Yealy D, Meckler G, Stapczynski J, Cline D, Thomas S, eds.*Rosen's Emergency Medicine: Concepts and Clinical Practice.* 9th ed. Philadelphia: Elsevier; 2018:1743-1754.e3; and the American Heart Association.

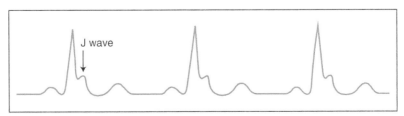

Fig. 59.2. Osborn wave. *(From Yentis S, Hirsch NP, Ip J.* Anaesthesia, Intensive Care and Perioperative Medicine A-Z: An Encyclopaedia of Principles and Practice. *6th ed. Philadelphia: Elsevier; 2019.)*

5. Which illnesses can mimic hypothermia?
See Table 59.7.

6. What are the nonfreezing tissue injuries, how do they present, and how are they treated?
See Table 59.8 and Figs. 59.3–59.5.

Table 59.7. Clinical Mimics of Cold-Related Illnesses

CONDITION	CLINICAL CLUES
Sepsis	Sepsis due to gram-negative pathogen infection is most commonly associated with hypothermia. History of recent illness or sick contacts.
Severe hypothyroidism (myxedema coma)	Inability to increase the body's basal metabolic rate to generate heat. History of hypothyroidism. Look for delayed relaxation of reflexes and nonpitting edema of the lower extremities. Patient may have ptosis, thin hair, and dry skin.
Adrenal insufficiency	Glucocorticoid and/or mineralocorticoid deficiency. History of fatigue, malaise, weight loss, nausea, vomiting, diarrhea. Skin hyperpigmentation. Hypotension. Possible hypoglycemia on POC blood glucose assessment.
Brain tumor, stroke, acute head trauma	Hinder interpretation of thermoregulatory signals. Question the patient regarding previous medical history, morning headaches, unintended weight loss, night sweats, vision alterations. Look for acute trauma.

POC, Point of care.
Data from Stephen R. Hypothermia and frostbite. In: Adams J, Barton E, Collings J, DeBlieux P, Gisondi M, Nadel E, eds. *Emergency Medicine: Clinical Essentials*. 2nd ed. Philadelphia: Saunders; 2010:1142-1147.e1; Leikin J, Leikin S, Korley F, et al. Disturbances due to cold. In: Kellerman R, Rakel D, eds. *Conn's Current Therapy*. Philadelphia: Elsevier; 2019:1253-1259; and Zafren K, Danzl D. Accidental hypothermia. In: Tintinalli J, Ma J, Yealy D, Meckler G, Stapczynski J, Cline D, Thomas S, eds. *Rosen's Emergency Medicine: Concepts and Clinical Practice*. 9th ed. Philadelphia: Elsevier; 2018:1743-1754.e3.

Table 59.8. Nonfreezing Tissue Injuries

CONDITION	MECHANISM	PRESENTATION	TREATMENT
Frostnip	Superficial, nonfreezing cold injury associated with vasoconstriction	Frost formation on the surface of the skin. Transient numbness. Tingling. Pallor. Erythema and edema develop with rewarming.	Self-resolving: move the patient to a warm environment. Remove wet clothing. Insulate the affected area. Do not use dry heat to warm (increases risk of tissue injury due to burns). Transport per protocol.
Pernio (chilblains)	Vasculitis resulting from repeated, intermittent exposure to cold, wet conditions	Burning paresthesias and itching. Erythema, edema, and skin lesions (nodules, plaques) involving the dorsum of the hands and the feet. Lesions appear within 12 hours of exposure.	Remove wet clothing. Insulate, splint, and elevate the extremity. Do not warm with dry heat. Provide analgesia as indicated. Nonsteroidal anti-inflammatories advised. Transport.
Cold immersion (trench foot)	Ischemic injury from sustained vasoconstriction	Paresthesias, skin mottling. Extremity insensate and possibly pulseless. Upon rewarming: severe, burning pain. Edema, blisters.	

Data from Stephen R. Hypothermia and frostbite. In: Adams J, Barton E, Collings J, DeBlieux P, Gisondi M, Nadel E, eds. *Emergency Medicine: Clinical Essentials*. 2nd ed. Philadelphia: Saunders; 2010:1142-1147.e1; Leikin J, Leikin S, Korley F, et al. Disturbances due to cold. In: Kellerman R, Rakel D, eds. *Conn's Current Therapy*. Philadelphia: Elsevier; 2019:1253-1259; and Zafren K, Danzl D. Accidental hypothermia. In: Tintinalli J, Ma J, Yealy D, Meckler G, Stapczynski J, Cline D, Thomas S, eds. *Rosen's Emergency Medicine: Concepts and Clinical Practice*. 9th ed. Philadelphia: Elsevier; 2018:1743-1754.e3.

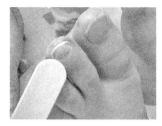

Fig. 59.3. Frostnip. *(From Ferri FF. Diseases and disorders. In: Ferri F, Studdiford J, Tully A, eds.* Ferri's Fast Facts in Dermatology. *2nd ed. Philadelphia: Elsevier; 2019).*

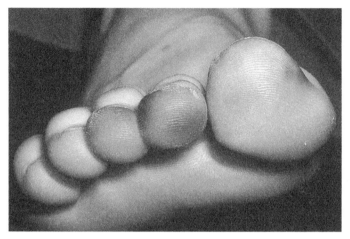

Fig. 59.4. Pernio (chilblains). *(From James WD, Elston DM, Treat JR, et al. Dermatoses resulting from physical factors. In: James WD, Elston DM, Treat JR, et al., eds.* Andrews' Diseases of the Skin. *13th ed. Philadelphia: Elsevier; 2020.)*

7. What is frostbite, how does it present, and how is it treated?
   See Table 59.9 and Fig. 59.6.

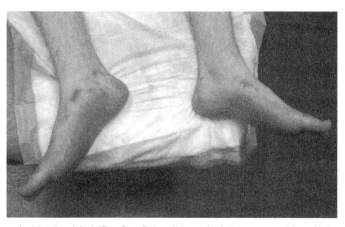

Fig. 59.5. Cold immersion injury (trench foot). (*From Olson Z, Kman N. Immersion foot: a case report.* J Emerg Med. *2015;49(2):e45.)*

Table 59.9. Presentation and Treatment of Frostbite.

CONDITION	MECHANISM	PRESENTATION	TREATMENT
Frostbite	Deposits of ice crystals cause cellular damage and activate the clotting cascade. Vessel thrombosis leads to tissue hypoperfusion, ischemia, and necrosis.	Dusky or white extremity. Insensate. Absent capillary refill. Possible hemorrhagic or clear blisters and tissue necrosis.	Move the patient to a warm environment. Remove wet clothing. Apply dry, sterile dressings (separate involved digits). Splint and elevate the extremity. Do not rewarm with dry heat. Administer analgesia. Transport.

Data from Stephen R. Hypothermia and frostbite. In: *Emergency Medicine: Clinical Essentials.* 2nd ed. Philadelphia: Saunders; 2010:1142-1147.e1; Leikin J, Leikin S, Korley F, et al. Disturbances due to cold. In: *Conn's Current Therapy.* Philadelphia: Elsevier; 2019:1253-1259; and Zafren K, Danzl D. Accidental hypothermia. In: *Rosen's Emergency Medicine: Concepts and Clinical Practice.* 9th ed. Philadelphia: Elsevier; 2018:1743-1754.e3.

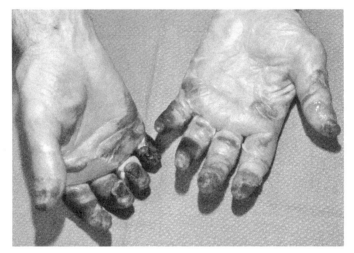

Fig. 59.6. Frostbite. *(From James WD, Elston DM, Treat JR, et al. Dermatoses resulting from physical factors. In: James W, Berger T, Elston D, eds.* Andrews' Diseases of the Skin. *13th ed. Philadelphia: Elsevier; 2020.)*

KEY POINTS

- Heat stroke can be differentiated from heat exhaustion by the presence of altered mental status.
- In the setting of cold-related injuries, do not rewarm the tissues with dry heat as this may lead to burns.
- As physiologic temperatures alter the effectivity of defibrillation and medications, BLS and ALS are modified in the setting of moderate and severe hypothermia.

BIBLIOGRAPHY

Balmain BN, Sabapathy S, Louis M, et al. Aging and thermoregulatory control: the clinical implications of exercising and heat stress in older individuals. *Biomed Res Int.* 2018;8306154. eCollection.

Cleland P, Heat-related illness. In: Kellerman R, Rakel D, eds. *Conn's Current Therapy.* Philadelphia: Elsevier; 2019:1259-1262.

Ferri F, Heat exhaustion and heat stroke. In: Ferri F, Studdiford J, Tully A, eds. *Ferri's Clinical Advisor 2020.* Philadelphia: Elsevier; 2020:637-638. e1.

Guidelines 2000 for cardiopulmonary resuscitation emergency cardiovascular care. Part 8: advanced challenges in resuscitation: section 3: special challenges in ECC. The American Heart Association in collaboration with the International Liaison Committee on Resuscitation. *Circulation.* 2010;102(8 suppl):12229-21252.

Leikin J, Leikin S, Korley F, et al. Disturbances due to cold. In: Kellerman R, Rakel D, eds. *Conn's Current Therapy*. Philadelphia: Elsevier; 2019:1253-1259.

Lipman GS, Gaudio FG, Eifling KP, et al. Wilderness Medical Society practice guidelines for the prevention and treatment of head illness: 2019 update. *Wilderness Environ Med*. 2019;S1080-6032(18):30199-30206.

Stephen R, Hypothermia and frostbite. In: Adams J, Barton E, Collings J, DeBlieux P, Gisondi M, Nadel E, eds. *Emergency Medicine: Clinical Essentials*. Philadelphia: Saunders; 2010:1142-1147. e1.

Zafren K, Danzl D, Accidental hypothermia. In: Tintinalli J, Ma J, Yealy D, Meckler G, Stapczynski J, Cline D, Thomas S, eds. *Rosen's Emergency Medicine: Concepts and Clinical Practice*. Philadelphia: Elsevier; 2018:1743-1754. e3.

CHAPTER 60

LIGHTNING AND ELECTRICAL EMERGENCIES

Andrew T. Krack and Selena Hariharan

QUESTIONS AND ANSWERS

Case: Four utility workers are assessing damage to a high-voltage power line transformer. One worker drops a wrench, creating an arc flash, with resultant flash of light and explosion. They are thrown. EMS arrives 7 minutes after the explosion to find three of the men in various stages of distress and a fourth man in cardiopulmonary arrest.

1. Which of the men should be the first to receive medical care?
   The man in cardiopulmonary arrest should be attended to first. In mass casualty incidents involving electrical injury, especially for lightning strike injuries, which are particularly amenable to resuscitation, reverse triage may be appropriate.

2. What are the priorities for a first responder prior to transport?
   First, an EMS provider must ensure personal safety by making sure they are not personally exposed to the electrical charge. Contrary to popular lore, standard rubber boots or jackets are not grounding or protective. Once the first responder has ensured their safety and discontinued electrical exposure for the victim, they should start resuscitation. EMS providers should assess circulation and cardiac rhythm as electrical forces may induce dysrhythmia or cardiac arrest. This can be done with a formal electrocardiogram (EKG) or with an automated external defibrillator (AED) to facilitate defibrillation and cardiopulmonary resuscitation (CPR). Simultaneously, while maintaining cervical spine stability given the risk of spinal cord injury even without obvious trauma, a first responder should maintain the airway and provide ventilatory support if needed. While fractures and other injuries are stabilized, fluids can then be started given the significant risk of rhabdomyolysis.

3. What factor(s) contributed to the current state of these men?
   A. Thermal burns
   B. Blast/blunt traumatic injury
   C. True electrical injury
   D. Both A and C
   E. All of the above
   Answer: E
   Electrical injury victims can suffer from both primary electrical injuries and burns and secondary traumatic injuries. Prehospital providers should be aware of several potential mechanisms of injury: thermal (heat burns), mechanical (blast or blunt traumatic), and true electrical (with a component of both thermal heat and nonthermal electrical forces).
   The degree of true electrical injury is predicted by (1) Kouwenhoven's factors: current type (direct current [DC] vs. alternating current [AC]), strength of current (amperage, I), voltage (V), duration of exposure, body resistance (R, Ohms), and the pathway the current takes through the body; and (2) electrical field strength: the intensity of electricity across the area to which it is applied. Joule's law explains why tissues with higher resistance sustain more significant injuries: as electrical current passes through tissues with high resistance (e.g., tendons), heat is produced.
   Arc flash, AC or DC currents, and, rarely, lightning can all result in thermal injuries, either superficially, through skin contact with superheated objects (metal, moisture, blast fragments) or burning clothing, or internally, due to body tissues acting as resistors and being heated to supraphysiologic temperatures.
   Nonthermal true electrical injuries occur in the presence of high electric field strength. Cell membranes of muscle fiber myocytes and nerves of both the central and autonomic nervous systems seem to be most susceptible to these nonthermal forces.
   Arc flash, high-voltage DC, and lightning exposure can also result in blast or traumatic injuries from compressive shock waves (e.g., thunder) or patients being thrown into or from objects.

4. Is electrical shock from a high-voltage DC or low-voltage household AC source more dangerous?
   It depends. Voltage is related to current through Ohm's law, $I = V/R$, where I is the current through the conductor (body tissues), V is the potential voltage difference measured *across* the conductor, and R is the resistance of the conductor (the various tissues).

Voltage is classified as low ($\leq$1000 V) or high (>1000 V). Voltage exposures as low as 24 V could be lethal. Theoretically, increased dose of voltage exposure increases risk of serious injury. However, high-voltage DC exposure tends to induce a singular forceful muscular contraction throughout the victim's body, often throwing them from the source, shortening exposure time. Low-voltage AC exposure (household circuits, 120 V or 240 V) is more likely to induce tetany. Because the flexors of the forearm are stronger than the extensors, grasping a frayed electrical cord can result in a "no-let-go" phenomenon, prolonging source exposure time.

Ultimately, the degree of true electrical injury is dependent on the amount and location of current exposure.

5. You are called to a construction worksite to evaluate a patient who "received an electrical shock" from a 240 V high-powered appliance. When you arrive, he is alert, talking, and refuses transport. He has no visible burns and states that if he leaves the job site, he will be replaced, and he needs the money. Which of the following statements is accurate?
   A. You should do an ECG, and if it is normal, you can feel safe leaving and tell him to call back if he feels unwell.
   B. You do not need to do any testing because this was not a lightning strike or a power line, rather a wall outlet injury and he has no risk.
   C. You should encourage him to accept transport because there is a risk of delayed arrhythmia or myocardial injury.
   D. You should check his urine for gross blood, and if it is normal, allow him to return to work.
   E. You should report him to his union representative.

Answer: C

While it is true that most well-appearing patients with a normal exam and EKG who have experienced a low-voltage electrical injury can be safely observed for a short period and discharged, even people who have not experienced a significant shock that results in muscle tetany and causes prolonged exposure to an electrical current may experience significant injury. If the electrical current arc crosses the myocardium, either from hand to hand (horizontal) or from head or hand to foot (vertical), it can cause multiple types of cardiac injury.

The first injury is an arrhythmia. The type of arrhythmia can vary from sinus tachycardia and premature ventricular contractions that self-resolve all the way to ventricular defibrillation that results in cardiac arrest. While the arrhythmia, especially if catastrophic, usually occurs proximate to the injury, there are cases where the arrhythmia presents hours later; these patients responded well to antiarrhythmic therapy.

The second injury is direct insult to the myocardium itself. Speculation as to the cause of the injury is rampant and the findings are nonspecific as T-wave and ST-segment changes may be harbingers of arrhythmia. Creatine kinase (CK) elevations are also seen with muscle injury from the described tetany, and ischemia from cardiac arrest can cause organ failure.

Ultimately, while the patient in this case cannot be forced to accept transport, he should be encouraged to seek care as he is at risk of cardiac complication given the higher-voltage injury and the risk for delayed complications. If he refuses, he should sign a refusal to transport. If he agrees, he should be transported with cardiac monitoring in place.

6. You are called to a summer camp for a potential lightning strike victim. A group of boys were hiking in the woods when they were caught in a pop-up thunderstorm. They took shelter under a grouping of trees. Without warning, there was a flash of lightning and one boy was thrown about 4 feet. His friends rushed to him and helped him stand up. Since then, he has complained of dizziness and "weakness and tingling" in the arms and hands. As the first responder, you immediately immobilize the patient because you are worried about what type of injury?
   A. Central cord syndrome
   B. Anterior cord syndrome
   C. Brown Sequard syndrome
   D. Complete spinal cord transection
   E. Epidural hematoma

Answer: A

Central cord syndrome is the most common incomplete cervical spinal cord injury. It causes disproportionate motor and sensation loss in the arms (though some loss can occur in the lower extremities also) and bladder function changes. Several described spinal cord syndromes each present with varying combinations of motor and sensory deficits.

People who are struck by lightning are susceptible to various injuries. People often think that if a person escapes cardiac arrest or burn, they are safe. Unfortunately, that is not true. While there are characteristic burns like punctate local burns and partial thickness burns, severe burns are relatively uncommon due to limited contact of the lightning with the victim. Significant burns usually occur at the site of jewelry or other metal on the body. Instead, victims are at risk of blunt force trauma from falls, being thrown, falling debris, electrocution from contact with water during the strike, or muscle injury. Some victims may also demonstrate significant autonomic dysfunction with paralysis and fixed dilated pupils, coined keraunoparalysis, which mimics death but is a transient state.

Given the significant risk of spinal cord injury, even without obvious deficit, first responders must maintain spinal precautions during all phases of resuscitation to avoid secondary injury while simultaneously maintaining circulation, airway, and breathing.

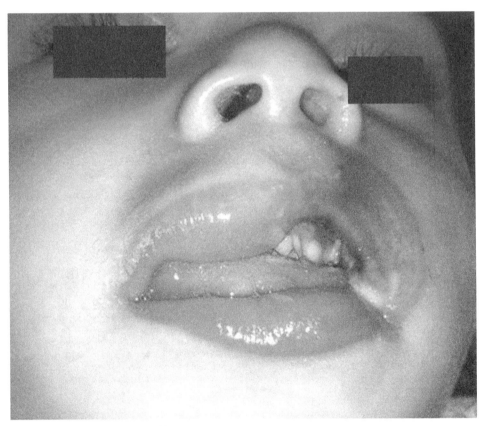

Fig. 60.1. An oral commissure burn in a toddler.

7. A curious, teething toddler exploring her home finds a weathered extension cord that serves to soothe her aching gums. The girl sustains burns to the lips and left oral commissure (Fig. 60.1). The parents heard an immediate cry with no witnessed loss of consciousness. They also note a slight burn to her left palm.
   What complications should be considered?
   A. Rhabdomyolysis
   B. Bleeding
   C. Airway compromise
   D. All of the above
   Answer: D
   Children with oral burns are at risk of exsanguination and airway compromise due to delayed labial artery bleed at the time of eschar separation. Historically, these children were admitted for up to 2 weeks until eschar separation with a dental device created to attempt to minimize contracture; this practice has been more recently liberalized, with a focus on strict return precautions.
       Equally concerning but easily dismissed is the burn on the hand. With any electrical injury, it is possible to have minimal external signs of injury with significant internal thermal/nonthermal electrical injuries. For this same reason, the Parkland formula/Rule of Nines tends to underestimate fluid requirements in electrical burn patients; these patients should be managed similarly to crush injury patients. This patient should also be evaluated for multisystem injury (cardiac, respiratory, nervous, integumentary, musculoskeletal, renal, and ophthalmologic) and may need to be admitted for observation.

8. What injuries are associated with Tasers?
   Touch stun exposure with a Taser (direct contact with the end of the device) of <15 seconds in the awake, alert patient does not require EKG, prolonged cardiac monitoring, ECHO, labs (troponin, CK, or electrolytes), prolonged emergency department (ED) observation, or hospitalization. Minor, clinically insignificant burns may occur at

contact sites. For probe stun exposure (propelled metal projectiles), penetrating barbs may cause injury to the eyes or superficial soft tissue structures (skin, vessels, nerves, bones), and muscle contractions can result in spinal compression fractures. Blunt trauma may also result from falls due to neuromuscular incapacitation.

KEY POINTS

- Consider reverse triage for mass casualty electrical injuries, especially lightning strikes, with a focus on dysrhythmias.
- Initiate ATLS, ACLS, ABLS, and PALS protocols, even with seemingly innocuous injuries.
- There may be minimal external signs of electrical injury even in the setting of severe internal injuries.
- Body location and amount of delivered current, dependent on not only voltage and resistance but also exposure time, are the best predictors of injury severity.
- Be aware of delayed arrhythmia and myocardial injury. Transport is encouraged for even innocuous appearing injuries.

BIBLIOGRAPHY

Arnoldo BD, Purdue GF. The diagnosis and management of electrical injuries. *Hand Clin.* 2009;25(4):469-479.

Jensen PJ, Thomsen PEB, Bagger JP, Norgaard A, Baandrup U. Electrical injury causing ventricular arrhythmias. *Br Heart J.* 1987;57(3):279-283.

Kang S, Kufta K, Sollecito TP, Panchal N. A treatment algorithm for the management of intraoral burns: a narrative review. *Burns.* 2018;44(5):1065-1076.

LeCompte EJG, Goldman BM. Oral electrical burns in children—early treatment and appliance fabrication. *Pediatric Denistry.* 1982;4(4):333-337.

Lubin J. Electrical injuries. In: Cone D, Brice J, Delbridge T, Myers B, eds. *Emergency Medical Services: Clinical Practice and Systems Oversight, Volume 1.* West Sussex, UK: Wiley; 2015:243-248.

ten Duis HJ, Klasen HJ, Reenalda PE. Keraunoparalysis, a 'specific' lightning injury. *Burns Incl Therm Inj.* 1985;12(1):54-57.

Waldmann V, Narayanan K, Combes N, Jost D, Jouven X, Marijon E. Electrical cardiac injuries: current concepts and management. *Eur Heart J.* 2018;39(16):1459-1465.

Zafren K, Durrer B, Herry JP, Brugger H, ICAR and UIAA MEDCOM. Lightning injuries: prevention and on-site treatment in mountains and remote areas. Official guidelines of the International Commission for Mountain Emergency Medicine and the Medical Commission of the International Mountaineering and Climbing Federation (ICAR and UIAA MEDCOM). *Resuscitation.* 2005;65(3):369-372.

CHAPTER 61

DROWNING AND SUBMERSION INJURY

Stephanie Lareau and Christopher Davis

QUESTIONS AND ANSWERS

1. What is drowning?

   Drowning is "the process of experiencing respiratory impairment due to submersion or immersion in liquid." Depending on outcomes, drowning can further be divided into drowning with morbidity, drowning with mortality, or drowning with neither morbidity nor mortality. Terms such as *near drowning*, *dry drowning*, and *delayed drowning* should be avoided as they are outdated and are not clinically based.

2. What causes mortality or morbidity in drowning?

   Drowning causes respiratory impairment, which leads to hypoxia. Cardiac arrest is typically secondary to hypoxia. Therefore, in resuscitation, focus should be placed on providing rescue breaths, positive pressure ventilation, and oxygen.

3. What is shallow water blackout?

   Typically, respiratory drive is initiated by hypercarbia. Often, when people are free diving or having breath-holding contests underwater, they will hyperventilate beforehand, lowering their carbon dioxide load. They can then become hypoxic before their carbon dioxide levels rise enough to give the sensation of needing to take a breath and they pass out.

4. Who is most at risk for drowning?

   Risk factors for drowning include male sex, pediatrics (<14), alcohol use, low socioeconomic status, lack of supervision, and risky behavior. Drowning is the second leading cause of injury-related death in children ages 1–4 in the United States. Underlying medical conditions, especially epilepsy, can increase the risk of drowning. Epileptic patients have a 15–19 times higher risk of drowning.

5. What comorbidities should be considered in drowning?

   Seizure disorders increase the chances of drowning as during seizure activity, patients are unable to maintain their posture in the water and, subsequently, their airways. Cardiac conditions such as prolonged QT syndrome or acute coronary syndrome can lead to drowning. Also consider low blood sugar. Trauma and spinal injury from diving injuries can also lead to drowning. Resuscitation of drowning should not be delayed assessing for these conditions, but they should be assessed for and managed concurrently.

6. What is in water resuscitation and when is it effective?

   In water resuscitation (IWR) consists of rescue breaths; chest compressions are ineffective in the water. IWR is advocated for trained professionals in shallow water or when a flotation device is available. One retrospective case series of patients rescued with IWR by trained lifeguards in Brazil shows significant survival benefit and decrease in neurological injury. IWR may increase the likelihood of favorable outcome by threefold. As drowning is a respiratory process, in which cardiac arrest occurs due to hypoxia, the concept is that limiting the hypoxia time should improve survival.

7. What should the priority be in resuscitation?

   As cardiac arrest in drowning is due to profound hypoxia from respiratory impairment, focus should be on establishing an airway and providing oxygen. Unlike the current layperson cardiopulmonary resuscitation (CPR) guidelines, which focus on hands-only CPR, rescue breaths and establishing an airway are of utmost priority in the drowning patient. Ongoing hypoxia leads to worse neurological outcomes and decreased survival. The European Resuscitation Council emphasizes the importance of airway/breathing by recommending five initial rescue breaths instead of the typical two. This emphasizes the importance of reversing respiratory impairment and acknowledges that air exchange may be limited due to aspiration.

8. Should the abdominal thrust be performed in drowning?

   The abdominal thrust was suggested in drowning resuscitation as a way to force aspirated water out of the lungs. There is no conclusive evidence that this technique is effective, and there is concern that it may delay oxygenation, leading to further harm from hypoxia. The abdominal thrust is not recommended.

9. Should all patients with drowning have their cervical spine immobilized?

The incidence of cervical spine injuries in patients with drowning is very low (0.5%–5%) and is typically associated with diving injuries. Cervical spine immobilization should be performed per local protocol or considered in the setting of blunt trauma with significant mechanism for injury, altered mental status (Glasgow Coma Scale [GCS] score <15), focal neurological deficit, or significant distracting injury.

Cervical spine immobilization can make airway management more challenging and increase aspiration in vomiting, so it should be used only when clinically indicated.

10. How should you deal with frothy sputum?

In drowning patients, airways are often obstructed with copious secretions. Extra time should not be wasted trying to suction out all the secretions. Ventilation and oxygenation are paramount, so oropharyngeal or suctioning from the endotracheal tube should not delay attempts at ventilation. The suction-assisted laryngoscopy airway decontamination (SALAD) methods for the drowned airway algorithm are described, in which intubation is attempted using a large-bore suction catheter. The catheter can be parked near the esophagus while direct or video laryngoscopy can be performed or alternatively the suction catheter can be used to intubate, then a bougie can then be placed through the suction catheter, using a Seldinger technique to establish a definite airway.

11. Who should be transported to a hospital or observed?

You should have a low threshold for transport to a hospital or at minimum observation for a drowning patient. Patients with cardiac arrest, respiratory distress, altered mental status, trauma, or abnormal vital signs should be immediately transported to the hospital. Observation can be considered for patients with no respiratory symptoms and completely normal respiratory exam.

12. How long should someone with a drowning event be observed?

Patients with very mild symptoms and a normal exam should be observed for 4 to 6 hours. After this time period, it is highly unlikely further symptoms will develop. The entity of delayed drowning, which is often mentioned in the media, is not well described in the medical literature.

13. What steps should be taken to rescue someone from the water?

Rescuer safety is paramount in drowning events. The only thing worse than one victim is multiple victims. Unless you have specialized training, you should first try to reach the victim with your voice and guide them to safety. Next, consider reaching with a long object (pole, tree limb, or paddle) to pull them to safety. Next, consider throwing a rope (never tie ropes around anything as this poses an entrapment hazard) or flotation device. Finally, consider going to the person only with proper training and some form of flotation.

KEY POINTS

- *Drowning* is a term than encompasses all respiratory impairment from immersion or submersion in water.
- Cardiac arrest due to drowning is a respiratory process, so initial resuscitation attempts should focus on immediate airway management.
- Comorbidities or the cause of drowning such as hypoglycemia, seizures, or cardiac events should be considered in the medical management of patients.
- Unless there is history of or mechanism suggestive of trauma, cervical spine immobilization does not have to be performed in all drowning patients.

BIBLIOGRAPHY

Farkas J. PulmCrit—Drown Airway Algorithm: Cut to the chase. https://emcrit.org/pulmcrit/drowned-airway-algorithm/.
Schmidt AC, Sempsrott JR, Hawkins SC, Aristos AS, Cushing TA, Auerbach PS. Wilderness Medical Society practice guidelines for the prevention and treatment of drowning. *Wilderness Environ Med.* 2016;27(2):236-251.
Szpilman D, Bierens JJ, Handley AJ, Orlowski JP. Drowning. *N Engl J Med.* 2012;366:2102-2110.

CHAPTER 62

INTERFACILITY TRANSPORT, INCLUDING GROUND CRITICAL CARE TRANSPORT

Philip S. Nawrocki and Matthew Poremba

QUESTIONS AND ANSWERS

1. What is an interfacility transport?

   Interfacility transport is the movement of a patient from one healthcare facility to another by licensed EMS personnel.

2. What are the reasons patients may need to be transferred between healthcare facilities?

   Interfacility transports in the healthcare industry take place for many reasons. They may be as simple as a wheelchair van transport of a patient from a long-term care facility to a scheduled appointment or as complex as the transfer of a critically ill intubated patient on multiple drips and advanced devices by rotor-wing aircraft to a quaternary care center. The decision for transfer should always be based upon the benefits of care versus the risks involved.

3. What does the term "regionalization of care" mean, and what are the implications for EMS?

   Regionalization of care is a method to provide high-quality, cost-efficient healthcare to the largest number of patients. In 2006, the Institute of Medicine (IOM) supported the process of regionalization of emergency care services in their white paper entitled "Emergency Medical Services: At the Crossroads". This paper defined regionalization as the "process of improving patient outcomes by directing patients to facilities with experience and optimal capabilities for any given type of illness or injury." The benefits of this strategy include improved outcomes through increased volumes and decreased costs through economies of scale. One challenge of this strategy has been an increased strain on the EMS system through increased numbers of interfacility transports.

4. How should hospitals without specialty services plan for interfacility transport of critically ill or injured patients?

   Hospitals that transfer critically ill or injured patients with time-sensitive conditions should have preexisting transfer agreements with EMS agencies and receiving hospitals to minimize the time necessary for transfer. For example, a local hospital without trauma services should have agreements with regional air medical transport services and trauma centers to ensure that critically injured patients have rapid access to critical care transport and definitive care. This requires that EMS agencies must ensure adequate capability to perform such transfers, and receiving facilities must ensure availability of sufficient personnel and resources to rapidly receive these patients.

5. Is there a federal law that requires the provision of emergency medical care in the United States and provides rules for interfacility transport?

   Enacted by Congress in 1986, the Emergency Medical Treatment and Labor Act (EMTALA) requires that anyone presenting to an emergency department to be stabilized and treated regardless of their insurance status or ability to pay. This was designed to prevent hospitals from not treating uninsured patients or transferring them to other hospitals for care based upon the ability to pay. EMTALA also provides specific rules for how patients are transferred from one hospital to another.

6. You respond to a local community hospital for a 57-year-old male who has had intermittent chest pain today. His cardiologist would like him transferred to the university hospital for possible surgery. What are the rules regarding EMTALA that must be followed when transferring a patient from one healthcare facility to another?

   If a patient does not have an emergency medical condition or the referring physician determines the patient is stable, meaning no risk of material deterioration during transfer, then EMTALA does not apply. In most cases, patients will have an emergency medical condition or at least some degree of risk of deterioration during transport. In these cases, the referring physician is required to:
   - Certify that the benefits of transfer outweigh the risks.
   - Inform the patient (or person acting on their behalf) of the risks and benefits of transfer to another facility.
   - Continue to treat the patient within the hospital's capabilities and capacity.
   - Obtain consent from the receiving hospital to accept transfer and ensure that they have the capacity to handle the transfer.
   - Ensure that the transport is effected through qualified personnel and transport equipment.

7. Your EMS service responds to an eight-bed community hospital with no obstetrics capabilities, for a 24-year-old female patient who is 34 weeks pregnant and in active labor. Can patients who are unstable or in active labor be transferred from one facility to another?

Active labor is defined by EMTALA as an "emergency medical condition." As long as the referring physician attests that the benefits of transfer outweigh the risks, AND the patient requests transfer to a higher level of care, a transfer can be initiated. This includes critically ill and injured patients who may be at risk of dying during transport as long as the previous criteria are met. The risks and benefits of transporting unstable patients, including those in active labor, should be weighed by the referring physician in consultation with the EMS transport service medical director as well as other specialists. EMS providers should discuss the case with their medical director prior to transport if they feel a patient is too unstable for transfer or is acutely deteriorating.

8. Can a patient who is unconscious or incapacitated and unable to provide informed consent be transferred?

In situations where the patient is not able to provide informed consent, attempts should be made to reach the power of attorney, healthcare proxy, or next-of-kin to obtain consent. If these persons cannot be contacted, providers should act in the best interest of the patients and proceed with transport if a "reasonable person" in a similar situation would elect to be transferred.

9. What vehicles may be used to transport a patient between healthcare facilities?

The decision of which mode of transport to utilize is complex and should be based on patient acuity, the time-sensitive nature of the patient's condition, available hospital and EMS resources, and patient preference. For stable patients that do not have a time-sensitive illness and without immediate life threats, transfer by taxi or private vehicle may be reasonable. This may be appropriate for a pediatric patient with an isolated minor fracture, or for patients with other non-life-threatening injuries. These types of transfers help reduce costs to patients and demand on the EMS system. Other vehicles that may be utilized include ground ambulances, rotor-wing aircraft, fixed-wing aircraft, and specialized vehicles such as watercraft or all-terrain vehicles.

10. Who provides medical oversight for EMS providers during interfacility transport?

EMTALA does not specify who provides "medical command" to the transporting EMS service. This decision should be made between the referring and receiving centers prior to transport, although it generally involves the medical director of the EMS transport service.

11. You are transporting a trauma patient from a critical access hospital to a trauma center. His condition becomes acutely worse, requiring placement of a definitive airway, and has uncontrolled hemorrhage of a previously stable extremity injury. What should be your next steps?

Clinically significant events during interfacility transport are infrequent but do occur. The existing literature suggests that such events occur during 6.5%–17.1% of interfacility transports. Common events include hemodynamic instability, need for vasopressor medication, and respiratory events. EMS crews should consider contingency plans for such events prior to initiating transport. This plan may include diversion to the nearest emergency department or en-route intercept with additional resources such as a rotor-wing aircraft.

12. What is the definition of "critical care transport?"

The US Department of Transportation's National Highway Traffic Safety Administration is the government agency that promotes the development and quality of EMS systems and defines critical care transport as "the level of transport care that is provided to patients with an immediate life-threatening illness or injury associated with single or multiple organ systems. This level of care requires an expert level of provider knowledge and skillset, a setting providing necessary equipment, and the ability to handle the added challenge of transport." Critical care transport generally refers to the level of clinical care provided in the prehospital environment.

13. How does this differ from "specialty care transport?"

Specialty care transport is defined by the Centers for Medicare and Medicaid Services (CMS) as the "provision of medically necessary supplies and services at a level of service beyond the scope of an EMT-Paramedic" and "requires ongoing care furnished by one or more professionals in an appropriate specialty (such as emergency or critical care nursing, emergency medicine, respiratory or cardiovascular care, or an EMT-Paramedic with additional training." Specialty care transport refers to the level of service provided with implications for billing and reimbursement by CMS.

14. What personnel typically make up a "critical care transport" team?

Most critical care transport services use a crew comprised of a nurse and paramedic, who each have additional training and experience in critical care medicine. Certain transports may require additional specialized crew members such as respiratory therapists, neonatal providers, EMS physicians, or perfusionists.

Table 62.1. Advantages and Disadvantages of the Different Modes of Interfacility Transport

	ADVANTAGES	DISADVANTAGES
Ground	More space for additional equipment and providers More available than aircraft Less expensive than aircraft	May be slower than air medical transport Dependent on road conditions, traffic, and weather
Rotor-wing aircraft	Can rapidly deliver advanced resources and providers to a critically ill patient Can transport patients medium distances with greater speed	May be limited by weather Challenging environment: limited space, excess noise and vibration, limited equipment Increased cost Weight restrictions (particularly in hot temperatures)
Fixed-wing aircraft	Can transport patients long distances with greater speed Generally provides more space than a rotor-wing aircraft	Requires ambulance transport to and from a fixed runway Challenging environment: limited space, excess noise and vibration, limited equipment Increased cost

15. What additional training, certification, or qualifications do critical care transport providers generally have?
    Although CMS stipulates that specialty care transport can be provided by a paramedic with "additional training," specific education and training qualifications are not defined at the federal level. The additional training required and scope of practice for critical care paramedics are defined at the state level. The training and qualifications needed by other healthcare providers to provide critical care transport services are generally defined at either the state or local level.

16. What are the advantages and disadvantages of the various modes of transport used for interfacility transport?
    Each mode of transport has specific advantages and disadvantages. See Table 62.1.

17. What specific challenges do pediatric and neonate patients present to the EMS provider during interfacility transport?
    A disproportionate amount of interfacility transports involve pediatric or neonatal patients due to the regionalization of pediatric emergency and specialty care at dedicated pediatric hospitals. Specific challenges include the need for specialized personnel and equipment to manage such patients, as well as the potential for long transport distances due to the small number of pediatric specialty centers.

18. I am interested in becoming more involved with interfacility and critical care transport. What other resources will help me learn more?
    There are many organizations that promote quality, safety, and best practices for interfacility and critical care transport. A list of several such organizations is provided here.
    • Commission on Accreditation of Medical Transport Systems (CAMTS)
      • CAMTS is a peer review organization dedicated to improving patient care and transport safety by providing a dynamic accreditation process through the development of standards, education, and services.
      • https://www.camts.org/
    • International Association of Flight & Critical Care Paramedics (IAFCCP)
      • The mission of the IAFCCP is to provide advocacy, leadership, professional development, and education opportunities for specialty care paramedics.
      • https://www.iafccp.org/
    • Air & Surface Transport Nurses Association (ASTNA)
      • ASTNA is a nonprofit member organization whose mission is to advance the practice of transport nursing and enhance the quality of patient care through commitment to safety and education
      • https://www.astna.org/
    • The Association of Critical Care Transport (ACCT)
      • ACCT is a nonprofit patient advocacy organization committed to ensuring that critically ill and injured patients have access to the safest and highest quality critical care transport system possible.
      • https://www.acctforpatients.org/

KEY POINTS

- Regionalization of EMS will likely lead to an increased volume and acuity of patients requiring interfacility transport.
- Successful interfacility transport depends on thorough patient preparation and planning, including a contingency plan for unexpected clinically significant events.
- EMS providers should confirm that the requirements specified in EMTALA, the regulatory body for interfacility EMS transports, are met prior to transport.
- EMS providers should reference specific local and state guidelines that define the training, qualifications, and certification needed to function as critical care transport providers.

BIBLIOGRAPHY

Centers for Medicare and Medicaid Services. Ambulance fee schedule and Medicare transports. 3 https://www.cms.gov/Outreach-and-Education/Medicare-Learning-Network-MLN/MLNProducts/Downloads/Medicare-Ambulance-Transports-Booklet-ICN903194.pdf.

Institute of Medicine Committee on the Future of Emergency Care in the U.S. Health Care System. *Emergency Medical Services: At the Crossroads.* Washington, DC: National Academy Press; June 2006.

National Highway Traffic Safety Administration. Guide for Interfacility Patient Transfer. 2000 https://www.ems.gov/pdf/advancing-ems-systems/Provider-Resources/Interfacility_Transfers.pdf.

Singh JM, Ferguson ND, MacDonald RD, Stewart TE, Schull MJ. Ventilation practices and critical events during transport of ventilated patients outside of hospital: a retrospective cohort study. *Prehosp Emerg Care.* 2009;13(3):316-323.

Singh JM, MacDonald RD, Ahghari M. Critical events during land-based interfacility transport. *Ann Emerg Med.* 2014;64(1):9-15.

State Operations Manual. Appendix V – Interpretive Guidelines – Responsibilities of Medicare Participating Hospitals in Emergency Cases. https://www.cms.gov/Regulations-and-Guidance/Guidance/Manuals/Downloads/som107ap_v_emerg.pdf.

CHAPTER 63

BARIATRIC EMERGENCIES

William C. Ferguson, Jr.

QUESTIONS AND ANSWERS

1. How is obesity defined?
   Body mass index (BMI) is a measure of body fat based on height and weight.

   BMI = body weight (in kg) ÷ height (in meters) squared

   Using BMI, obesity is then classified as follows:
   - Overweight = BMI $\geq$ 25.0 to 29.9 kg/m^2.
   - Class I obesity = BMI of 30.0 to 34.9 kg/m^2.
   - Class II obesity (formerly known as morbid obesity) = BMI of 35.0 to 39.9 kg/m^2.
   - Class III obesity (formerly known as severe obesity) = BMI $\geq$ 40 kg/m^2.

2. What is the prevalence of obesity in the United Sates and why is it a health problem?
   Obesity is a major health problem worldwide, with over 604 million adults defined as obese. In the United States, 37% of the population is considered obese, and 7% is classified as morbidly obese. Obesity is a major contributor to overall morbidly and mortality. There is a strong correlation with insulin resistance and obesity, with 80% of all type 2 diabetics being classified as obese. Obstructive sleep apnea (OSA) also plays a large role in chronic health problems and is associated with BMI $>$ 30. Obesity strains all the major organ systems. From a cardiovascular standpoint, for example, it leads to heart failure, cardiac enlargement, venous stasis, deep vein thrombosis, hypertension, and early cardiovascular disease, stroke, and kidney disease.

3. What is the difference between total body weight and ideal body weight? Does it matter in managing an obese patient clinically?
   Total body weight (TBW) is what the patient weighs, and we use this weight for the calculation of the BMI. Ideal body weight (IBW) is a calculation based upon their height. There are several formulas available for the calculation of IBW, with the Devine formula or Hamwi method used most commonly. The additional adipose of obese patients affects pharmacokinetics, and dosing of weight-based medications should be modified. The same is true for volume resuscitation and tidal volume calculation. For example, in a hypotensive septic patient, a routine volume of isotonic fluid resuscitation would be 30 cc/kg. If a patient was 5 foot 2 inches and had a weight of 220 kg, their IBW would be roughly 60 kg. So, 1800 cc of fluid would be used. If you used TBW, it would be closer to 6 L, which may be somewhat overzealous. Using an online calculator for IBW, or having a quick reference guide readily available, is essential.

4. How does obesity alter the way we manage the airway?
   Obese patients have excess soft tissue in the neck and upper airway, because of this upper airway obstruction with supine positioning is common. Basic airway maneuvers may start with simple positioning in a semi-Fowlers position. If the supine position is required, a towel roll under the shoulders or between the shoulder blades is preferred. The goal is not to hyperextend or flex the neck but improve airway positioning. A simple way to assess good position is to have the external auditory canal line up horizontally with the sternal notch when supine.

   A nasopharyngeal airway is a reasonable approach to assist with opening an airway. The obese patient should not need modifications for sizing of these (or oropharyngeal airways) as airway length and diameter are not affected by body mass. Definitive airway control with endotracheal intubation will be difficult due to excessive soft tissue anatomy, limitations in extending the neck, a relatively large tongue, and more anterior airway. Use of video laryngoscopy and/or bougie has greatly decreased failed intubation rates. This is particularly reassuring as a surgical airway on these patients is extremely difficult and problematic for even the most advanced practitioners.

5. How does obesity affect the way we provide assisted ventilations?
   With decreased pulmonary reserve, increased intra-abdominal pressure pushing up on the diaphragm, and decreased chest wall compliance related to overlying soft tissue, morbidly obese patients are often in a state of mild respiratory distress at baseline. OSA is a common occurrence, and even while awake, there can be a propensity for impaired ventilation and underlying hypercapnia. As even minor insults to the respiratory system can lead to significant respiratory compromise, early intervention to assist ventilations and prevent hypoxia or hypercarbia (retention of carbon dioxide) is paramount. After adequate positioning, early use of continuous positive airway pressure (CPAP) or bilevel positive airway pressure (BiPAP) is prudent. This positive pressure ventilation will increase alveolar recruitment and both oxygenation and ventilation. The additional pressure support will also help to maintain an open airway around redundant upper airway tissue. Preload and afterload will be reduced as

the blood pressure is lowered. This may improve cardiac output and help with any component of heart failure, common in obesity. If the patient becomes apneic or requires assisted ventilations, using the tight seal/mask that was used for CPAP/BiPAP along with an oropharyngeal or nasopharyngeal airway is prudent, especially if a single person is assisting ventilations. The common theme of assessing ventilation by watching chest rise and fall will be of little value in the obese patient, but the use of end-tidal capnography along with SpO_2 monitoring can yield valuable data on the adequacy of supportive ventilations. Keep in mind that when calculating tidal volumes, IBW, not TBW, should be used.

6. How does obesity alter the way we assess and manage emergencies related to circulation?
Obesity can pose many challenges to the assessment of the circulatory system. For example, it is not uncommon for heart and lung sounds to be muffled or distant, capillary refill to be delayed, and extremity pulse palpation to be extremely difficult, if not impossible, forcing you to use central pulses alone. An adequately sized blood pressure cuff may not be available. The key is to do the best assessment possible by adapting your techniques to the size of the patient. You may need to place the blood pressure cuff on the patient's forearm and auscultate over the radial artery or just obtain a systolic blood pressure with palpation. You may have to adopt the use of other cues such as mental status as a surrogate for perfusion.

Several routine interventions become difficult when the patient is obese, such as placing an intravenous or intraosseous line because of the excess adipose tissue at the insertion site. Consider using a longer needle than you would normally use for your selected site, particularly with intraosseous insertions. Defibrillation and external pacing are also adversely affected by excess adipose tissue. Higher energy levels may be necessary to achieve therapeutic effects and anterior posterior placement may be more effective. If CPR is necessary, automatic devices are unlikely to fit, and excessive mass will limit the effectiveness of manual CPR.

7. What are some techniques used to stabilize extremity fractures in the obese patient?
Extremity fractures can be difficult to manage in morbidly obese patients due to lack of access to bariatric splints and supplies. These items are expensive and hard to store, unless an agency has a bariatric response unit. EMS personnel may find it necessary to improvise and modify splints from tarps or other materials. Lifting and movement of some patients on power stretchers are often contraindicated due to weight and/or girth limits. The use of man sacks, heavy-duty tarps, ancillary vehicles, or event flatbed trucks has been utilized. Proper on-scene planning and bariatric action plans in place to assist with bariatric emergencies are paramount.

8. What is the biggest risk to healthcare providers in providing care for the obese patient?
Back injuries from lifting patients are the most common cause of occupational injury to EMS providers. This risk is multiplied when dealing with morbidly obese patients. Moving obese patients should be done with the safety of both the patient and provider in mind. It is frequently appropriate to delay moving an obese patient until an adequate number of providers are on the scene to assist with the proper equipment.

Obese patients should generally be moved using commercially produced soft stretchers that are rated at or above the patient's weight. These devices allow for multiple providers to share the weight when lifting and moving. There are also commercially available pneumatic bag systems that can be used to move the patient from a supine position to a seated position. These types of techniques are much safer and effective if the EMS providers train for such events prior to real-world execution.

9. Do you have to transport a morbidly obese patient that has a medical emergency?
Consideration should always be given to the risks of transporting a patient versus the risks of not transporting a patient. This is especially true for obese patients. Moving, standing, rolling, and sliding cause an obese patient to consume additional oxygen. This may be the tipping point for the patient to progress into a worse physiological state. Many times, acute medical issues can be resolved on the scene by EMS providers in consultation with medical command without necessitating moving the patient. Even severe medical emergencies should be mitigated by taking reasonable steps to stabilize the patient prior to moving. These suggestions do not apply to patients with serious traumatic injuries or time-sensitive emergencies such as stroke, severe trauma, or heart attack. Early medical command assessment and guidance are paramount, as weight restrictions may even limit the ability to intervene with cardiac catheterization and/or computed tomography (CT) imaging for strokes. Do not take big risks to accomplish small gains as the benefits should always outweigh the risks.

KEY POINTS

- Obesity is a national epidemic that is a major player in the health of the general population.
- Obesity alone is an independent risk factor for cardiovascular disease, sleep apnea, diabetes, and kidney disease.
- Obesity causes significant alterations to anatomy and physiology that can impact healthcare needs and hinder normal resuscitative interventions.

BIBLIOGRAPHY

Alabama EMS Challenge. Core Content. 2019. Alabama EMS Challenge on Facebook. Available from: https://bremssaemsc.wordpress.com/

Schumann R. Anesthesia for the obese patient. UpToDate. August 2019.

Collopy KT. How obesity impacts patient health and EMS. *EMS Today*; April 2012.

Brown CA. Emergency airway management in the morbidly obese patient. UpToDate. May 2019.

O'Donnell CP, Holguin F, Dixon AE. Pulmonary physiology and pathophysiology in obesity. *J Appl Physiol*. 2010;108(1):197-198.

Perreault L, Laferrère B. Overview of Health Consequences of Obesity. UpToDate. Sept 2019.

CHAPTER 64

GERIATRIC EMERGENCIES

Sarah A. Gibson

QUESTIONS AND ANSWERS

1. Who is considered a "geriatric patient" and why does that matter?

   Geriatric patients are classified as persons over the age of 65 years. This is the fastest-growing segment of the population in the United States. The US Census Bureau estimates that by the year 2040, there will be 80 million older adults, making up 21% of the population.

   The chronological age is the actual number of years that an individual has lived, whereas the physiologic age describes the actual functional capacity of the patient's organ systems in a physiologic sense (Fig. 64.1). Disease states such as diabetes mellitus, coronary artery disease, renal disease, arthritis, and pulmonary disease can decrease the physiological reserve. This makes it more difficult for elderly patients to recover from a traumatic injury or illness. There are significant physical and physiologic changes that occur with aging (Table 64.1).

2. What are the top mechanisms of injury for geriatric patients?

   Falls and motor vehicle collisions (MVCs) are the leading mechanisms of injury that bring elderly patients to a trauma center in the United States.

3. What are the neurological findings you may see when you assess a geriatric trauma patient?

   As the brain ages, the overall mass decreases, and as a result, there is greater stretching of the bridging vessels that pass from the brain to the dural sinuses. This puts the geriatric population at a higher risk for sheer injury with a low mechanism of action (resulting in a higher incidence of subdural hematomas). Altered mental status is common, and it can be difficult to determine acute versus chronic changes. When possible, talk with caregivers and family to determine baseline and obtain an initial Glasgow Coma Scale (GCS) score at the time of transport.

4. What are the respiratory findings you may see when you assess a geriatric patient?

   Elderly patients have a reduction in pulmonary compliance, total lung surface area, and decreased ability to cough. These changes result in greater risk for elderly patients to develop infectious processes and greater injury from pulmonary and thoracic traumas. Calcium deposits begin to form where the ribs meet the sternum, making the rib cage less flexible and placing the patient at an increased risk for injury. The lungs lose elasticity, the muscles used in breathing lose strength and coordination, and gas exchange becomes impaired, resulting in low oxygen (hypoxia) and elevated carbon dioxide (hypercapnia) levels.

5. What are the common spinal changes and resultant injuries that are seen in geriatric trauma?

   Cervical spine injury has been found to be twice as great in geriatric patients than in the general population. The most common cervical fracture in the elderly population is the odontoid fracture (fracture of the C2 vertebra). Spinal precautions are extremely important in the geriatric patient. In general, the tissues of the spine become more rigid and fibrotic. This is important to recognize because the spine is less flexible during a trauma, leaving it at risk for significant injury with low force applied. Significant pathology can occur even with just a ground-level fall.

   Geriatric patients have a dulled pain response as well. Therefore, with mechanisms of action including falls, MVCs, or other blunt force trauma where a cervical injury is possible, applying a cervical collar for stabilization and transport is extremely important.

6. What are the cardiovascular findings you may see when you assess a geriatric patient?

   The most important cardiac changes include stenosis (narrowing) of the cardiac and peripheral vessels, increased thickening of the heart muscle, and underlying dysrhythmias. During an assessment, you may note murmurs, muffled heart sounds, or irregular rhythm. There is a progressive stiffening of the heart muscle (myocardium) with age that results in a decreased pumping mechanism. This results in a decreased ability to respond to catecholamines and other "stress" hormones that are released during trauma or infection, with less ability to raise the heart rate to meet increased demand from infection, shock, respiratory distress, or injury. Patients may also be taking medications, such as beta-blockers that mask tachycardia and hinder complete evaluation.

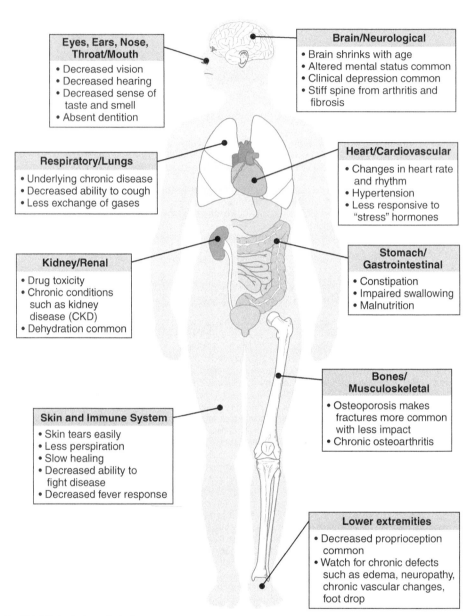

Eyes, Ears, Nose, Throat/Mouth
- Decreased vision
- Decreased hearing
- Decreased sense of taste and smell
- Absent dentition

Brain/Neurological
- Brain shrinks with age
- Altered mental status common
- Clinical depression common
- Stiff spine from arthritis and fibrosis

Respiratory/Lungs
- Underlying chronic disease
- Decreased ability to cough
- Less exchange of gases

Heart/Cardiovascular
- Changes in heart rate and rhythm
- Hypertension
- Less responsive to "stress" hormones

Kidney/Renal
- Drug toxicity
- Chronic conditions such as kidney disease (CKD)
- Dehydration common

Stomach/Gastrointestinal
- Constipation
- Impaired swallowing
- Malnutrition

Bones/Musculoskeletal
- Osteoporosis makes fractures more common with less impact
- Chronic osteoarthritis

Skin and Immune System
- Skin tears easily
- Less perspiration
- Slow healing
- Decreased ability to fight disease
- Decreased fever response

Lower extremities
- Decreased proprioception common
- Watch for chronic defects such as edema, neuropathy, chronic vascular changes, foot drop

Fig. 64.1. Effects of aging on the body.

7. What are the common findings of the eyes, ears, nose, mouth, and throat that come with aging?
Eyesight becomes compromised with aging, which not only sets patients up for traumatic injury risk but can also make it difficult for the provider to assess for an acute deficit. The patient may have sluggish pupillary response and changes consistent with cataracts or prior surgery, making acute conditions difficult to assess. Hearing decreases as well. Look for signs of a hearing deficit, such as hearing aids. Speak loudly but respectfully when indicated, and

Table 64.1. Effects of Aging on the Body

Brain/Neurological	Eyes/Ears/Nose/Mouth/Throat	Lungs/Respiratory
• The brain shrinks with age • Altered mental status common • Clinical depression common • Spine stiffens from arthritis and fibrosis	• Decreased vision • Decreased hearing • Decreased sense of taste and smell • Absent dentition • Difficulty swallowing	• Underlying chronic disease • Decreased ability to cough • Less exchange of gasses
Heart/Cardiovascular	Stomach/Gastrointestinal	Bones/Musculoskeletal
• Narrowing of heart valves • Changes in heart rate and rhythm • Hypertension common • Less responsive to "stress" hormones	• Constipation common • Impaired swallowing • Malnutrition	• Osteoporosis makes fractures more common • Chronic osteoarthritis increases fall risk
Kidneys/Renal	Skin/Integumentary	Lower Extremities
• Drug toxicity can easily occur • Chronic kidney disease at baseline • Dehydration common	• Skin tears easily • Less perspiration • Slow healing • Decreased ability to fight disease • Decreased fever response	• Diminished proprioception • Chronic underlying disease such as edema, neuropathy, chronic vascular changes, and prior evidence of stroke (weakness)

look for signs of trauma during your assessment. Smelling and taste decrease with age, which is why there is an increased risk for malnutrition. And swallowing becomes more difficult, which increases the risk of aspiration.

8. **What are the musculoskeletal findings you may see when you assess a geriatric trauma patient?**
Musculoskeletal fractures are common in the elderly population during traumatic events, specifically long bone fractures. Even with low-velocity mechanisms of action, such as a ground-level fall, they can commonly suffer hip fractures and pelvic fractures, which can quickly result in hypovolemia and signs of shock. Geriatric patients often have underlying osteoporosis (weakening of the bones) and osteoarthritis (degenerative changes). Look for deformity, feel for pulses, assess skin breakdown, and assume that fractures are present. With aging also comes decreased proprioception, the receptors in your body that tell your brain where you are located. Combine this with chronic conditions such as neuropathy, peripheral vascular disease, chronic edema, or underlying deficits from prior injury or stroke and you get an increased risk for geriatric falls.

9. **What are the gastrointestinal findings you may see when you assess a geriatric patient?**
Patients may complain of abdominal pain, but due to decreased ability to sense pain, the pain scale for small bowel obstruction or abdominal perforation may look similar to that seen with constipation. A decreased sense of taste and smell can lead to malnutrition. The opening between the esophagus and stomach (pyloric sphincter) loses elasticity, resulting in conditions such as heartburn. Constipation is a common complaint in this population.

10. **What are the renal findings you may see when you assess a geriatric patient?**
Geriatric patients are often dehydrated and can have underlying chronic kidney disease. The kidney itself loses nephrons and becomes fibrotic, which results in decreased renal blood flow and, therefore, decreased filtration ability. Due to the decreased function of the kidneys, patients are more susceptible to drug toxicity. Pain can often be controlled with acetaminophen, and rehydration should be slow and monitored for signs of fluid overload when possible.

11. **What are the integumentary findings you may see when you assess a geriatric trauma patient?**
Geriatric patients have very thin skin, which can make them more susceptible to skin tears and cause difficulty with thermoregulation. This is why hypothermia is more common in the elderly. They do not have as many sweat glands and therefore may not mount a perspiration response to acute illness. Skin injuries often heal very slowly, and the sense of touch and proprioception is diminished. This can lead to skin breakdown and a tendency for sores and skin infections to worsen rapidly.

12. **What are the most important questions to ask at the scene in a geriatric trauma setting?**
Obtain a history from the patient and witnesses regarding the mechanism of injury, blood loss at the scene, the degree of damage to any vehicles, and descriptions of weapons used, similar to your approach with the general population. However, the age of the patient, underlying chronic medical conditions, and medications are crucial in the geriatric assessment. Specific use of anticoagulants or other blood-thinning agents must be determined

and relayed to the accepting facility. Patterns of injuries and expected physiological responses can be obtained by collecting information regarding the circumstances of the event: single versus multiple vehicle crash, fall from a specific height, smoke inhalation, ingestion of intoxicants, preexisting medical conditions, and current medications.

13. **How do I know if a finding is chronic or acute? Medical or traumatic?**
With geriatric patients, it is often difficult to determine if a finding is chronic or acute. The history will often lead you toward a medical or traumatic cause; however, sometimes, a traumatic event (such as a fall) can happen because of a medical cause (such as a heart attack or stroke).

One-third of patients over the age of 75 years can have some form of coronary artery disease, and heart attacks are often unrecognized. The typical "chest pain" presentation may not be the main symptom and you may need to dig deeper and note findings of syncope, confusion, epigastric pain, or shortness of breath to indicate an acute myocardial infarction.

Elderly patients are at an increased risk for pneumonia and may not present with typical complaints such as cough, fever, and shortness of breath. Weakness or confusion may be the presenting complaint, and further in the disease process, you may see tachypnea or hypoxia.

Stroke may present as a "migraine"; however, as we age, migraine headaches are much less common. Headache in the elderly is much more likely to hold the diagnosis of a significant medical disease, such as a tumor, intracranial hemorrhage, or stroke, than seen in younger cohorts.

And lastly, shortness of breath in the elderly is a common complaint that can represent a wide range of diagnoses, from fluid overload to pulmonary embolism. Monitoring respiratory rate and oxygen saturation will help determine the best supportive care during transport (Table 64.2).

14. **What are the main considerations for the transport of the geriatric patient?**
Remember that elderly patients have inherently less reserve, so they may deteriorate more rapidly than the younger population, especially with a traumatic injury. The mainstays of transportation are similar to that of the general population. Special considerations may need to be made for airway insertion and patient positioning.

Airway insertion can be complicated by the presence of false dentition and limited range of motion of the cervical spine. A decreased gag reflex can predispose this population to aspiration and choking episodes.

When positioning the patient for transport, it is often different for medical vs. traumatic etiology. If the complaint seems to be medical, and the patient is protecting their airway, an upright (Fowler's) position is often best tolerated. This position has the patient seated in a semisitting position (45–60 degrees) with knees bent or straight.

If the patient has an altered mental status and cannot protect their airway, a left lateral (recovery) position is best to avoid aspiration.

Use backboard positioning only when absolutely necessary, due to risk for skin breakdown. However, if used, add additional padding as needed to protect from any further injury. For example, patients with severe kyphosis (curved spine) can be injured if forced to lie flat. When possible, a vacuum mattress may be the safest option.

15. **What is elder abuse and how can I spot it?**
Elder abuse can occur anywhere, from care centers to independent living. Patients most commonly at risk include those with a caregiver who is stressed or has poorly controlled mental health disease. Types of abuse include neglect, physical, sexual, emotional, and financial and can look similar to pediatric abuse cases (Table 64.3).

Talk directly with the patient when possible to maintain respect and prevent any perceived discrimination against elderly individuals. Each state typically has Elder Abuse Hotlines open 24 hours a day to report any concerns.

Table 64.2. Considerations When Taking Geriatric Vital Signs

- Resting heart rate is typically higher in the geriatric population, around 90 bpm.
- Respiratory rate is typically higher at baseline; around 20 rpm is normal.
- Skin is dry and produces very little sweat.
- Fever is less common, even with active infection.
- Blood pressure is usually elevated at baseline, specifically systolic pressure, which can mask hypovolemia.
- Pupils are sluggish at baseline and may be distorted due to cataract surgery, eye-drop medications, or other chronic conditions.

Table 64.3. Elder Abuse Overview

General Considerations	Behavioral Signs	Abuse Risk Factors	Signs of Abusive Caregivers
• Malnourished • Poor hygiene • Untreated bedsores • Medication errors	• Depression • Withdrawn • Anxiety, agitation, or fear • Confusion • Unwillingness to talk freely • Injuries inconsistent with mechanism of action	• Any living situation, demographic, race, or culture • Most commonly in homebound elders, women, over the age of 80 years, and isolated living conditions • Caretaker with substance abuse or mental health issues	• History of mental illness, substance abuse, family violence, or criminal behavior • Failing to show affection toward the older person • Keeping the elderly person from talking to visitors alone • Being indifferent, angry, or aggressive toward the elderly person • Speaking about the elder as if they were a burden • Withholding affection from the elderly person • Having conflicting explanations of physical incidents
Physical or Sexual Abuse • Unexplained broken bones • Welts • Bruises, cuts, sores, or burns • STDs • Bruising on inner thighs and around genitals • Bleeding, pain of the genitals or anus	Financial Abuse • Lack of amenities within the home that they can afford • Providing extravagant gifts or excessive money in exchange for care or companionship • Caregiver has control over finances but does not provide for basic needs	Emotional Abuse • Patient is withdrawn • Caregiver will not leave them alone with medical personnel or other family members • Caregiver is demeaning or verbally aggressive	Neglect • Lack of basic hygiene • Lack of proper clothing for the season/weather • Lack of food within the home • Missing medical aids and devices (walker, hearing aids) • Being left in bed for an extended period of time • Cluttered and dirty living space • Lack of basic amenities within the living space (refrigerator, heating, electricity) • Severe pressure ulcers or bedsores

From https://www.nursinghomeabusecenter.com/elder-abuse/signs/

- Geriatric patients are those over the age of 65 years; however, significant differences are noted between physiologic age and chronologic age based on underlying medical health.
- Significant changes occur to the body with aging that can predispose the geriatric population to different injuries than the younger cohort.
- Baseline vital signs will typically look different in the geriatric population and may not be a reliable indicator of underlying pathology or worsening disease process.
- Have a high index of suspicion even with low-velocity injuries.
- Look for signs of elder abuse.
- Gain information from family members, caregivers, and the scene, but be sure to speak with the patient whenever possible to show respect and concern.

BIBLIOGRAPHY

American Trauma Society. *ATLS: Student Course Manual*. Chicago, IL: American College of Surgeons; 2008. www.amtrauma.org/page/traumalevels.

Carpenter MD, Avidan CR, Wildes T, Stark S, Fowler SA, Lo AX. Predicting geriatric falls following an episode of emergency department care: a systematic review. *Acad Emerg Med*. 2014;21(10):1069-1082.

Centers for Disease Control and Prevention. Glasgow Coma Scale. www.cdc.gov/masstrauma/resources/gcs.pdf.

EMS zone. emt.emszone.com/docs/CH33_AEC_Table.pdf.

Henry MC, Stapleton ER, Edgerly D. *EMT Prehospital Care*. St. Louis, MO: Mosby JEMS/Elsevier; 2012.

Kartiko S, Jeremitsky E, Cripps MW, Konderwicz I, Jarosz E, Minshall CT. Fall prevention initiative: a fall screening and intervention pilot study on the ambulatory setting. *J Trauma Acute Care Surg*. 2019;10(1097).

Mistovich JJ, Karren KJ. *Prehospital Emergency Care*. 11th ed. New York: Pearson; 2014.

Murdoch I, Turpin S, Johnston B, MacLullich A, Losman E. *Geriatric Emergencies*. Wiley Blackwell; 2015.

Nursing Home Abuse Center. *Signs of Elder Abuse*. www.nursinghomeabusecenter.com/elder-abuse/signs/.

Pollak AN, Edgerly D, McKenna K, Vitberg DA. *Emergency Care and Transportation of the Sick and Injured*. Burlington, MA : Jones & Bartlett Learning, 2017.

Söz G, Karakaya Z. The evaluation of geriatric patients who presented with trauma to the emergency department. *Arch Med Sci*. 2019;15(5.):1261–1268.

AEROMEDICAL TRANSPORT

Ryan Kelly

CHAPTER 65

QUESTIONS AND ANSWERS

1. What is aeromedical transport?

   Aeromedical transport was born out of the need to move wounded service members during World War I. Injured soldiers could be transported to more definitive care in a shorter time, increasing survivability. Throughout the 20th and 21st centuries, the US Military advanced the field of aeromedical transport and battlefield evacuation to include point of injury care with rotor-wing aircraft and transfer to major theater hospitals with fixed-wing aircraft. During the Vietnam war, helicopters were used extensively to pick up wounded soldiers and transport them back to high levels of care, which greatly improved their chances of survival. The idea of flight to rapidly move patients to specialty care was not a strictly American idea; programs were developed in places like Australia, Canada, and Germany. The United States opened its first civilian hospital-based helicopter program in 1972 at St. Anthony's Hospital in Denver, CO; this program remains open to this day. Since that time, hundreds of rotor-wing patient transport programs have opened in the United States and abroad.

   One should not forget that fixed-wing aircraft are also used to move patients. Although less likely to be used for point of injury transport, airplanes have a much longer range, can fly at higher altitudes, and can fly much faster than rotor-wing aircraft. The military model for patient transport illustrates this well when one compares the UH60 "Blackhawk" to the C-130 "Hercules." The Blackhawk can only transport a handful of injured patients a short distance, but they can be picked up on the battlefield and brought to Combat Surgical Hospital for initial stabilization. Those patients can then be grouped with other injured patients and placed on a waiting Hercules aircraft that can hold 70+ patients depending on configuration and transport them several hours by air to more definitive medical care at a large theater hospital.

2. Who should be considered for transport by air?

   Air transport has some unique challenges that come with it. There are not a lot of hard exclusions for transport, but care should be taken in selecting the mode of transport. To start, it should be noted that violent and overtly aggressive or suicidal patients should not be transported by air without chemical or physical restraints. Also, patients who have been exposed to hazardous materials should not be flown without proper decontamination. Beyond these situations, most patients will qualify for transport by flight. The limiting factor for transport usually rests more with the crew abilities, weight and balance, and en-route weather. Ultimately, the clinician that is making the call for transport should weigh the risk and benefits of air versus ground transport. Time, distance, weather, patient condition, and possible complications should all be part of the equation when deciding on the transport method. For example, a patient who is involved in a high-speed motor vehicle collision on a highway and has a significant traumatic injury to the abdomen may only be 10 minutes from the nearest trauma center, but because of traffic caused by the accident, ground transport will take 45 minutes while air transport will only take 15 minutes. Transport by air, in this case, will save critical time as long as weather permits flight. Another example to consider is an American that gets ill or injured while in another country and needs to be transported back to the United States for more definitive care. Fixed-wing air transport is the most likely resource to transport this patient unless they are close to a US border in either Mexico or Canada.

3. What kind of equipment and capabilities do air transport teams have?

   Crew complement, equipment, and abilities vary based on the platform and the type of transport requested. Generally, you should expect the medical crew to consist of one flight paramedic and one flight nurse. The nurse and medic should ideally have critical care experience, but that is not always required. Their monitoring abilities and equipment will usually be on par with intensive care unit (ICU) level patients including invasive blood pressure monitoring, ventilator support, multiple IV infusions, suction equipment, and even extracorporeal membrane oxygenation (ECMO) in some cases. The US Air Force, which handles the majority of patient movement throughout the military system, has a standard crew complement of two flight nurses and three aeromedical evacuation technicians (flight medics) to allow for larger and longer distance fixed-wing transport missions. When requesting air transport, it is essential to discuss what the patient will need so that the transporting agency can ensure that the crew will have the equipment and training needed to safely transport the patient.

4. What kind of stresses of flight should be considered when thinking about air transport?

   The stresses of flight vary based on altitude and airframe, but generally, you should be thinking about the following:
   - The decreased partial pressure of oxygen (Dalton's law)—the law of partial pressure. Oxygen concentration in the atmosphere remains constant regardless of altitude. The oxygen actually available decreases with altitude because oxygen molecules are farther apart, resulting in hypoxia.

- Barometric pressure changes (Boyle's law)—the principle of gas expansion. As altitude increases, gasses expand. Consider how a sealed balloon would expand as the altitude climbs.
- Temperature variations—Temperature can fluctuate greatly from the ground level to the cruise level of an aircraft. Critically ill, burn patients, and infants are especially susceptible to hypothermia in flight.
- Fatigue—Long distance travel over several days and time zones can disrupt the normal circadian rhythm of a patient.
- G-forces—Gravitational forces involve concepts related to exerted forces, speed, velocity, weight, mass, and the laws of motion. Patients with risk for increased intracranial pressure, pregnant patients, and patients with unstable fractures are at high risk for G-force related issues.
- Decreased humidity—As the air cools, its ability to hold moisture decreases. At high altitudes over a long period of time, humidity can drop significantly in flight. Fluid balance can be affected and should be monitored closely, especially in renal, cardiac, and respiratory compromised patients.
- Noise and vibration—Not all aircraft are equipped with noise dampening materials, making communication and assessments very difficult. Likewise, vibrations are not usually dampened either, which can increase metabolic rate and oxygen demand in a patient.

5. How can I best prepare a patient for air transport?
   The most important thing that you can do is make sure they are as stable as you can get them on the ground. Remember that inside the airplane or helicopter is a very small work area and movement can be limited. Obtaining two large-bore IVs prior to flight is ideal in any patient, but especially the critically ill. Additionally, it is not uncommon for a flight crew to intubate a patient prior to flight if there is any concern that the patient may decompensate while in the air, since placing an endotracheal tube at altitude is not ideal. If a patient is already intubated, or there is concern for gastric distention, a gastric tube should be placed to prevent increased gastric distention or vomiting (because of Boyle's law). If the patient's condition and time allow, it would be beneficial to explain to the patient why you think they need air transport and what they can expect while in the air. This can help reduce the anxiety and fear that inherently comes with the high-stress environment of air transport.

6. Is this a cost-effective mode of transport?
   It depends. Unfortunately, many helicopter systems have high operating costs but low call volumes, making it one of the most expensive ways to be transported. Flights can range from a few thousand dollars to over half a million dollars. Insurance will sometimes pay a portion of that cost, but a significant portion of that burden may fall on the patient. Hospital-based flight programs usually have some ways to help offset the cost, but private companies generally need to collect the bills to keep their program running. With regard to patient outcome, there is not a significant amount of research available comparing the difference between ground and air transport, and it would be nearly impossible to perform a randomized controlled trial for air versus ground transport. That said, survivability on the battlefield for US servicemembers has significantly improved since helicopters were introduced.

7. Where can I get more information about aeromedical transport?
   The Air and Surface Transport Nurse Association has several publications and courses available for those wanting to explore the aeromedical world. The *Air Medical Journal* is a publication that contains practical how-to articles, debates on controversial industry issues, legislative updates, case studies, and peer-reviewed original research articles covering all aspects of the medical transport profession. Also, the US Air Force is a global leader in patient movement via air, with 30+ Aeromedical Evacuation Squadrons across the globe. Find the aeromedical resources that are closest to you and it may even be possible to get a ride-along to see what the aircrew does on their missions.

KEY POINTS

- Aeromedical transport enlists rotor-wing and fixed-wing aircraft to transport ill and injured patients to a higher level of care with significantly less time than ground transport.
- There are far fewer accidents involving aeromedical assets than ground vehicles, but aircraft accidents have a higher likelihood of fatalities.
- Patient condition, weather, terrain, and medical personnel capabilities all factor into the decision to transport a patient by air.

BIBLIOGRAPHY

Bedi S. *The Evolution of Aeromedical Evacuation Capabilities Help Deployed Medicine Take Flight.* Air Force Medical Service. March 15, 2008. https://www.airforcemedicine.af.mil/News/Display/Article/1466825/the-evolution-of-aeromedical-evacuation-capabilities-help-deployed-medicine-tak/.
Holleran RS. *ASTNA Patient Transport Principles and Practice.* St. Louis: Elsevier; 2010.
Loyd JW, Swanson D. *Aeromedical Transport.* Stat Pearls. June 16, 2019. https://www.ncbi.nlm.nih.gov/books/NBK518986/.
US Air Force. Air Force Instruction 48-307, Volume 1. *En Route Care and Aeromedical Evacuation Medical Operations.* January 9, 2017. https://static.e-publishing.af.mil/production/1/af_sg/publication/afi48-307v1/afi48-307v1.pdf.

COMMUNITY PARAMEDICINE

Brandon Wattai

CHAPTER 66

QUESTIONS AND ANSWERS

1. What is community paramedicine?

   The healthcare landscape is changing rapidly. Hospitals, health systems, and insurers are increasingly focusing on efforts to expand access to care for a wider population. There is an accelerating shift toward the concept of *value-based healthcare*, where providers and facilities are paid based on patient outcomes, rather than the traditional fee-for-service healthcare delivery model.[1] As these movements grow, there is an expanding need for innovative programs and solutions that can fill significant gaps that have come to exist in the larger healthcare system. Community paramedicine (CP) is emerging as such a solution.

   CP, also known as mobile integrated healthcare, has existed on a small scale in varying formats throughout the country for over 15 years. The underlying theory is simple: utilize paramedics or EMTs outside of traditional emergency response and transport roles to address some unmet need in a community or for a partnered healthcare element. For many EMS agencies, the application may be as simple as providing an additional service to help reduce inappropriate utilization of the 911 system or an emergency department, an issue that has long been a major challenge for the industry.

   However, what is rapidly coming into focus is that community paramedicine's impact can extend far beyond EMS operations. In the era of value-based healthcare, a collaborative and comprehensive approach to patient care is critical. Consequently, community paramedicine programs are increasingly being created to provide a significant enhancement to ongoing postdischarge support for high-risk patients.[2]

2. What is the scope of community paramedicine?

   What makes the community paramedicine concept so compelling is its versatility. These programs can target a wide range of historically challenging problems. In addition to addressing inappropriate system utilization, CP elements may seek to address specific clinical or social issues. Partnerships or integration with hospitals and health systems allow for significant enhancements to acute and chronic disease management and may significantly reduce the occurrence of readmissions or other negative outcomes. These partnerships may also provide for a significant ability to extend primary care to the home of the patient, improving medical access in underserved populations.

   As a result of this versatility, operations and interventions will vary from program to program. In general, a community paramedicine assessment will consist of medical evaluation and education, as well as a thorough social assessment. While EMS is highly trained in managing medical needs, a comprehensive approach to addressing social barriers may require additional training or a new perspective. However, it is increasingly obvious that the value of addressing these needs cannot be overstated, and this plays a huge role in improving outcomes.[3]

3. What does a community paramedicine home visit consist of?

   In general, most community paramedicine home visits will feature:
   - A history review
   - Patient education
   - Medication reconciliation
   - Physical exam
   - Social assessment
   - Interventions
   - Documentation

4. What does a community paramedicine history review require?

   Not unlike emergency calls, a patient's history of present illness is crucial for a community paramedicine contact. It is important to assess a patient comprehensively, and performing a deep dive into a patient's medical and social history will accomplish this. Doing so will highlight for the provider obvious and hidden challenges that may have been resulting in recent 911 calls, hospitalizations, or other complications. For example, we might learn that a complex heart failure patient had attended a cookout that featured heavily salty foods prior to a recent admission. We now know that a focus on reinforcing disease education and self-care parameters will be very important for this individual.

You should also evaluate how a patient is affected by comorbidities. Those with heart failure, stroke, chronic obstructive pulmonary disease (COPD), and others are at least as likely to be readmitted for factors outside of those conditions as they are for a primary exacerbation. For instance, a COPD patient may ultimately be readmitted for diabetic complications rather than respiratory distress. An evaluation of patient history should include consideration of these secondary conditions to identify trends or behaviors that place your patient at increased risk.

5. What kind of education should community paramedicine provide?
Few things will make a more substantial impact on a patient's ability to care for themselves than adequate education. This will include an understanding of a specific disease process and related self-care directions. For those that progress through an acute inpatient hospital setting, ongoing care needs can often be quite overwhelming. In many cases, a new diagnosis of a high-risk condition results in the need for a "new normal," which dramatically alters lifestyles. If this change is complex or unpleasant, patients may struggle to fully appreciate how to care for themselves or maintain consistency. This places patients at increased risk for hospitalization and other complications.

A community paramedic is often in a unique position to either introduce or reinforce critical education for the patient. For instance, heart failure patients have extremely particular diets requiring a maximum of 2000 mg of sodium and 64 oz of fluid to be consumed daily. Even an isolated deviation from these parameters can lead to a sequence of events that results in hospitalization. A standard overview of self-care directives should be a component of every visit.

6. Why is it important to perform a medication reconciliation?
A common cause of complications for patients of all types is prescription medication error. Studies have indicated that upward of 30% or more of hospitalized patients have one or more discrepancies when medication lists are reconciled.[4] These errors translate to billions of dollars of healthcare costs annually in addition to varying clinical ramifications. For community paramedicine, it becomes critical to evaluate each patient's current medication list and compare it to bottles or boxes that are present while ascertaining a patient's understanding of what they are to take and when.

7. How does a physical exam for community paramedicine differ from a traditional EMS assessment?
A thorough physical exam is a critical component of any EMS patient contact. In the context of a nonemergency Community Paramedicine assessment, this will be an important means of evaluating a patient's current state of health as well as disease progression. This exam may provide evidence of an early exacerbation of an underlying condition, and relaying this information to partnered clinical providers allows for real-time changes to a patient's care plan that may prevent negative outcomes.

Medical directors are able to work with community paramedicine teams to expand assessment skills while remaining consistent with scope-of-practice considerations. Through this, disease-specific evaluations may be performed that can provide critical and comprehensive information that may not have been possible via a traditional prehospital physical assessment. For instance, a National Institutes of Health Stroke Scale (NIHSS) may be performed by a community paramedic in a patient's home post hospital discharge to assess ongoing progression. This and similarly focused exams around other high-risk conditions are important to consider for home visits, as these assessments can fill a significant gap between clinical appointments.

8. Why is it important to perform a social assessment?
One of the most important things that community paramedicine can provide for patients is a thorough assessment of their home environment and social needs. The social determinants of health describe the factors and conditions that exist in a patient's life that may either support or hinder positive health outcomes and are at the heart of this consideration.

The social determinants of health include factors such as availability of transportation, education, clinical access, family support, financial stability, access to community resources, etc. These are considerations that are often noted by prehospital providers as being an apparent challenge, but it is becoming increasingly clear that addressing any gaps that exist in this area is often critical to a patient's long-term health. For instance, an acute heart failure patient may receive outstanding prehospital and inpatient care as well as obtaining all appropriate prescriptions and education to manage his or her condition going forward. However, if this individual is discharged to a compromised environment where they cannot reliably afford all medications or appropriate dietary options, the likelihood of negative outcomes increases dramatically.

A community paramedicine home visit provides a unique opportunity to identify many of these potential challenges that may not have been known to the hospital or outpatient providers. Helping a patient to navigate these challenges can itself dramatically improve outcomes. This application highlights the substantially expanded role that EMS providers may have on the wider healthcare landscape in the future.

9. What interventions can community paramedicine perform?

    EMS is, by design, a highly solution-oriented field. This remains true for the role of a community paramedic. The concept of an "intervention" becomes much broader in the nonemergency environment, as these will range from clinical procedures to social assistance.

    Clinically, many potential interventions are very familiar to EMS providers. Blood draws and medication administration remain options that can provide timely diagnostics and support to prevent a negative outcome. These may be performed based on standing orders established by medical direction, and potentially at a request by partnered healthcare elements based on patient need.

    Socially, interventions will be any action taken to overcome an identified social barrier. For instance, if reliable transportation is a clear challenge, working with a patient to utilize a ride-sharing service or some other available option is a crucial measure. Similarly, if a patient is under a considerable financial strain, you may be able to assist with securing medical assistance via a primary care provider's office or hospital resources.

    Ultimately, there is a significant amount of "social work" in community paramedicine, which initially is unfamiliar to many prehospital providers. However, establishing an array of resources to address social barriers will be a powerful means of improving the outcome for your patients.

10. What should be documented for a community paramedicine contact?

    Community paramedicine documentation needs will vary as much as programs themselves. In general, it will be important to document a patient's history, social assessment, medication reconciliation, physical exam, interventions, and ideally a care plan for the next steps you will be taking to further assist your patient. This documentation may occur in either traditional EMS documentation software or a hospital's electronic health record, if possible.

KEY POINTS

- Community paramedicine is an effective solution to a rapidly changing healthcare landscape.
- Community paramedicine programs are able to adapt to meet the needs of a community, hospital, or health system.
- Prehospital providers are able to make a considerable impact on healthcare beyond traditional emergency operations.
- Community paramedics should assess both a patient's clinical and social condition.
- Multidisciplinary collaboration is an approach that is critical to community paramedicine services and patient care.

REFERENCES

1. Gray M. Value based healthcare. *BMJ.* 2017;356:j437.
2. Roeper B, Mocko J, O'Connor L, Zhou J, Castillo D, Eric B. Mobile integrated healthcare intervention and impact analysis with a Medicare advantage population. *Popul Health Manage.* 2018;21(5):349-356.
3. Williams DR, Costa MV, Odunlami AO, Mohammed SA, Moving upstream: how interventions that address the social determinants of health can improve health and reduce disparities. *J Public Health Manage Pract.* 2008;14(suppl):S8-S17.
4. Da Silva B, Krishnamurthy M. The alarming reality of medication error: a patient case and review of Pennsylvania and national data. *J Community Hosp Intern Med Perspect.* 2016;6(4.).

CHAPTER 67

INTIMATE PARTNER VIOLENCE, SEXUAL ASSAULT, AND CHILD MALTREATMENT

Carolina Pereira

QUESTIONS AND ANSWERS

INTIMATE PARTNER VIOLENCE

Case: EMS is called to a 29-year-old female who "fell down the stairs." Upon arrival, EMS notices that the patient's partner answers questions for her and jokes about how clumsy his partner is. The astute EMT notes the home has only three steps leading into the living room, and the patient has extensive injuries that include a deformity to her wrist, bruising about the eyes and neck, severe pain to her chest wall, and blood coming from the right ear. The EMT whispers to the paramedic that he is concerned that these injuries are too extensive for the reported mechanism.

1. What patterns should EMS watch for in trying to identify intimate partner violence?
   - Mismatch in the explanation of the injury and the reported mechanism, a delay in seeking care, or a pattern of repeated EMS use.

2. What patient symptoms should EMS watch for that can be suggestive of intimate partner violence?
   - Bruises in various stages of healing, particularly over nonbony surfaces like the abdomen or trunk, bite marks, abrasions, and defensive injuries over the forearms.
   - Pregnant women are at higher risk of being victims of intimate partner violence, with rates as high as 9% of all pregnant women experiencing violence. This number is even higher for single, pregnant women of low social economic status.

3. How should EMS approach a case where intimate partner violence is suspected?
   - Prehospital personnel should attempt to build rapport with all involved and normalize separating the patient and the suspected abuser to allow questioning of the victim without the suspected abuser in the same space. This can often be accomplished by saying that some part of the exam needs to be performed privately.

4. I am worried my patient will immediately shut down if I ask about intimate partner violence. How do I bring up the subject?
   - Try normalizing the question by saying, "I don't know if this is a problem for you, but many of my patients are dealing with abusive relationships. Some are too uncomfortable to bring it up themselves, so I've started asking routinely." Framing the question as if it is a question asked of every patient helps break through the stigma associated with intimate partner violence as, frequently, patients are embarrassed to come forward themselves as a feeling of isolation is inherent to the cycle of abuse.
   - Remember that EMS is in a unique position to see into the lives of our patients that clinic and hospital staff usually do not get to see. Trust your instincts, and ask regularly.

5. What should I do if I suspect intimate partner violence, but the patient denies that they are being abused?
   - Respond with supportive language. Remember that your patient may not be ready to ask for help yet, but your response can be instrumental in building their confidence in healthcare providers for future interactions with the healthcare system.
   - Avoid judgmental responses such as "I don't know why you'd stay in a relationship like that," as this may further dissuade the patient from asking for help during this and future encounters.
   - You may consider discussing local resources anyway by framing intimate partner violence as a common problem that a friend may face.

6. How should I respond when a patient does admit that they are a victim of intimate partner violence?
   - Respond with supportive language such as "no one deserves to be treated this way," "you are not alone," or "thank you for telling me."
   - Gently encourage transport to the hospital particularly if the patient is unsafe at home, and avoid criticizing their willingness to stay with the partner.

7. Why do victims of intimate partner violence often stay with their abuser?
   - Frequently, victims of intimate partner violence have been systematically victimized. They have been victims of verbal, financial, and emotional abuse even prior to physical abuse. This often leaves them socially and financially isolated from friends and family so that leaving their abuser is incredibly difficult and even dangerous as they have no one to turn to or resources with which to leave.

8. What is mandatory reporting?
   - Mandatory reporting is when certain occupations are required by law to report types of abuse. This varies drastically from state to state, so be familiar with your local and state laws to see if prehospital personnel are mandatory reporters for intimate partner violence.

9. Are prehospital personnel considered mandatory reporters?
   - In most states, the answer is yes, but this is not always the case.

10. Is there mandatory reporting for intimate partner violence?
    - Mandatory reporting for intimate partner violence remains controversial as it is widely believed to increase the likelihood that the victim will experience further violence and escalation of the danger from the violence. The American Medical Association and American College of Emergency Physicians oppose mandatory reporting for intimate partner violence for this reason.

11. When should EMS seek law enforcement involvement for intimate partner violence?
    - Again, this varies from state to state, but it is common that if the violence is life threatening and/or involves a deadly weapon such as a gun or a knife, this must be reported to law enforcement. Know your local laws and statutes to understand what must be reported.
    - It is important to maintain the rapport that you have built with the patient (remember they may have told you something they have never told anyone before), so be honest with them. Do not promise confidentiality if this is not something you will be able to keep given your state's mandatory reporting laws.

SEXUAL ASSAULT

Case (continued): Once in the back of the ambulance, the patient admits that her partner has been getting mad at her with increasing frequency and hitting her when frustrated. She reports that he pushed her into a cabinet, breaking her arm, choked her, and forcibly had sex with her against her will while hitting her repeatedly about the face.

1. What is sexual assault?
   According to the US Department of Justice, sexual assault is "any type of sexual contact or behavior that occurs without the explicit consent of the recipient."

2. Is it still sexual assault if it is perpetrated by her partner?
   - Yes, absolutely! Eighty percent of sexual assaults are committed by someone known to the victim, and 33% are committed by a current intimate partner.

3. What can I actually do for a victim of sexual assault?
   - Prehospital providers play a large role in the treatment of sexual assault as they are the first healthcare providers to come in contact with a victim following the attack.
   - Naturally, EMS providers should, first and foremost, provide high-quality medical care for any life-threatening conditions present.
   - While less obvious, prehospital providers should also provide emotional first aid (caring for the emotional injuries in addition to the physical ones) and avoid revictimization of the patient while encouraging the patient to seek medical care at the hospital. The hospital will have a way to contact a sexual assault response team that is specially trained in sexual assault counseling and evidence collection.

4. How can I make sure I do not revictimize the patient?
   - Believe and support the patient. Everyone accused of a crime deserves to be held innocent until proven guilty in a court of law. Your ambulance is not that court. This is a great time to use the patient's own words in direct quotes in your documentation as it is important to document impartially.
   - Additionally, it is rarely necessary to perform a sexual assault exam in the prehospital environment. Pay special attention to the patient's comfort level, particularly as they were recently victimized, and accommodate whenever possible. For example, your patient may not feel comfortable alone with a male if she was recently sexually assaulted by one.

5. What to advise the victim of sexual assault?
   - As with intimate partner violence, laws and resources governing sexual assault vary widely from state to state. Familiarize yourself with your local laws and resources for victims of sexual assault, as well as the process that sexual assault victims may have to go through. Letting the patient know what to expect in the hospital and with follow-up will be reassuring.
   - Encourage the patient, if at all possible, to avoid any actions that can lead to destruction of evidence, such as taking a shower, urinating, and wiping their genitals.
   - Refer to the Rape, Abuse, & Incest National Network (RAINN) for further resources for the patient and for educational materials including information on your state's law's.

CHILD MALTREATMENT

Case: A crew gets a call for a 2-month-old male infant who is fussy after a fall off the bed. The patient's mother says she did not see the fall. The crew sees a child in visibly dirty clothes who is inconsolably crying. The paramedic examines the child and notes no obvious signs of trauma but that the child appears to be extremely lethargic and much smaller than a typical 2-month-old child. The paramedic is concerned about the fall given that the child would not be able to move on their own at that age.

1. What is considered child abuse?
   - Child abuse is the action or inaction that results in putting a child at risk of harm, including physical, verbal, or psychological harm. This can include intentional physical injury, neglect, knowingly permitting others to endanger the child, and sexual abuse.

2. What are the signs/symptoms of child maltreatment?
   - Similar to intimate partner violence, look for injuries that do not fit the story. While this child does not have obvious injuries, his dirty clothing, small size, and suspicious "fall" all point toward child maltreatment, including physical abuse and neglect.

3. What do I do when the child is not old enough to report the abuse?
   - Remember that your examination and intuition are going to be much more important with a child as they may not be able to describe the danger they are in or even recognize it as danger if they are old enough to talk. Look more closely for signs and symptoms of child maltreatment.

4. Is there mandatory reporting for child maltreatment?
   - All states have some mandatory reporting due to the fact that children are considered a vulnerable population; however, who is listed among those required to report child abuse is not uniform across all states. (Often, the elderly and disabled are considered vulnerable populations, as well.)

5. What should I do if the parents refuse care?
   - Attempt to build rapport with those involved in the case as encouraging the family to seek medical care is easier. However, it may become necessary to involve law enforcement particularly in cases where the child may be in danger by staying in the home or there are other siblings at risk. Be familiar with the laws in your state and local resources for dealing with child maltreatment.

KEY POINTS

- Know your local regulations and resources with regard to intimate partner violence, sexual assault, and child abuse.
- Trust your instincts and be on the lookout for injury patterns that do not match with the reported mechanism of injury.
- Be supportive and nonjudgmental in your questioning so that victims can feel as comfortable as possible opening up to you about these traumatic events.

BIBLIOGRAPHY

Bailey BA, Daugherty RA. Intimate partner violence during pregnancy: incidence and associated health behaviors in a rural population. *Matern Child Health J.* 2007;11:495-503.

Child Welfare Information Gateway. Mandatory reporters of child abuse and neglect. 2019. https://www.childwelfare.gov/pubPDFs/manda.pdf.

Martin SL, Mackie L, Kupper LL, Buescher PA, Moracco KE. Physical abuse of women before, during, and after pregnancy. *JAMA.* 2001;285:1581-1584.

Mason R, Schwartz B, Burgess R, Irwin E. Emergency medical services: a resource for victims of domestic violence?. *Emerg Med J*. 2010;27(7):561-564.

RAINN. The nation's largest anti-sexual violence organization. Rainn.org. 2019. https://www.rainn.org/.

Sachs C. Mandatory reporting of injuries inflicted by intimate partner violence. *AMA J Ethics*. 2007;9(12):842-845.

Sawyer S, Coles J, Williams A, Williams B. A systematic review of intimate partner violence educational interventions delivered to allied health care practitioners. *Med Educ*. 2016;50(11):1107-1121.

Stanford Medicine. Child abuse. 2019. http://childabuse.stanford.edu/.

US Department of Justice. Sexual Assault. Justice.gov. 2019. https://www.justice.gov/ovw/sexual-assault.

CHAPTER 68

END-OF-LIFE ISSUES

Carolina Pereira

QUESTIONS AND ANSWERS

HEALTHCARE DECISION MAKERS AT THE END OF LIFE

Case: EMS receives a call for an 85-year-old female who had an unwitnessed fall at a skilled nursing facility. The patient has a past medical history of lung cancer with metastasis, chronic obstructive pulmonary disease (COPD), and dementia. The nurse assigned to the patient called 911 after she heard a loud noise from this patient's room and ran in there to find the patient getting up off of the floor with a small laceration to her forehead. The patient states that she "feels fine" but does not remember falling despite the laceration to her forehead and is only oriented to person, but not place, time, or context. The patient's daughter, who was also called after this event, arrives and asks that her mother not be taken to the emergency department, stating that the patient has a durable power of attorney for healthcare that designates her as the attorney-in-fact.

1. What is capacity?
   Capacity refers to the determination that a person has the ability to make decisions for themselves. The four elements of capacity are having an understanding of the decision to be made, having an appreciation of the possible outcomes of said decision and how it applies to one's circumstances, having the reasoning ability to deliberate between the options, and the ability to express a choice. Capacity is dynamic and may change with time such as patients with dementia or advanced medical illness.

2. How is this different than competence?
   Competence also refers to the ability to make decisions but is decided upon by a judge as a legal decision. As determinations of competence are made within the court system, they are less dynamic than capacity. In the prehospital and other healthcare fields, we evaluate for capacity rather than competence.

3. What is a durable power of attorney?
   Power of attorney is a legal order designating a person (designated as the attorney-in-fact) to make decisions for another person (referred to as the principal) in the case that they become incapacitated. This can be for all decisions in a person's life including financial or business decisions. This may also be only specifically for healthcare decisions.

4. What is a healthcare proxy or healthcare surrogate?
   A healthcare proxy or surrogate is someone who is appointed by you to make medical decisions. This can be someone that is designated by the patient themselves when they had the ability to make decisions such as in a power of attorney. This can also be someone appointed after they lose the capacity to make decisions. The process of who becomes designated as the healthcare proxy varies widely from state to state. Some states have a set hierarchy of people that become the default healthcare proxy if one isn't designated by the patient prior to incapacitation.

DNR AND ADVANCED DIRECTIVES

Case (continued): The patient is deemed to not have capacity to make decisions currently as she does not understand her current situation and the ramifications of her choices. Shared decision-making is done with the patient's daughter (and power of attorney) who understands the risks, benefits, and alternatives to refusing transport to the emergency department.
   Three days later, EMS is again called back to the same skilled nursing facility for the same patient who has now developed severe respiratory distress. The patient is found obtunded with labored respirations at 35 breaths/minute. Her oxygen saturations are 75% on 4L via nasal cannula, which was increased from her baseline 2L via nasal cannula. The nurse states that the daughter has been contacted and will meet them at the hospital with a copy of the DNR.

1. What is a DNR?
   A DNR (do-not-resuscitate) is a legal order that allows a patient to forego cardiopulmonary resuscitation (CPR) and usual advanced cardiovascular life support (ACLS) care in situations of cardiopulmonary arrest.

2. When does a DNR apply?

   A DNR order only applies in cases involving cardiopulmonary arrest, which would typically require CPR as standard treatment.

3. Does a DNR mean "do not treat?"

   Absolutely not! Simply because a patient has a DNR does not mean they should not get treatments for other conditions short of cardiopulmonary arrest. For example, a patient in severe respiratory distress can get noninvasive positive pressure ventilation (bilevel positive airway pressure [BiPAP]/continuous positive airway pressure [CPAP]) to help with their breathing, hospitalizations, and other standard medical therapies.

4. Does DNR mean "do not intubate" as well?

   Not necessarily. Remember that the DNR only goes into effect once the patient is in cardiac arrest. This does not mean that patients who are in respiratory failure only should not be intubated as cardiac arrest makes up <2% of the indications for intubation. However, if you feel that a patient requires intubation this may prompt further discussion with the patient and family regarding their goals of care and patient wishes prior to intubation.

5. What constitutes a valid DNR?

   There is significant variability on what constitutes a DNR within different countries and from state to state in the United States. It is of the utmost importance to understand your local laws regarding what makes a DNR valid and what is accepted as documentation for a DNR.

CHALLENGES IN PREHOSPITAL END-OF-LIFE CARE

Case (continued): The patient is placed on CPAP by EMS and transported to the hospital is initiated. During transport, the patient's condition worsens and progresses to cardiac arrest despite high-quality care. The crew does not initiate ACLS care with CPR due to having a copy of the patient's DNR as a part of the previously electronic patient care report. They arrive at the hospital and the patient is pronounced dead by the emergency physician upon arrival.

1. Should DNRs be honored in prehospital emergency care?

   Yes. However, that is dependent on following prehospital protocols from medical direction, and having a valid DNR presented within the relatively short time that prehospital providers care for a patient often makes this challenging. EMS personnel often begin CPR by acting in the best interest of the patient when in doubt of a patient's DNR status. This may be difficult or impossible to confirm in the prehospital setting as family are not always available to confirm the patient's wishes or present the appropriate DNR documentation.

2. What is an advanced directive?

   Advanced directives are a set of instructions from a patient or healthcare surrogate to healthcare providers regarding end-of-life care. This includes but is not limited to a DNR or healthcare proxy. Advanced directives can be very general like a DNR or specific, like the desire to not have particular procedures or forms of medication.

3. Should advanced directives be honored in prehospital emergency care?

   Yes. However, this can be even more challenging than honoring a DNR in the prehospital environment as advanced directives may be lengthy, specific, and in direct conflict with EMS protocols. Medical direction should be contacted to clarify if questions arise, but prehospital personnel should act with the best interest of the patient in mind.

4. How do I start the discussion about the death and dying process with families?

   Admittedly this is a difficult discussion for anyone, but EMS gets a rare glimpse into patient's lives that most people in healthcare never do. Be honest and empathetic with the patient and family, give information at a pace dictated by the patient/family, and anticipate for and answer questions calmly. Remember that everyone processes end-of-life issues in variable speeds and in a variety of ways.

KEY POINTS

- Patients at the end of their life may have difficulty with the ability to make medical decisions for themselves, and it is important to determine if the patient has the capacity to do so.
- Powers of attorney or a healthcare proxy may make decisions on a patient's behalf if they are not able to regarding their medical care.
- A DNR or advanced directive may limit the types of care that a patient or their proxy would like them to receive at the end of their life.

BIBLIOGRAPHY

Breu A, Herzig S. Differentiating DNI from DNR: combating code status conflation. *J Hosp Med.* 2014;9(10):669-670.

DeMartino E, Dudzinski D, Doyle C, et al. Who decides when a patient can't? Statutes on alternate decision makers. *N Engl J Med.* 2017;376(15):1478-1482.

Iserson K. A simplified prehospital advance directive law: Arizona's approach. *Ann Emerg Med.* 1993;22(11):1703-1710.

Marco C, Brenner J, Kraus C, McGrath N, Derse A. Refusal of emergency medical treatment: case studies and ethical foundations. *Ann Emerg Med.* 2017;70(5):696-703.

Marco C, Schears R. Prehospital resuscitation practices: a survey of prehospital providers. *Ann Emerg Med.* 1999;34(4):S81.

Ptacek J. Breaking bad news. *JAMA.* 1996;276(6):496.

Reuter P, Agostinucci J, Bertrand P, et al. Prevalence of advance directives and impact on advanced life support in out-of-hospital cardiac arrest victims. *Resuscitation.* 2017;116:105-108.

CHAPTER 69

POISONINGS AND TOXIC EXPOSURES

Robert N.E. French

QUESTIONS AND ANSWERS

Case: EMS responds to a home where an 18-month-old child may have ingested some of his grandmother's medications. The child is found awake and alert. The child was under the care of the grandparents who were babysitting. While briefly unattended, he got into his grandmother's purse. The contents of the purse are scattered. Pills from a medication organizer are spilled. It is unclear if any are missing. There are no labels. The grandmother does not know the names of her medications but can tell you that she has diabetes and hypertension and is being treated for chronic pain and depression. You decide to transport the patient to the hospital for medical evaluation.

1. What is the phone number for the Poison Control Center?
   According to the American Association of Poison Control Centers, the Poison Help hotline, 1-800-222-1222, connects callers to their local poison control center anywhere in the United States and its territories. An interactive online tool is also available at www.poisonhelp.org. The Poison Control Center can help with pill identification.

2. Name some drugs and household products that, when taken in small quantities, are potentially lethal to small children.
   - Antimalarials
   - Antidysrhythmic drugs
   - Benzocaine
   - Beta-blockers
   - Calcium channel blockers
   - Camphor
   - Clonidine and similar pharmaceuticals
   - Diphenoxylate with atropine
   - Lindane
   - Methanol
   - Methyl salicylate
   - Opioids
   - Sulfonylureas
   - Theophylline
   - Tricyclic antidepressants

Case: EMS is called for an altered mental status case. The family reports that the patient may have overdosed on medication or used a recreational drug.

3. Where does one start when evaluating an overdose patient?
   One starts by examining the patient. Particular attention is paid to the vital signs (blood pressure, heart rate, respiratory rate, and temperature) and to other physical exam findings such as the mental status (depressed, agitated, hallucinating), pupil size (pinpoint or dilated), skin (dry vs. moist axillae), mucous membranes (dry vs. moist), gastrointestinal (GI) system (presence or absence of bowel sounds, presence of diarrhea), and urinary system (presence of a distended bladder or evidence or urinary incontinence).

4. What is a "toxidrome?"
   The group of physical exam findings and symptoms that are characteristically associated with a certain type of toxicant is known as a toxidrome. Thus, one does not necessarily need to know the specific toxicant when providing initial care to the poisoned patient.

Case (continued): The patient has a depressed mental status. His pupils are noted to be small. He is breathing 4–6 times a minute. A belt is around the left arm and there is an empty syringe nearby.

5. What toxidrome does this describe? What is the antidote and what are the indications for use?
   The opioid toxidrome is classically characterized by the triad of miosis, mental status depression, and respiratory depression. These signs are not always consistently present. The most important sign is respiratory depression, which can progress to apnea, hypoxia, and death. Naloxone should be given to those who are suspected of having

overdosed on an opiate AND have respiratory depression. Those who have been exposed to a substance that is suspected to be an opiate who have nonspecific symptoms without respiratory depression should not be treated with naloxone.

Case: *The patient appears to be having visual hallucinations, he has mumbling speech, and he is picking in the air and at his clothing. He is tachycardic and hypertensive. His axillae and mucous membranes are dry and his skin is hot and flushed. His pupils are markedly dilated. An empty bottle of over-the-counter allergy medication is found nearby.*

6. What toxidrome does this describe?
   The anticholinergic (antimuscarinic) toxidrome occurs when the effect of acetylcholine at the muscarinic receptor is antagonized. It is characterized by anhidrosis (dry skin), mydriasis (dilated pupils), flushing, hyperthermia, and delirium. Urinary retention is common and may contribute to a patient's agitation. Features are variably present. There are several medications that can cause anticholinergic toxidrome, including atropine, hyoscyamine, and scopolamine. Anticholinergic features are common in overdose of antihistamines, antipsychotics, and tricyclic antidepressants. BZ (3-quinuclidinyl benzilate) was developed as a potential anticholinergic incapacitating agent.

Case: *The patient is agitated, tachycardic, and hypertensive. He is markedly diaphoretic. He reportedly was smoking a crystalline substance.*

7. What is this toxidrome? What substances can cause it and how is it treated?
   Sympathomimetic toxicity is characterized by elevated blood pressure, tachycardia, tachypnea, and hyperthermia. Other physical findings include agitation, dilated pupils, and diaphoresis.
   Toxicants include amphetamine, methamphetamine, cocaine, and caffeine. Treatment involves preventing self-harm from agitation and prevention of the development of hyperthermia. Hyperthermic patients should be rapidly cooled.

Case: *The patient has a depressed mental status. His respirations are sonorous, raising concerns about his ability to protect his airway. There is a nearly empty bottle of a brown liquid at his side.*

8. What is this toxidrome? What substances can cause it and how is it treated?
   Sedative hypnotic toxicity is characterized by a depressed mental status. Blood pressure, heart rate, and respiratory rate may be depressed. Toxicants include ethanol, benzodiazepines, and barbiturates. Treatment is generally supportive care.

Case: *Rescue is called for a "person down." Upon arrival, three people are found unconscious and unresponsive at the bottom of a stairwell leading into a basement. A fourth states that two collapsed when they descended the stairs to assist the first who collapsed at the bottom of the stairwell.*

9. Describe the knockdown toxidrome.
   The knockdown toxidrome is characterized by a sudden loss of consciousness. This is caused by cellular asphyxia caused by inadequate ambient oxygen, by impaired delivery of oxygen to the tissues, or by impaired use of oxygen by the tissues.

10. What is a simple asphyxiant?
    A simple asphyxiant acts by displacing oxygen. Displacement of oxygen by a gas that is heavier than air is a hazard of the confined space environment even if that gas has no other effect on the body.

11. What is a systemic asphyxiant?
    A systemic asphyxiant interferes with oxygen transport or with oxygen utilization.
    In the case of carbon monoxide and toxicants that induce methemoglobinemia, oxygen transport by hemoglobin is impaired. In the case of cyanide and hydrogen sulfide, oxygen utilization in the mitochondria is impaired by binding to cytochrome-c-oxidase in the electron transport chain.

12. What are the recommendations for hyperbaric therapy in the setting of carbon monoxide poisoning?
    Carbon monoxide impairs the transport of oxygen by binding to hemoglobin. Hyperbaric oxygen therapy shortens the duration of this binding. The Undersea and Hyperbaric Medicine Society recommends that hyperbaric oxygen therapy be considered for all cases of acute symptomatic CO poisoning. You may go to their website at www.uhms.org to locate a list of accredited hyperbaric chamber facilities.

13. What is methemoglobinemia (MetHb)? Name some potential inducers of MetHb. What medication can be used to reverse MetHb and what are contraindications to this treatment?
    MetHb occurs when the iron in hemoglobin is oxidized from the Fe^{2+} form to the Fe^{3+} form. Methemoglobin is not capable of carrying oxygen; thus, oxygen transport is impaired. Methemoglobin causes the blood to have a brown color; the patient may appear blue or cyanotic.

Occupational/environmental hazards that can cause MetHb include nitrates, aniline dyes.

Pharmaceuticals that can cause MetHb include amyl nitrite, sodium nitrite, benzocaine, dapsone, and phenazopyridine. Methylene blue can be used to treat MetHb. It is contraindicated in those with known glucose-6-phosphate dehydrogenase deficiency.

14. What is the mechanism of cyanide poisoning? What treatments are available? How do they work?

Cyanide blocks the electron transport chain by binding to iron atoms that are in the Fe^{3+} form in cytochrome-c-oxidase. This prevents the utilization of oxygen and the production of adenosine triphosphate (ATP).

Two treatments are available in the United States, hydroxocobalamin and the three-drug cyanide antidote kit. Hydroxocobalamin contains a cobalt atom. Cyanide has a higher affinity for the cobalt atom than it does for the Fe^{3+} atom in cytochrome-c-oxidase. Cyanide binds to hydroxocobalamin, forming cyanocobalamin, which is not toxic and is eliminated in the urine. The cyanide antidote kit contains three drugs: amyl nitrite, sodium nitrite, and sodium thiosulfate. Amyl nitrite and sodium nitrite work by oxidizing the iron atom in hemoglobin from Fe^{2+} to Fe^{3+} causing MetHb. Since a far greater amount of iron in the body is in hemoglobin than in cytochrome-c-oxidase, cyanide moves from the Fe^{3+} in the bound cytochrome-c-oxidase to the Fe^{3+} in MetHb. Sodium thiosulfate facilitates the conversion of cyanide to the far less toxic thiocyanate.

Case: *In 1995, a religious cult released sarin, a nerve agent, on the Tokyo Metro. Twelve people were killed, and over 5000 were injured.*

15. Describe the cholinergic toxidrome. What groups of toxicants cause the cholinergic toxidrome? What are the treatments for cholinergic poisoning? How do they work?

The cholinergic toxidrome occurs with organophosphate or carbamate insecticide exposure or with exposure to the so-called "nerve agents." These toxicants inhibit acetylcholinesterase, which breaks down acetylcholine. Acetylcholine accumulates in the synapse, leading to overstimulation of acetylcholine receptors. This causes several signs and symptoms that are easily recognizable in patients. Overstimulation at peripheral muscarinic receptors leads to salivation, lacrimation, urination, diarrhea, diaphoresis, miosis, bronchorrhea, bronchospasm, and bradycardia. Overstimulation at peripheral nicotinic receptors induces fasciculations and muscle weakness. Overstimulation at CNS receptors causes confusion, seizures, and coma.

Atropine is used to treat peripheral muscarinic symptoms. It works by competitively antagonizing the accumulated acetylcholine at muscarinic receptors. Pralidoxime "reactivates" acetylcholinesterase inhibited by organophosphate insecticides or nerve agents if it is given before "aging" occurs, where the inhibition becomes permanent.

16. What is the CHEMPACK program?

The CHEMPACK program provides prepositioned atropine and pralidoxime, an antidote for nerve agent poisoning, to state, local, and/or tribal authorities. There are two types of containers: EMS containers, which are geared to first responders and are 85% autoinjectors, and hospital containers, which are geared to the clinical care environment and are 85% multidose vials.

COMMON OVER-THE-COUNTER MEDICATIONS

1. What are the characteristics of salicylate (aspirin) overdose?

Salicylate poisoning is characterized by hyperventilation, tinnitus, and GI irritation.

Salicylates stimulate respiration, and patients will have an increased rate and/or depth of ventilation. In addition, they may have metabolic acidosis. Nothing should be given that could depress the respiratory drive as this could worsen the metabolic acidosis and lead to rapid deterioration and death. Patients may notice that sounds are muffled or they may have a ringing sensation; unable to hear, they may come across as confused.

2. What are the characteristics of diphenhydramine (Benadryl) overdose?

Diphenhydramine is an antihistamine. In overdose, patients develop anticholinergic symptoms including anticholinergic delirium. Cardiac sodium channel blockade can also be seen, which can manifest as a wide QRS complex and ventricular dysrhythmia.

3. What are the characteristics of dextromethorphan overdose?

Dextromethorphan is an over-the-counter cough suppressant that can cause disassociation in overdose similar to ketamine or Phencyclidine (PCP).

4. What are the characteristics of acetaminophen overdose?

Acetaminophen overdose is common and it is a leading cause of liver failure. Acetaminophen is available alone as well as in combination with other over-the-counter medications such as diphenhydramine and dextromethorphan or in combination with opiate pain medications such as codeine, hydrocodone, or oxycodone. Overdose is often intentional but can also occur unintentionally when people take combination medications without realizing that they contain acetaminophen.

KEY POINTS

- The Poison Help Hotline, 1-800-222-1222, connects callers to the local poison control center.
- A toxidrome is a group of physical exam findings and symptoms that are characteristically associated with a certain type of toxicant.
- Simple asphyxiants displace oxygen, whereas systemic asphyxiants interfere with oxygen transport or utilization.
- Overdose of commonly available, over-the-counter medications can cause life-threatening toxicity.

BIBLIOGRAPHY

Abdi A, Rose E, Levine M. Diphenhydramine overdose with intraventricular conduction delay treated with hypertonic sodium bicarbonate and IV lipid emulsion. 7, September. *Western Journal of Emergency Medicine*. 2014;15:855-858.

American Association of Poison Control Centers June 19, 2019. https://www.aapcc.org/.

Arens AM, et al. Safety and effectiveness of physostigmine: a 10-year retrospective review. *Clinical Toxicology*. 2018;56(2):101-107.

Borron S. Asphyxiants. In: Walter FG, ed. *Advanced Hazmat Life Support Provider Manual*. s.l: Arizona Board of Regents; 2014.

Borron SW, Babarta VS. Asphyxiants. *Emerg Med Clin N Am*. 2015;33:88-115.

Boyer EW. Management of opioid analgesic overdose. *N Engl J Med*. 2012;367(2):146-155.

Ciotonne GR. Toxidrome recognition in chemical-weapons attacks. *N Engl J Med*. 2018;378(17):1611-1620.

Dawson AH, Buckley NA. Pharmacological management of anticholinergic delirium—theory, evidence, and practice.3. *Br J Clin Pharmacol*. March 2015;81:516-524.

Eldridge DL, Van Eyk J, Kornegay C. Pediatric Toxicology. *Emerg Med Clin N Am*. 2007;25(2):283-308.

Hall AH, Borron SW. Antidote: hydroxocobalamin. In: Walter FG, ed. *Advanced Hazmat Life Support Provider Manual*. s.l: Arizona Board of Regents; 2014.

Hall AH, Walter FG. Antidote: methylene blue. In: Walter FG, ed. *Advanced Hazmat Life Support Provider Manual*. s.l: Arizona Board of Regents; 2014.

Hall AH, Walter FG. Antidote: amyl nitrite. In: Walter FG, ed. *Advanced Hazmat Life Support Provider Manual*. s.l: Arizona Board of Regents; 2014.

Hall AH, Walter FG. Sodium nitrite. In: Walter FG, ed. *Advanced Hazmat Life Support Provider Manual*. s.l: Arizona Board of Regents; 2014.

Hodgeman MJ, Garrard AR. A review of acetaminophen poisoning. *Crit Care Clin*. 2012;28(4):499-516.

Hoffman RS, Howland MA, Lewin NA, Nelson L, and Goldfrank LR. Initial evaluation of the patient: vital signs and toxic syndromes. *Goldfrank's Toxicologic Emergencies*. New York: McGraw Hill Education; 2015:26-29.

Holstege CP, Borek HA. Toxidromes. *Crit Care Clin*. 4, October 2012;28:479-498.

Mofenson HC, Greensher J. The unknown poison. *Pediatrics*. 3, September 1974;53:336-342.

O'Malley, Gerald F. Emergency department management of the salicylate-poisoned patient. *Emerg Med Clin N Am*. 2007;25(2):333-346.

Romanelli F, Smith KM. Dextromethorphan abuse: clinical effects and management. *Journal of the American Pharmacy Association*. 2, March-April 2009;49:e20-e25.

Tokuda Y, et al. Prehospital management of sarin nerve gas terrorism in urban settings: 10 years of progress after the Tokyo subway sarin attack. *Resuscitation*. 2006;68:193-202.

US Department of Health and Human Services. Chemical Hazards Emergency Management. *CHEMPACK*. June 20, 2019. https://chemm.nlm.nih.gov/chempack.htm.

US Department of Health and Human Services. Public Health Emergency. June 19, 2019. https://www.phe.gov/about/sns/Pages/default.aspx.

US Department of Health and Human Services. Toxic Syndromes/Toxidromes. Chemical Hazards Emergency Medical Management. June 20, 2019.https://chemm.nlm.nih.gov/toxicsyndromes.htm.

US Department of Health and Human Services. Guidance on Diagnosis and Treatment for Healthcare Providers. Radiation Emergency Medical Management. June 19, 2019. https://www.remm.nlm.gov/.

US Department of Health and Human Services. Strategic National Stockpile. Public health emergency. June 19, 2019. https://www.phe.gov/about/sns/Pages/default.aspx.

US National Library of Medicine. *WISER*. June 19, 2019. https://wiser.nlm.nih.gov/.

Weaver LK. Carbon Monoxide Poisoning. *Undersea and Hyperbaric Medical Society Hyperbaric Oxygen Therapy Indications*. North Palm Beach: Best Publishing Company; 2014:47-55.

White CC, DeBaltz G. One pill can kill. *JEMS*. 2015;40(9):56-59.

AIRWAY MANAGEMENT, OXYGENATION, AND VENTILATION

Jeffrey L. Jarvis and John Gonzales

CHAPTER 70

QUESTIONS AND ANSWERS

1. What is the point of airway management in the prehospital setting?

The point is the same regardless of setting: to ensure adequate oxygenation and ventilation while protecting the patient from aspiration.

Oxygenation is the process of oxygen diffusing to cells down a concentration gradient, while ventilation is the process of gas movement down a pressure gradient. It is possible to have oxygenation without ventilation (passive or apneic oxygenation) and to have ventilation without oxygenation (movement of oxygen-depleted gas). Both are critical. Likewise, oxygenation and ventilation are both dependent on an unobstructed path from the exterior environment to the alveoli. If that path is obstructed by vomitus, blood, excessive secretions, teeth, or the tongue, neither oxygenation nor ventilation can occur.

2. What are the indications for providing airway management?

Interruptions in oxygenation or ventilation, i.e., some type of respiratory failure, or the need to protect the patient's airway from obstruction.

Acute respiratory failure can roughly be broken into two groups: hypoxic and hypercapnic. If a patient is not maintaining sufficient oxygenation, increased inspired oxygen must be provided. If the patient is not moving sufficient gas to remove carbon dioxide, ventilatory support must be provided. Often, these two overlap, but it is helpful to think of why a patient needs airway support.

3. How can oxygenation and ventilation be assessed?

There are direct and indirect approaches to assessing oxygenation and ventilation. The direct approach involves measurement. Pulse oximetry (SpO_2) uses infrared light projecting through a tissue bed to measure the oxygen saturation of hemoglobin, while end-tidal carbon dioxide ($EtCO_2$) measures the partial pressure of expired CO_2. SpO_2 directly measures oxygenation and $EtCO_2$ measures ventilation.

Indirectly, oxygenation should be assessed through the patient's mental status (oxygen is required for proper cognitive function), skin color, work of breathing, and degree of dyspnea (the sensation of not being able to breathe). Ventilation can be assessed by estimating the patient's tidal volume (V_t). V_t is the volume of air moved in a single breath. It can be assessed by looking at chest rise and fall and, roughly, at the amplitude of the $EtCO_2$ waveform. Minute volume (V_m) is the amount of gas moved in a minute and is calculated by multiplying the V_t by the respiratory rate. If the respiratory rate is too slow, there will be inadequate gas exchange.

Respiratory rate is under complex physiologic control. Tachypnea (rapid respiratory rate) is often a response to hypoxia or increased metabolic need for either more oxygen or more CO_2 off-loading.

Auscultation of breath sounds can provide useful information about ventilation. The presence of wheezing can indicate bronchospasm of the small airways, crackles can indicate increased interstitial fluid seen in pulmonary edema or presence of pneumonia, while the absence or decreased breath sounds can indicate obstruction of the airways or collapse of the lung.

4. How is oxygenation assisted?

Patients with inadequate oxygenation can be supported by providing supplemental oxygen by a variety of means including nasal cannula, face mask, nonrebreather mask, venturi mask, or bag-valve mask. Each of these requires a patent airway to allow for unimpeded movement of oxygen as well as an adequately ventilated patient. Each delivers a different concentration of oxygen (fraction of inspired oxygen, FiO_2). In general, patients should receive the minimum concentration of oxygen needed to ensure adequate oxygenation. Just as hypoxia is harmful, so is excessive oxygen administered for anything other than short periods.

Inadequate tissue oxygenation can also occur in the presence of plenty of oxygen reaching the lungs. This can occur when there is a mismatch between ventilation (movement of gas) and perfusion (movement of blood). Since the vast majority of oxygen is transported attached to hemoglobin molecules and these hemoglobin molecules are transported in blood, obstructions to the movement of blood, as seen in pulmonary embolism, can cause hypoxia even when a patient is breathing 100% oxygen. Additionally, even if there is plenty of oxygen and no obstruction to blood movement, inadequate amounts of hemoglobin (anemia) can cause tissue hypoxia. Anemia from chronic blood loss from a slow gastrointestinal bleed is often first noticed by a patient because they get short of breath.

5. **How is ventilation assisted?**
First, adequate ventilation requires the presence of a patent airway allowing for unimpeded gas movement. If this is not present, a patent airway must first be provided. Ventilation can then be assisted with NIPPV devices such as continuous positive airway pressure (CPAP) or bilevel positive airway pressure (BiPAP or bilevel). These assist a patient's ventilation by decreasing the work of breathing, recruiting additional alveoli, and keeping smaller airways open.

6. **How can airway patency be maintained?**
Proper airway positioning is an important first step in maintaining an open airway. Opening the airway using a head-tilt-chin lift or jaw thrust (in suspected trauma patients) can clear an airway by moving the tongue away from the back of the throat, thus opening the airway.
Clearing the airway of debris such as vomitus, blood, or other foreign bodies will also help maintain a patent airway. Suction assisted laryngoscopy and airway decontamination (SALAD) is highly effective in clearing an airway.
If the airways are obstructed, they can be held open by airway adjuncts. Oral and nasal pharyngeal airways (OPA and NPA) are inserted into either the mouth or the nose and are designed to keep the tongue and soft tissues of the upper airway from falling backward and obstructing air movement. NPAs are typically better tolerated by patients with some level of gag reflex, while OPAs are typically more noxious and require more obtunded patients. Neither of these will protect against liquid obstruction such as vomit or blood, however.
More invasive devices are typically required to protect against aspiration of liquid airway contaminants. Blind insertion airway devices (BIADs) are a group of airways designed to be blindly inserted into the upper airway. These include the King laryngeal tube (LT) and various types of laryngeal mask airway (LMA). These protect the airway and allow for assisted ventilation and typically require less skill to insert.
Endotracheal tube insertion (ETI) has classically been considered the "gold standard" of airway management. It involves placing a tube into the trachea under visualization with a laryngoscope. It requires substantial training to acquire and maintain this skill.

7. **What is the best type of advanced airway to use in cardiac arrest?**
This is an ongoing and controversial question. The classic answer has been an ETI; however, several recent large, well done randomized controlled trials (RCTs) have questioned this dogma. The PART trial was an American multicenter trial comparing ETI to the King LT airway and found a 2.9% mortality benefit with the LT insertion. The AIRWAYS-2 trial was a British multicenter trial comparing ETI with the iGel airway and found no difference in mortality. Both were limited by poor ETI performance. What is still unclear is the impact that well-performed ETI with no compression interruption has on mortality. What is clear, however, from these trials is that a strategy using either LT or iGel as the primary airway management strategy is an acceptable strategy and requires less training and quality improvement effort than ETI.

8. **What are the potential risks of endotracheal intubation?**
While ETI placement offers several benefits (airway protection, ability to place patients on ventilators for long periods), there are risks involved.
The most important interventions for patients in cardiac arrest are rapid defibrillation and minimally interrupted chest compressions. Early and poorly done ETI can interrupt both of these.
For patients not in cardiac arrest, the biggest potential risks are peri-intubation hypoxia and hypotension. This is most well documented in patients with traumatic brain injury where even one episode of hypoxia or hypotension can raise the odds of death by over fourfold. Profound peri-intubation hypoxia is common and harmful, leading to bradycardia and cardiac arrest in between 2% and 3% of all intubations.
Once the patient is intubated, overventilation can be very harmful. Overinflation of the lungs increases intrathoracic pressure, which decreases cardiac preload (blood returning to the heart), leading to a drop in cardiac output and blood pressure. Hyperventilation also leads to cerebral vasoconstriction, which decreases cerebral blood flow and increases mortality.

9. **What can be done to mitigate the potential risks of endotracheal intubation?**
For patients in cardiac arrest, it has long been assumed that compressions must be interrupted to successfully perform intubation. This is not true, but successful intubation without compression interruption requires deliberate practice and may be aided by adjuncts such as a Bougie or video laryngoscopy. Most importantly, though, it requires a well-choreographed and preplanned team approach to resuscitation where every team member recognizes that compressions must not be interrupted to intubate.
For nonarrest patients, awareness, attention, and adequate preparation go a long way to preventing peri-intubation hypoxia, hypotension, cardiac arrest, and hyperventilation. The highest rates of first-pass success occur with the use of sedation and neuromuscular blocking drugs in a procedure known as rapid sequence intubation

(RSI). This involves inducing complete muscle relaxation to enable tube placement but also involves a period of apnea. Adequately raising preintubation oxygen saturation will allow longer periods of safe apnea, allowing for less rushed and more successful intubation. Adequate preoxygenation typically requires 3 minutes of normal V_t breathing at 100% oxygen levels. Several studies show that starting an intubation attempt with oxygen saturations less than 93% is almost always associated with peri-intubation hypoxia which may be profound. Raising preintubation saturations above 93% for at least 3 minutes replaces inert nitrogen with oxygen and is associated with lower risk of hypoxia during the intubation attempt. Provision of apneic oxygenation (high-flow oxygen administered through a nasal cannula during the intubation attempt while the patient is apneic) can prolong the safe apneic period and decrease the rates of peri-intubation hypoxia.

Proper patient positioning, with the head and shoulders elevated ("ramping") and the neck in extension ("sniffing") places patients in an "ear-to-sternal notch" position, which has been associated with improved intubating conditions, improved preoxygenation, and longer periods of safe apnea prior to desaturation.

Delayed sequence intubation (DSI) is a process of giving ketamine to patients to allow optimal preoxygenation to occur, and then administering a neuromuscular blocking agent in a delayed fashion to facilitate intubation. DSI has been associated with improved preoxygenation and lower rates of peri-intubation hypoxia.

Together, proper positioning, mandatory preoxygenation for 3 minutes, apneic oxygenation, and DSI were associated with a 40% absolute reduction in peri-intubation hypoxia.

10. What are the best performance measures for an airway management quality improvement effort?
The best measures are those that focus on patient-oriented outcomes, such as avoidance of harm or improvement in mortality. These are often more challenging to measure, however, because they require more patients to see a difference and many EMS agencies are hampered by a lack of patient follow-up data from hospitals.
Useful and achievable measures include the proportion of:
a. hypoxic patients with improved SpO_2 from first to last measurement,
b. intubated patients with First Pass Success without hypoxia or hypotension,
c. patients with ETI or supraglottic airway (SGA) insertion with $EtCO_2$ placement confirmation,
d. advanced airway placed without interruption of compressions in cardiac arrest.

KEY POINTS

- The purpose of airway management is to ensure adequate ventilation and oxygenation.
- The indications for airway management are hypoxic respiratory failure, hypercapnic respiratory failure, and inability to protect one's airway.
- Oxygenation and ventilation can be supported with oxygen administration, NIPPV, or advanced airways such as endotracheal intubation or supraglottic airways.
- The role of advanced airways in cardiac arrest management is not clear but should not detract from establishing good-quality compressions and early defibrillation.
- If providers are going to intubate, they should pay close attention to physiologic optimization of oxygen saturation and blood pressure before, during, and after the intubation, as well as avoiding overventilation.

BIBLIOGRAPHY

Benger JR, Kirby K, Black S, et al. Effect of a strategy of a supraglottic airway device vs tracheal intubation during out-of-hospital cardiac arrest on functional outcome: the AIRWAYS-2 randomized clinical trial. *JAMA*. 2018;320:779-791.

Jarvis JL, Barton D, Wang H. Defining the plateau point: when are further attempts futile in out-of-hospital advanced airway management. *Resuscitation*. 2018;130:57-60.

Jarvis JL, Gonzales J, Johns D, Sager L. Implementation of a clinical bundle to reduce out-of-hospital peri-intubation hypoxia. *Ann Emerg Med*. 2018;72:272-279.

Jarvis JL, McClure SF, Johns D. EMS intubation improves with King vision video laryngoscopy. *Prehosp Emerg Care*. 2015;19:482-489.

Jarvis JL, Wampler D, Wang HE. Association of patient age with first Pass Success in out-of-hospital advanced airway management. *Resuscitation*. 2019;141:136-143.

Prekker ME, Delgado F, Shin J, et al. Pediatric intubation by paramedics in a large emergency medical services system: process, challenges, and outcomes. *Ann Emerg Med*. 2016;67:20-29.

Spaite DW, Hu C, Bobrow BJ, et al. The effect of combined out-of-hospital hypotension and hypoxia on mortality in major traumatic brain injury. *Ann Emerg Med*. 2017;69:62-72.

Wang HE, Donnelly JP, Barton D, Jarvis JL. Assessing advanced airway management performance in a national cohort of emergency medical services agencies. *Ann Emerg Med*. 2018;71:597-607.

Wang HE, Lave JR, Sirio CA, Yealy DM. Paramedic intubation errors: isolated events or symptoms of larger problems? *Health Aff (Millwood)*. 2006;25:501-509.

Wang HE, Mann NC, Mears G, Jacobson K, Yealy DM. Out-of-hospital airway management in the United States. *Resuscitation*. 2011;82:378-385.

CHAPTER 71

ANALGESIA

Colby Redfield

QUESTIONS AND ANSWERS

Case: *You are dispatched to a local athletic field for a player down on the field with a leg injury. A 21-year-old male was playing soccer when he was tackled from behind, causing him to have ankle pain. You arrive on scene to find him with a deformed right ankle and screaming in pain. He is otherwise uninjured and is neurovascularly intact in the right foot.*

1. What do studies suggest about pain control in the prehospital setting?
    Studies have suggested that pain is undertreated in the prehospital setting. The National Association of EMS Physicians (NAEMSP) currently recommends that EMS agencies have a policy in place to address adequate pain control. Obviously, the methods of pain control available will differ depending on the level of provider responding to the call. The options for pain control range from oral acetaminophen or ibuprofen to parenteral narcotics depending on level of certification of the provider and local protocols.

2. What are the desirable properties of opioids in the prehospital setting?
    Opioids are useful for controlling severe pain. They have several desirable properties, including rapid onset, high potency, reversibility, titratability, and relative safety when used per protocol. When using parenteral narcotics, all patients must be closely monitored. This monitoring should include pulse, blood pressure, oxygen saturation, and possibly end-tidal CO_2 monitoring.

3. What are some of the side effects of opioids that prehospital providers must be aware of?
    Opioids may lead to respiratory depression and hypotension and they may cause nausea. Each of the opioids tends to have a "typical" side effect profile that the provider must be aware of and prepared to manage.

4. What are common opioids used by EMS crews?
    Morphine, hyrdomorphone (Dilaudid), and fentanyl are commonly used in the prehospital setting. Depending on your local and/or state protocols, and availability, you may have access to a combination of these medications. Each of these medications has a unique profile regarding time to onset of action, hemodynamic effects, and side effects. The practitioner must be aware of the idiosyncrasies of each of these medications and take them into account when administering them.

5. What are alternative routes of medication administration besides the intravenous (IV) route?
    Various routes of administration including intramuscular (IM), intraosseous, intranasal, and oral have been used for opioid medications. The administration route will influence the time to onset and the side effect profile. For instance, medication given IM will have a slower onset of action than one given IV push. The route of administration may also influence the side effect profile of the medication. Intranasal medication administration is hampered by unpredictable absorption and total volume of medication that can be administered.

6. After assessing your patient and determining his level of distress, you decided to administer 6 mg of morphine IV for pain control. Shortly afterward, your patient begins to become hypoxic. How is an opioid overdose reversed?
    Opioid overdose can be successfully reversed with naltrexone. Naltrexone is a competitive antagonist at the μ-opioid receptor that will reverse the effect of an opioid medication. Depending on the dose of naltrexone given, reversal may range from improvement of respiratory depression to causing the patient to go into opioid withdrawal. It is generally advised to titrate the administration of naltrexone to effect by giving small doses (0.4 mg IV) until the respiratory depression resolves. During this time, respirations should be supported by basic life support (BLS) airway maneuvers such as head tilt/jaw thrust, nasopharyngeal/oropharyngeal airway insertion if needed, and bag-valve mask ventilation. Rapid administration of large doses of naltrexone may lead to noncardiogenic pulmonary edema.

7. Which opioid does not cause a release of histamine?
    Fentanyl is a synthetic opioid and does not cause a release of histamine. Due to this feature, it reduces the chance of significant hemodynamic effects. Fentanyl is very lipid soluble, which allows for quick crossover of the blood-brain barrier, making it faster acting compared with other opiates.

8. Which are the expected changes in vital signs with opioid administration?

Opioids have the potential to cause hypotension, decrease respiratory drive, and decrease in mental status. Studies suggest that hypotension is less common with the administration of fentanyl. Slow administration of medication may also limit some of the side effects.

9. Are there alternative pharmacologic options to opiates for prehospital analgesia?

Multiple options exist to opiates for pain control. Commonly available options include nonsteroidal anti-inflammatory drugs (NSAIDS), acetaminophen, ketamine, and nitrous oxide.

10. What dose of ketamine is used for control of acute pain?

Typical pain dosing of ketamine is 0.1–0.3 mg/kg IV. This may be guided by local protocol. Some protocols call for this medication to be diluted in a 10-cc bag of saline and then run over a period of 5 to 10 minutes rather than as an IV push. Administering an opioid before giving ketamine may provide improved pain relief.

11. Which are common vital sign changes with ketamine?

Ketamine can cause an increase in blood pressure and heart rate. If the dose is given as a rapid IV push, there can be transient respiratory depression. Slow administration of the medication will generally avoid this side effect. Recent studies have debunked the myth that ketamine causes an unsafe increase in intracranial pressure.

12. Which IV NSAIDs are typically used in EMS?

Because of concern with opiate abuse and misuse, there has been push to seek nonopioid alternatives for pain control. Ketorolac has been demonstrated to be safe in most instances in the prehospital setting. The onset of action of ketorolac is longer than that of opioids, about 15 minutes. Again, administration of this medication is likely subject to local protocol.

13. Does acetaminophen have a role in pain management in the field?

Traditionally, acetaminophen has not been used in the prehospital setting for pain control. It has typically been used as an antipyretic for children. However, over the last several years, some EMS agencies have started using IV acetaminophen as an alternative to opioids. The cost of this medication may limit use in the prehospital setting as a single 1000-mg dose costs about $40.

14. Is the use of nitrous oxide safe?

Nitrous oxide has been demonstrated to be safe and effective in several studies.

The major advantage of nitrous oxide is the lack of serious side effects. Nitrous oxide has a relatively fast onset of action and the analgesic effect is lost about 3 to 5 minutes after cessation of administration. Administration of nitrous was added to the Advanced Emergency Medical Technicians (AEMT) scope of practice more than 10 years ago.

15. What are the contraindications to the use of nitrous oxide?

Contraindications to nitrous oxide administration include obvious intoxication, altered mental status, pregnancy, suspected pneumothorax, decompression sickness, suspected bowel obstruction, systolic blood pressure (SBP) <90 mm Hg, or respiratory rate <8/min. Again, close monitoring of the patient, as would be done if you were administering an opioid, should be in place when administering nitrous oxide.

16. Are there modalities besides medication that can reduce pain in the prehospital setting?

There are several nonpharmacologic approaches to help alleviate pain. Applying ice to the area and splinting the extremity involved has been shown to help control pain. Elevation of the extremity to above the level of the heart may also help in pain reduction.

It is important that we keep our patients informed about any movement that may cause them discomfort. Sometimes, it is necessary to move patients with painful orthopedic injuries before we can provide pharmacologic pain relief. Telling patients that we have to move them and that it may cause pain may actually help lessen the pain.

17. How can providers assess the effectiveness of our pain control efforts?

The perception of pain varies from person to person considerably. What one person finds exquisitely painful, another may tolerate rather well. Thus, it is crucial to assess the pain level of each patient that you are going to treat. One size does not fit all regarding pain control.

When assessing an individual with pain, you need to ascertain their perception of the pain. Ask them to rate the pain on a numeric scale and use this as a guide to treatment and effectiveness of any medication that you have administered. There are many adult and pediatric versions of these scales available for use.

KEY POINTS

- Pain has been undertreated in the prehospital setting and should be a focus of care.
- Opioids have been traditionally first line for pain management due to many desirable properties that they have.
- Alternatives to opioid medication include ketamine, NSAIDS, acetaminophen, and nitrous oxide. All of them have been used in the prehospital setting and have proven safety records.

BIBLIOGRAPHY

Bronsky E, Koola C, Orlanod A, et al. Intravenous low-dose ketamine provides greater pain control compared to fentanyl in a civilian prehospital trauma system: a propensity matched analysis. *Prehosp Emerg Care.* 2019;23(1):1-8.

Ducassé JL, Siksik G, Durand-Béchu M, et al. Nitrous oxide for early analgesia in the emergency setting: a randomized, double-blind multicenter prehospital trial. *Acad Emerg Med.* 2013;20(2):178-184.

Hilton MT, Paris P. Analgesia. In: Cone D, Brice JH, Delbridge TR, Myers B, eds. *Emergency Medical Services: Clinical Practice and Systems Oversight.* 2nd ed. Hoboken, NJ: John Wiley & Sons; 2015:470-475.

Walsh B, Cone DC, Meyer EM, Larkin GL. Paramedic attitudes regarding prehospital analgesia. *Prehosp Emerg Care.* 2013;17(1):78-87.

CHAPTER 72

CARE OF THE AGITATED/SUICIDAL PATIENT

Michelle A. Fischer

QUESTIONS AND ANSWERS

Case: A 911 call comes in for a suicidal patient. The basic life support (BLS) unit is dispatched. They arrive at a residence where police are already on the scene. You learn that the mother called for assistance when she arrived home from work 30 minutes ago to find her 18-year-old daughter locked in the bathroom after discovering a suicide note on the kitchen table. She had last spoken with her daughter approximately 3 hours prior and provided additional information that her daughter has a history of bipolar disease and has been extremely depressed over the past week since her longtime boyfriend ended their relationship. Mom states that she could not get into the bathroom as the door is locked. When she tried to enter, the daughter "freaked out," then started yelling "just let me die" and sobbing hysterically. Mom believes that she may have tried to overdose because she found empty bottles of beer, vodka, acetaminophen, and fluoxetine near her note. The BLS unit on the scene has upgraded for advanced life support (ALS) support.

1. What is the best way to approach the care of this suicidal patient?

   The safety of EMS providers is always the top priority. If police or law enforcement are not yet on the scene, wait for them to arrive before engaging the patient to assist with maintaining a safe environment. It is extremely important to ensure that the suicidal patient is not in possession of any potentially harmful items including firearms, knives, medications, or toxic substances. When the scene is deemed safe, and any serious medical conditions or needs have been addressed, then you can then approach the patient and attempt to establish rapport by interacting in a calm, accepting, and supportive manner. Pay attention to the scene surroundings, looking for any evidence of alcohol, pill bottles, or drug paraphernalia. If substances have been identified, collect them to accompany the patient to the hospital to assist the medical staff in determining appropriate treatment. Supervise the patient constantly. Supplement your history from family and bystanders. Transport the patient to the closest emergency department.

2. Does a suicidal patient have the right to refuse medical care?

   Each state has its own legal statutes involving *involuntary* detention of patients with imminent risk of harm to self or others. This is in contrast to a *voluntary* refusal, where patients who are deemed competent to make decisions may refuse care but they must show no immediate risk of danger to themselves or others. In an emergency, medical personnel may provide involuntary treatment, such as medication administration, but only to control the emergency. In this case, the emergency is the "imminent danger to self or others"; therefore, the patient cannot refuse medical care.

3. Are there any medical conditions that may cause acute agitation?

   Multiple medical conditions may cause agitation; always consider these conditions when caring for the agitated patient. These are high-risk patients that cause anxiety to all personnel. It is essential to remember that pathology may be driving agitated (or altered) behavior, some of which may be life-threatening, and we need to try to calm the individual in order to investigate the underlying etiology. It is prudent to consider, identify, and treat the reversible causes of acute agitation (Table 72.1). EMS personnel should check vital signs on all agitated patients, including oxygen saturation, temperature, and blood glucose level and examine the patient for external signs of trauma or localizing neurological findings.

Table 72.1. Medical Causes of Acute Agitation	
Infection	Sepsis, meningitis, encephalitis
Metabolic	Hyper- or hypoglycemia, thyroid storm, electrolyte derangement
Temperature	Hyper- or hypothermia
Trauma	Head injury
Toxins	Drug overdose, withdrawal, or adverse reaction
Alcohol	Intoxication or withdrawal
Respiratory	Hypoxia or hypercarbia
Neurologic	Stroke, seizure, hemorrhage

4. What are the chances of me ever having to care for a suicidal patient?
   Suicide remains one of the leading causes of death overall in the United States according to the Centers for Disease Control and Prevention (CDC) in 2017. Among individuals aged 10 to 34 years of age, suicide is the second leading cause of death and suicide rates were two times higher than that of homicides. Firearms are the most common method used for suicide in the United States, with almost half of all suicide deaths. In 2017, 4.3% of adults 18 years or older in the United States had thoughts of suicide; this is approximately 9.8 million adults, with over 1 million making an attempt. Almost 500,000 people are seen in hospital emergency departments each for self-injury. Based upon these statistics, you will likely encounter numerous suicidal patients during your EMS career, so review your organization's protocols and procedures and be prepared to respond appropriately.

5. When do I need to call the medical command physician?
   In general, EMS providers are permitted to perform patient care within their scope of practice when following their statewide protocols *or* when following the order of a medical command physician. The universal goal is to provide safe, effective, and high-quality prehospital care. If you are ever in doubt, need clarification, or would benefit from physician direction, then contact medical command.

6. Is there an EMS protocol available to guide me on the prehospital management of this patient?
   Most states have protocols in place for the management of agitated behavior or psychiatric disorders. All of them share the principles of safety of EMS personnel and awaiting for law enforcement to assist. Patients who are at imminent risk of self-injury or harm to others may require immediate medication intervention.

7. What are some verbal de-escalation techniques that I can utilize when taking care of this patient?
   Verbal de-escalation is very effective but does require a calm, composed, and deliberate approach. It is best done by a single provider in a quiet environment. Maintaining an awareness of your speech tone and content in addition to your body language is of utmost importance. Your body stance should be unconfrontational and at least a leg length away, respectful, and unaggressive without crossed arms or clenched fists. Maintain indirect eye contact and avoid facial expressions. Be direct, empathetic, and honest to establish rapport and trust. Set clear limits and options. If uncertain on what to say you can always start with the mnemonic **SAVE: support, acknowledge, validate, and emotion naming**. For example, "Let's talk together (support), I know this has been hard for you (acknowledge), and I would probably be reacting in a similar fashion (validate), it's normal for you to be upset (emotion naming)."

8. How do I decide when I need to medicate or physically restrain this patient? Can I do this before discussing it with the medical command physician?
   It is helpful to classify patients into one of three categories according to their level of agitation:
   Mild = Agitated but cooperative
   Moderate = Disruptive without danger
   Severe = Dangerous to self and/or others *or* excited delirium
   Many scales exist to help classify a patient's degree of agitation, but they are often not practical in the EMS world. One tool that may be simple enough for application in the prehospital setting is the Broset Violence Checklist (Table 72.2). This tool is able to aid in the prediction of future violent or aggressive behavior. When applying this scale, patients may receive one point for the presence or absence of each of the following findings: confusion, irritability, boisterousness, physical threats, verbal threats, attacks on objects. The score then determines if

Table 72.2. Broset Violence Checklist

SCORE ALL COMPONENTS OF CHECKLIST	PATIENT VIOLENCE SCREENING ELEMENTS
(0 = absent, 1 = present)	Confusion
(0 = absent, 1 = present)	Irritability
(0 = absent, 1 = present)	Boisterousness
(0 = absent, 1 = present)	Physical threats
(0 = absent, 1 = present)	Verbal threats
(0 = absent, 1 = present)	Attacks on objects
0–6 total	**Total risk of violence score**
Risk of Violence Score	**Preventative Measures Advised**
Low = 0	None
Moderate = 1–2	Recommended
High = 3 or more	Required

preventative measures are necessary. A low score (0) will not need chemical or physical restraints. Scores of 1–2 may need chemical intervention and it should be considered in discussion with the medical command physician. Scores of 3 or higher are considered the highest risk for violence and intervention is typically required. This may be a combination of medication and/or physical restraints but it is best practice to defer to your state protocol.

9. What are the typical medications used by EMS personnel to assist with the agitated patient?
   Most EMS agitated behavior algorithms use some form of a benzodiazepine as a sedative agent. Commonly used initial medications and dosages are:
   Lorazepam 0.5-2mg intramuscular (IM), intravenous
   (IV), intraosseous (IO), oral (PO) or 0.1 mg/kg IN (intranasal) max dose 4mg
   Midazolam 2.5-5mg IM, IV, IO, PO or 0.2-0.5mg/kg IN max dose 10mg
   Diazepam 2-10mg IM, IV, IO, PO or 0.2mg/kg IN max 10 mg

10. What is excited delirium?
   This form of agitation has several distinctive features and can be considered a life-threatening medical emergency. Patients typically are extremely aggressive and agitated and have profound vital sign derangement with diaphoresis, tachycardia, tachypnea, and hyperthermia. Not only are they not directable, but they are also often incoherent and inattentive, display superhuman strength, and do not perceive pain. These extremely high-risk patients will require immediate attention. If you encounter this type of patient, immediately call for help. They will require chemical sedation. Some states have separate protocols for excited delirium and will require medical command for authorization before medication administration. One commonly utilized medication is ketamine 4–5 mg/kg IM or 2 mg/kg IV/IO.

Case (continued): *A paramedic from the ALS unit was able to promote discussion with the patient and build rapport by using the SAVE mnemonic (support, acknowledge, validate, and emotion naming). The patient agreed to unlock the door and allow the paramedic team to take her vital signs, with a pulse of 120, blood pressure of 120/70, respiratory rate of 20, oxygen saturation of 100% on room air, temperature of 37 °C, and a glucose level of 85. She did admit that she had attempted suicide by an overdose of alcohol, acetaminophen, and fluoxetine approximately 60 minutes ago. You are able to assess for future violence using the Broset Violence Checklist and give her a score of zero or low risk of violence. She is agreeable for transport to the local emergency department and you do not believe she will require any medications currently as she is cooperative and no longer agitated.*

KEY POINTS

- Always consider and rule out an acute medical etiology when caring for an acutely agitated patient.
- Approach suicidal patients with a calm, courteous, and empathic manner in order to establish rapport and trust.
- Attempt verbal de-escalation techniques as a first measure to calm agitated patients.

BIBLIOGRAPHY

Almvik R, Woods P, Rasmussen K. The Broset Violence Checklist: sensitivity, specificity, and interrater reliability. *J Interpersonal Violence.* 2000;15(12):1284-1296.
Dollops KT. Managing psychiatric emergencies. EMSWorld. May 2013. http://www.emsworld.com/article/10931747/managing-psychiatric-emergencies.
Helman A, Strayer R, Thompson M. Ep 115 Emergency management of the agitated patient. Emergency Medicine Cases. 2018 Sept:18-32. https://emergencymedicinecases.com/emergency-management-agitated-patient/.
Lipton L. Emergency responders management of patients who may have attempted suicide. *IJRDMS.* 2005;5(2):1-16. *http://ispub.com/IJRDM/5/2/5315.*
Nordstrom K, Zun LS, Wilson MP, et al. Medical evaluation and triage of the agitated patient: consensus statement of the American Association for Emergency Psychiatry Project BETA Medical Evaluation Workgroup. *West J Emerg Med.* 2012 Feb;13(1):3-10.
Pennsylvania Department of Health. EMS statewide ALS and BLS protocols. http://health.pa.gov/topics/Documents/EMS/2019%20PA%20ALS%20Protocols%20Final.pdf.
Richmond JS, Berlin JS, Fishkind AB, et al. Verbal de-escalation of the agitated patient: consensus statement of the American Association for Emergency Psychiatry Project BETA de-escalation workgroup. *West J Emerg Med.* 2012;13(1):17-25.
Scheppke KA, Braghiroli J, Shalaby M, et al. Prehospital use of I.M. ketamine for sedation of violent and agitated patients. *West J Emerg Med.* 2014 Nov;15(7):736-741.
Wilson A, Ritchie JD. Evaluation and management of psychiatric emergencies in the prehospital setting. *JEMS.* 2014 Jul;7(39):1-27. *http://www.jems.com/2014/07/10/evaluation-and-management-psychiatric-em/.*
Wilson MP, Pepper D, Currier GW, et al. The psychopharmacology of agitation: consensus statement of the American Association for Emergency Psychiatry Project BETA Psychopharmacology Workgroup. *West J Emerg Med.* 2012 Feb;13(1):26-34.

CHAPTER 73

CPR, AED, AND MECHANICAL COMPRESSION

Abagayle E. Renko and Chadd E. Nesbit

QUESTIONS AND ANSWERS

CPR AND MANUAL COMPRESSIONS

1. What is meant by cardiopulmonary resuscitation (CPR)?

   CPR is a lifesaving intervention performed when an individual's heart stops beating in order to maintain blood flow and promote oxygen delivery to one's vital organs. To most, "CPR" refers to basic life support (BLS), consisting of chest compressions and rescue breathing. To other healthcare providers, it can also encompass advanced cardiac life support (ACLS), pediatric advanced life support (PALS), and advanced trauma life support (ATLS).

2. What are the indications to perform CPR?

   In general, CPR should be started immediately on any patient who has become unconscious and is found to be pulseless. CPR is also indicated in any infant less than 12 months of age with a pulse rate of less than 60 beats per minute.

3. Explain the difference between a heart attack and a cardiac arrest.

   A **heart attack** is a problem with *circulation*, occurring when blood flow to one or more parts of the heart is blocked. A **cardiac arrest** is an *electrical* problem and occurs when the heart malfunctions and stops beating. While a heart attack can cause a cardiac arrest, they are *not* synonymous terms and should *not* be used interchangeably.

4. What are the most common reversible causes of cardiac arrest?

   The reversible causes of cardiac arrest can be remembered by the "6 H's" and "6 T's." Table 73.1 describes the 6 H's and 6 T's and offers some basic considerations that may help prehospital providers identify the cause of an arrest and expedite reversal (when appropriate, amidst a multiprovider resuscitation scenario). The causes of cardiac arrest in infants and children differ from those in adults; these causes include but are not limited to sepsis, hemorrhage, overdose, hypoglycemia or other electrolyte derangement, arrhythmia or heart block secondary to myocarditis, congenital heart disease, and pulmonary hypertension.

5. List the various links in the cardiac chain of survival.

   The six links of the *adult* chain of survival are recognition and activation of the emergency response system, immediate high-quality CPR, rapid defibrillation, basic and advanced emergency medical services, advanced life support, post–cardiac arrest care, and recovery. The six links of the *pediatric* chain of survival are arrest prevention, immediate high-quality CPR, prompt access to the emergency medical services system, advanced life support, and post–cardiac arrest care, and recovery. Strong chains increase the chances of survival for a victim of cardiac arrest—for every 1 minute that CPR and defibrillation are delayed, the victim's survival rate drops by approximately 10%.

6. What is the appropriate sequence for performing CPR?

   The 2015 AHA guidelines replaced the traditional "airway, breathing, compressions (ABC)" sequence with "compressions, airway, breathing (CAB)" in an effort to avoid delays in initiation of compressions and thus improve patient outcomes. However, certain exceptions to this generally accepted sequence do exist (such as in drowning victims), and it is recommended that providers tailor their sequence based on the etiology of the arrest.

Note: Most of the information in this chapter can be found in greater detail through the guidelines published and regularly updated by the American Heart Association (AHA), in conjunction with the International Liaison Committee on Resuscitation. Specifically, the website section on "CPR & ECC Guidelines" goes into great detail regarding highlights, summary of evidence, and recommendations. Of note, this chapter is targeted toward prehospital providers and therefore does not go into greater detail beyond the expected scope of practice of a basic emergency medical technician (EMT-B), advanced EMT (AEMT), or paramedic provider.

Table 73.1. Reversible Causes of Cardiac Arrest

6 H'S		6 T'S	
Hypovolemia/ hemorrhage	History of fluid or blood loss? Obvious source of blood loss?	Tablets (overdose)	History of overdose? Pupil size and reactivity? Narcan considered?
Hypoxia	Airway placed correctly? Bilateral breath sounds? Source of oxygen verified?	Tamponade	Jugular venous distention? Muffled heart sounds? Portable ultrasound available to assess contractility?
Hydrogen ions (acidosis)	Respiratory or metabolic? Ventilating properly?	Tension pneumothorax	Unequal breath sounds after verification of endotracheal tube placement?
Hyperkalemia	On dialysis? Visible arteriovenous fistula or dialysis port?	Trauma	Obvious signs of trauma?
Hypothermia	Temperature obtained? Rewarming measures (warm blankets, warm IV fluids) started?	Thrombosis (coronary)	Risk factors[a] present? EKG obtained?
Hypoglycemia	History of diabetes? Last oral intake? Fingerstick glucose obtained?	Thrombosis (pulmonary embolism)	History of shortness of breath? Unilateral leg swelling? Risk factors[b] present?

[a]Risk factors for acute coronary syndrome include history of chest pain brought on by exertion with associated diaphoresis, nausea or vomiting, arm or jaw radiation; ST depression or elevation on EKG not due to other factors; age 45 or older; history of hypertension, hyperlipidemia, diabetes, obesity, or smoking; previous myocardial infarction, coronary artery bypass graft surgery, transient ischemic attack, cerebrovascular accident, or peripheral artery disease; parent or sibling with cardiovascular disease before the age of 65.
[b]Risk factors for pulmonary embolism include states of hypercoagulability (current or recent pregnancy, malignancy); recent travel, prolonged immobilization, surgery, or trauma; prior deep venous thrombosis or pulmonary embolism; or hormone use (oral contraceptives, hormone replacement, or estrogenic hormone use in male or female patients).
EKG, Electrocardiogram; *IV*, intravenous.

Table 73.2. Central Pulse Locations

ADULT	CHILD	INFANT
Carotid artery (on side of neck) OR	Femoral artery (inner thigh in the crease between leg and groin)	Brachial artery (inside of the upper arm, between an infant's elbow and shoulder)

7. Are "pulse checks" still recommended? If so, how often, and in what anatomical location(s)?
   Although BLS CPR courses traditionally teach a pulse check for no longer than 10 seconds before initiating CPR, the AHA has since *deemphasized* these "pulse checks." Even experienced clinicians can have difficulty determining whether a pulse is present within 10 seconds, so it is better to initiate CPR on a patient who does in fact have a pulse than not provide or delay CPR to a truly pulseless patient. If you do check for a pulse, check in an appropriate location (Table 73.2) for no more than 10 seconds. Of note, a patient with a palpable carotid pulse has a systolic blood pressure of at least 60 mm Hg.

8. What are the most current guidelines for rate of compressions, compression-to-ventilation (C:V) ratios, expected depth of compressions, and appropriate hand positioning?
   See Table 73.3.

9. What reasons exist to *pause* compressions?
   The ultimate goal of CPR is to minimize the length of time that compressions are not delivered. The only time compressions should be paused is during defibrillation, although compressions should be continued just up until (and resumed directly after) the shock is delivered. Although, previously, some had advocated for rhythm check directly after defibrillation, it is no longer recommended to do so; compressions should be immediately resumed following delivery of shock. If the patient has no airway secured, or does not have an advanced airway, pausing compressions to allow for airway placement is also *not* recommended.

Table 73.3. Differences in BLS CPR for Adults, Children, and Infants

		C:V RATIO[a]	RATE	DEPTH	HAND POSITION
Adult	One rescuer	30:2	100 to 120/min	2–2.4 inches	Heel of one hand on the lower sternum of the chest (center); overlap in parallel with the heel of the other hand
	Two rescuers				
Child	One rescuer	30:2	100 to 120/min	2–2.4 inches	Same as in adults, but may only use one hand in certain situations (depending on the size of the child)
	Two rescuers	**15:2**			
Infant	One rescuer	30:2	100 to 120/min	**1.5 inches**	Two fingers on the center of the chest
	Two rescuers	**15:2**			Two thumbs with the hands encircling the infant's chest

[a]Ratios are based off the assumption that the patient does not have an advanced airway. Once an advanced airway such as an endotracheal tube is secured, rescuers should switch from standard ratios to continuous compressions with ventilations given through a bag valve mask every 6 seconds in adults and every 2-3 seconds (20-30 breaths per minute) in infants and children (a new recommendation per the 2020 AHA guidelines). The ratios for two rescuer CPR in children and infants are bolded to highlight the difference between the C:V ratio in adult and children/infant two rescuer CPR. Similarly, the depth of infant compressions is bolded to emphasize its difference from the recommended depth of compressions for adult and children.

BLS, Basic life support; *CPR*, cardiopulmonary resuscitation; *C:V ratio*, compression-to-ventilation ratio.

10. Are there instances in which you should *not* initiate CPR on a pulseless patient?

You should not start CPR on a pulseless patient in cases of penetrating or blunt trauma in which the victims will obviously not survive. Do not initiate CPR on patients who have injuries not compatible with life or who have signs of rigor mortis.

11. What is an active compression-decompression (ACD-CPR) device?

An ACD-CPR device is a mechanical device that not only performs chest compressions but also alternates those compressions with active decompression by a suction cup forcing the thorax back to its uncompressed volume. While various adjunctive devices to CPR have been devised in an attempt to eliminate (or at least minimize) the human fatigue component from a resuscitation scenario, the only automatic ACD-CPR device on the market is the LUCAS, which is manufactured by Jolife AB (a part of Stryker) in Lund, Sweden.

12. Which is more effective: mechanical or manual compressions during CPR?

Trick question—they are currently thought to be of equal efficacy, for studies have failed to show a survival benefit of the mechanical ACD-CPR devices when compared to manual compressions. The mechanical devices' utility lies predominantly in situations where the delivery of high-quality manual compressions is challenging or dangerous for the provider. For example, an automated device could be of use when limited rescuers are available; in situations of prolonged CPR including extrication scenarios, long transport times, or hypothermic arrest; in a moving ambulance; and during preparation for extracorporeal CPR.

13. What is an impedance threshold device (ITD)? Does the AHA recommend its use?

An impedance threshold device (ITD) such as a ResQPOD is a small device that attaches between a bag-valve mask and any airway adjunct (i.e., a face mask, supraglottic airway, or endotracheal tube). It was designed to occlude air entry into the lungs during the decompression phase of CPR when the thoracic pressure within the chest falls below atmospheric pressure. By doing so, it creates a vacuum within the chest and enhances both venous return and cerebral circulation. Although the AHA does not recommend the routine use of ITDs as adjuncts to conventional CPR, the combination of an ITD with an ACD-CPR device may be a reasonable alternative to conventional CPR in certain settings. If an ITD is used and a patient is successfully resuscitated, the device should be removed from the airway circuit to allow breathing without inspiratory resistance.

14. Describe the possible complications of CPR.

Ventilations can insufflate the patient's stomach, risking regurgitation, aspiration, and potentially gastric rupture. Closed chest compressions can cause rib and/or sternal fractures, separation of ribs from sternum, pulmonary contusions, pneumothoraxes, myocardial contusions, hemorrhagic pericardial effusions, and splenic or liver lacerations. Later complications include pulmonary edema, pneumonia, gastrointestinal hemorrhage, and recurrent arrest.

15. What is the most common cause of death in resuscitated patients?
    Anoxic brain injury secondary to prolonged hypoxia.

16. What indications, if any, exist to cease compressions?
    The only definitive indications to cease compressions are if the patient regains a pulse or upon receipt of a do not resuscitate (DNR) order (or similar advanced directive) specifying the patient's wishes *not* to be resuscitated. Various guidelines also suggest that cessation of resuscitation efforts is appropriate in the following situations:
    - After 20 minutes of CPR in an intubated patient, failure to achieve an end-tidal carbon dioxide ($EtCO_2$) level >10 mm Hg by waveform capnography
    - For an out-of-hospital cardiac arrest (OHCA) that was not witnessed by EMS personnel, if defibrillation did not occur and return of spontaneous circulation (ROSC) was not obtained prior to transport
    - After asystole of 20 minutes or longer
    - If the heart rate of a newborn has remained undetectable for approximately 20 minutes or longer
        In general, the decision to cease compressions in a multidisciplinary team scenario is made based on several factors, including the patient's age, suspected etiology of the arrest, and total time without return of spontaneous circulation.

17. If the scene becomes unsafe or a provider is fatigued, do circumstances exist for CPR cessation?
    First responders and general citizens are generally protected by Good Samaritan laws should they need to cease CPR due to scene safety concerns or due to physical exhaustion.

18. How should special considerations be addressed?
    See Fig. 73.1.

AED/DEFIBRILLATION

1. What does "AED" stand for? What role does an AED play in resuscitation?
   An "AED," or automated external defibrillator, is a portable electronic device that is able to automatically detect and treat shockable rhythms (see question 2 of this section) by administering electrical current through electrode pads placed on the patient's chest. Defibrillation, or administration of electrical current, can terminate the shockable rhythm underlying one's arrest and reestablish an effective rhythm.

2. What is the difference between "shockable" and "nonshockable" rhythms?
   Shockable rhythms refer to electrical disturbances that may benefit from defibrillation, such as **ventricular tachycardia** or **ventricular fibrillation**. With these rhythms, the heart is electrically active but is unable to effectively pump or circulate blood. **An AED can recognize only shockable rhythms.**
        Nonshockable rhythms, or "preterminal" rhythms, are electrical disturbances that would not benefit from defibrillation. These include **pulseless electrical activity** (presence of electrical complexes without any accompanying mechanical heart contraction) and **asystole** (complete absence of cardiac electrical activity).

3. When is it appropriate to defibrillate *before* starting compressions?
   If the cardiac arrest was *witnessed* and an AED *is* readily available, defibrillation should occur immediately; survival in victims with shockable rhythms is highest when defibrillation occurs within 3 to 5 minutes of collapse. If the arrest was *unwitnessed* or an AED *is not* readily available, compressions should be started while an AED is retrieved; as soon as the AED arrives, it should be applied and defibrillation should be attempted as soon as possible, if indicated. If two or more rescuers are present, one should immediately begin CPR while the other activates the emergency response system and gets a defibrillator.

4. What are the appropriate voltage settings for defibrillation?
   For adults and children older than 8 years old, unsynchronized defibrillation should occur at **200 Joules (biphasic)** or 360 Joules (monophasic). For children between 1 and 8 years old, an AED with a pediatric dose attenuator is preferred; for infants less than 12 months of age, a manual defibrillator is preferred. The recommended **initial** defibrillation strength for children and infants is at **2 Joules/kg**, followed by 4 Joules/kg for any additional defibrillation efforts.

5. Are adult and child/infant AED pads interchangeable?
   No. While adult pads (designed for anyone over the age of eight) may be used on children and infants if no smaller pads are available, child/infant pads should NOT be used on an adult.

6. What is double sequential defibrillation?
   Double sequential defibrillation is a technique that involves delivering two sequential shocks to patients in ventricular fibrillation, and is typically only utilized after several failed standard defibrillation attempts. However, studies have yet to suggest that the technique improves patient outcomes, so its routine use is not recommended by the 2020 AHA guidelines.

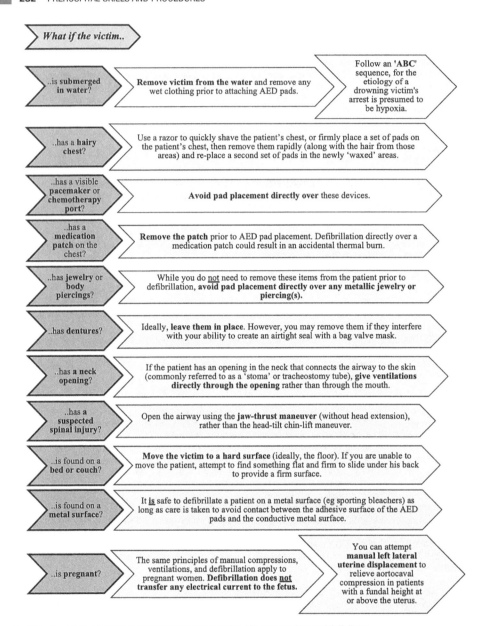

What if the victim..

..is submerged in water?	Remove victim from the water and remove any wet clothing prior to attaching AED pads.	Follow an 'ABC' sequence, for the etiology of a drowning victim's arrest is presumed to be hypoxia.

..has a hairy chest? — Use a razor to quickly shave the patient's chest, or firmly place a set of pads on the patient's chest, then remove them rapidly (along with the hair from those areas) and re-place a second set of pads in the newly 'waxed' areas.

..has a visible pacemaker or chemotherapy port? — **Avoid pad placement directly over** these devices.

..has a medication patch on the chest? — **Remove the patch** prior to AED pad placement. Defibrillation directly over a medication patch could result in an accidental thermal burn.

..has jewelry or body piercings? — While you do not need to remove these items from the patient prior to defibrillation, **avoid pad placement directly over any metallic jewelry or piercing(s).**

..has dentures? — Ideally, **leave them in place.** However, you may remove them if they interfere with your ability to create an airtight seal with a bag valve mask.

..has a neck opening? — If the patient has an opening in the neck that connects the airway to the skin (commonly referred to as a 'stoma' or tracheostomy tube), **give ventilations directly through the opening** rather than through the mouth.

..has a suspected spinal injury? — Open the airway using the **jaw-thrust maneuver** (without head extension), rather than the head-tilt chin-lift maneuver.

..is found on a bed or couch? — **Move the victim to a hard surface** (ideally, the floor). If you are unable to move the patient, attempt to find something flat and firm to slide under his back to provide a firm surface.

..is found on a metal surface? — It **is** safe to defibrillate a patient on a metal surface (eg sporting bleachers) as long as care is taken to avoid contact between the adhesive surface of the AED pads and the conductive metal surface.

..is pregnant?	The same principles of manual compressions, ventilations, and defibrillation apply to pregnant women. **Defibrillation does not transfer any electrical current to the fetus.**	You can attempt **manual left lateral uterine displacement** to relieve aortocaval compression in patients with a fundal height at or above the uterus.

Fig. 73.1. Special considerations of cardiopulmonary resuscitation. *AED,* Automated external defibrillator.

KEY POINTS

- Uninterrupted, high-quality compressions and early defibrillation are the keys to increasing your patient's chance of survival.
- Checking for a pulse can be difficult regardless of one's level of training and should not delay initiation of compressions in an unconscious patient suspected to need resuscitation efforts.
- While automated compression devices can be useful in certain scenarios, they do not provide any survival benefit to patients when compared to conventional, manual compressions.

BIBLIOGRAPHY

American College of Surgeons Committee on Trauma, American College of Emergency Physicians Pediatric Emergency Medicine Committee, National Association of EMS Physicians, American Academy Of Pediatrics Committee on Pediatric Emergency Medicine Policy statement: withholding or termination of resuscitation in pediatric out-of-hospital traumatic cardiopulmonary arrest. *Pediatrics.* 2014;133(4):e1104-e1116.

American Heart Association. CPR FAQs. 2016. https://ahainstructornetwork.americanheart.org/idc/groups/ahaecc-public/@wcm/@ecc/documents/downloadable/ucm_484812.pdf.

American Heart Association. *2020 AHA Guidelines Update for CPR and ECC.* 2020.

American Red Cross. CPR/AED for professional rescuers and health care providers. https://www.redcross.org/content/dam/redcross/training-services/handbooks-and-catalogs/CPRO-Handbook.pdf.

Aufderheide TP, Nichol G, Rea TR. A trial of an impedance threshold device in out-of-hospital cardiac arrest. *N Engl J Med.* 2011;365:798-806.

Baskett PJ, Steen PA, Bossaert L. European Resuscitation Council. European Resuscitation Council guidelines for resuscitation 2005. Section 8. The ethics of resuscitation and end-of-life decisions. *Resuscitation.* 2005;67:S171-S180.

Biarent D, Bingham R, Richmond S, et al. European Resuscitation Council. European Resuscitation Council guidelines for resuscitation 2005. Section 6. Paediatric life support. *Resuscitation.* 2005;67:S97-S133.

Kattwinkel J, McGowan JE, Zaichkin J. *Textbook of Neonatal Resuscitation.* 6th ed. American Academy of Pediatrics; 2011.

Morrison LJ, Kierzek G, Diekema DS, et al. Part 3: ethics: 2010 American Heart Association guidelines for cardiopulmonary resuscitation and emergency cardiovascular care. *Circulation.* 2010;122:S665-S675.

Parsons PE, Wiener-Kronish JP, Berra L, Stapleton RD. *Critical Care Secrets.* 6th ed. New York: Elsevier; 2018.

Tintinalli JE, Stapczynski JS, Ma OJ, Cline D, Meckler GD, Yealy D. *Tintinalli's Emergency Medicine: A Comprehensive Study Guide.* 8th ed. New York: McGraw-Hill Education; 2016.

CHAPTER 74

FIELD AMPUTATION

Michael Shukis and Chadd E. Nesbit

QUESTIONS AND ANSWERS

1. Who can perform a field amputation?
   Field amputation is a rare procedure; therefore, preplanning is necessary. EMS providers in some areas may be faced with the prospect of having to perform a field amputation. It would be desirable to be in contact with medical control to discuss the procedure before proceeding. Having multiple trained providers will also facilitate a smooth procedure. Additional providers may be needed to assist in sedation and airway management.
   Ideally, any field amputation should be performed by an appropriately trained provider from the nearest hospital. This may be an emergency physician, an orthopedic surgeon, or a trauma surgeon. Additional personnel might include an operating room (OR) scrub nurse and/or anesthesiologist. Having a preplanned "go team" is one way many hospitals have planned for these types of rare events. While hospital personnel may have medical expertise, they are not usually familiar with working on an uncontrolled scene. If available, emergency physicians trained in EMS would be an excellent resource as they are comfortable operating in a prehospital setting and managing complex trauma patients.

2. What are the indications for a field amputation?
   Field amputation is a true "life-over-limb" procedure. The most common indication for a field amputation is when the patient either cannot be extricated or the time to extricate the patient will be too lengthy given the extent of the patient's injuries. Another indication is the patient has life-threatening injury to an area of the body that cannot be accessed due to the manner in which the patient is entrapped. Field amputation should also be performed if the entrapped limb is mutilated, nonviable, or only hanging on by small amounts of tissue. The viability of a limb, however, is difficult to ascertain in a field, and as such, this indication should be utilized with caution. The environment the patient is in is also a factor. If the patient's life is in imminent danger secondary to the environment, including fire, extreme cold, submersion in water, structural collapse, or chemical exposure, a field amputation may also be indicated, if it is safe for the provider to do so. The final indication is if the amputation is being performed on a deceased patient who is blocking the ability to access other patients who may be injured.

3. What are the contraindications for a field amputation?
   The contraindications for performing a field amputation are relative if the indications earlier were met. The decision to perform a field amputation should only be made in conjunction with the technical rescue team, in order to ensure that all other options have been considered. Additionally, there are times when the patient can be extricated by cutting away any entangled clothing or by giving the patient enough analgesia to relax and loosen the entrapped limb. It is also possible that you only need to remove some soft tissue in the area to allow the remaining limb to be freed. If this is the case, a full-field amputation should not be performed.

4. What equipment is needed for a field amputation?
   The actual equipment necessary to perform a field amputation is not much more than what is already available on most ambulances; however, it is best to have all these items pulled together in one kit to ensure that all items are quickly available when needed. Table 74.1 outlines these items.

5. Which bone cutting device is preferred?
   The most commonly used devices include a Gigli saw, a Stryker bone saw, or a reciprocating saw. Other devices that have been discussed, but are less ideal, include a hack saw or a hydraulic cutting tool. Each of these devices has their own advantages and disadvantages, which are outlined in Table 74.2. It is recommended to have at least two different types of saw available, as the demands of the situation will vary, and having a backup method available will help ensure success.

6. What medications should I use for sedation, analgesia, and rapid sequence intubation?
   Any patient undergoing field amputation should at least have moderate sedation. Ideally, complete sedation with intubation is performed prior to the amputation. Ketamine 2 mg/kg intravenous (IV) or 4 mg/kg intramuscular (IM) is an ideal agent as it is not likely to cause hypotension. Fentanyl is also a good choice for pain management as it is fast and has less hemodynamic effects. Other medications, including Versed, morphine, propofol, and etomidate, can all be used as well, but care should be taken with regard to the patient's hemodynamic status. If the patient will require rapid sequence intubation, use of rocuronium instead of succinylcholine may help mitigate concerns for hyperkalemia.

Table 74.1. Items Needed for Field Amputation

ITEM	USE/ADDITIONAL COMMENTS
Tourniquet ×2	Used to occlude flow to the entrapped limb prior to amputation
Chlorhexidine/iodine	To sterilize the field prior to performing the amputation
#10 blade scalpel ×2	Cut through soft tissue (these dull quickly)
Combat gauze/blue towels	To retract the soft tissue
Kelly/Pean forceps	To get combat gauze behind the bone
ABD pad ×2/ACE wrap ×2	To cover the stump
ACE wrap ×2	To cover the stump
Sterile trauma shears	To cut away clothing and remaining soft tissue
Saline	To moisten gauze surrounding the entrapped limb
Biohazard bag	To transport the entrapped limb
Sharps container	
PPE including eye protection, surgical masks, and sterile gloves/gowns	Be sure to utilize FFP3 dust masks if utilizing a reciprocating saw
Bone cutting device including Gigli saw, Stryker saw, reciprocating saw, or hydraulic cutters	At least one primary and one backup method

PPE, Personal protective equipment.

Table 74.2. Types of Saws for Amputation

TYPE OF SAW	ADVANTAGES	DISADVANTAGES
Gigli saw	• Fast (approx. 90 seconds) • Easy to tell if you are through the bone • Compact, easy to store	• Requires two hands to operate • Requires elbow room to saw
Stryker saw	• Designed to cut bone in the operating room • One-handed operation	• Must be plugged in • Must have charged batteries if battery powered
Reciprocating saw	• Fast (approx. 20 seconds) • One-handed operation • Good for confined spaces • Readily available	• Saw tends to spray significant amounts of bio-material, making it difficult to see where you are cutting, and requires an FFP3 mask for protection • Difficult to tell when you have cut through the bone
Hack saw	• One-handed operation • Compact, easy to store • Readily available	• Blade easily gets jammed/gummed up with tissue • Requires a lot of elbow room
Hydraulic cutting tool	• Quick to cut through bone	• Causes crushing to soft tissue and splintering of the bone up to 5 cm away from the cut • Requires running a hydraulic line to the patient

7. What should be done before starting the field amputation?

Before performing a field amputation, treat the patient like any trauma patient. A rapid, thorough assessment for polytrauma is necessary. Address life-threatening issues. Providers should consider premedicating with analgesics, sedation, intubation, and resuscitating with either packed red blood cells or whole blood as available/needed prior to performing the procedure. Clothing should be cut away, and two tourniquets should also be applied proximal to the limb where the amputation will occur. Make sure not to place the tourniquets over a joint. A blood pressure cuff can also be used if tourniquets are not available. While the wound will likely already be dirty and contaminated, try to sterilize the area as best you can with chlorhexidine or Betadine before proceeding.

This is obviously a life-changing procedure. If the patient is conscious, you should discuss the plan with them and obtain informed consent, preferably with a witness.

8. How do I perform a field amputation?

   At the level where you will be performing the amputation, cut through as much of the exposed soft tissue as possible using long smooth strokes with your scalpel. Cut as far around the limb as possible in order to expose the bone. Once the bone is exposed, you will need to retract the soft tissue. Grab the middle of your combat gauze with your Kelly/Pean forceps and pass the gauze as close as possible behind the exposed bone. Place the ends of the combat gauze or towel through the loop that you just created and apply traction proximally to retract the soft tissue from where you will be cutting the bone. If using a reciprocating saw, Stryker saw, or hack saw, cut through the exposed bone at this time. If you are using a Gigli saw, pass the wire through the same tract that you created for the combat gauze. Attach the handles to the wire and bring them together to form a V-shape no greater than 90 degrees apart. Pull tension and saw back and forth until you have cut through the bone. Cut through the remaining tissue using sterile trauma shears or a scalpel.

   Now that the stump is exposed, place the remaining combat gauze on the end of the bone where the marrow will likely continue to leak. Elevate the stump, and place moist bandages along the end of the stump, followed by an ACE wrap to apply additional pressure. Reassess your tourniquets, and tighten as necessary. If possible, retrieve the amputated limb at this point, as it may be used for skin grafting. This should not hold up transport of a critically ill patient. The amputated limb should be wrapped with moist, sterile gauze, placed in a biohazard bag, and then placed in a cooler on wet ice for transport.

9. How do I manage a patient who has recently undergone limb amputation?

   At this point, the patient should either be moderately sedated, or sedated and intubated. Additional doses of sedatives and analgesia may be necessary. Keep the patient on end-tidal CO_2 to assess respirations. Resuscitation would include giving the patient whole blood or blood products if there is evidence of hemorrhagic shock, as well as the use of tranexamic acid (TXA) (1 g over 10 minutes), and reversal agents if the patient is anticoagulated. Many of these patients may require treatment for hyperkalemia as they are often victims of crush injury as well. If possible, there is likely no harm in starting antibiotics early as this has been shown to significantly reduce morbidity and mortality in open fractures. The antibiotic of choice would be cefazolin 2 g (25 mg/kg). If the patient is allergic to penicillin, an alternate choice would be clindamycin 600 mg IV (10 mg/kg). Gentamicin 1.5–2.5 mg/kg Ideal Body Weight (IDW) may be necessary as well. Tetanus should also be updated.

10. What is the morbidity associated with field amputations?

   There are not enough data to reliably say what the outcomes are from a field amputation. Many of these patients will require intensive care and will likely require revision of the amputation site. Because of this, it is always better to err on the side of leaving the most material possible for the surgeon to revise the amputation in the future. Also, having additional fractures proximal to the amputation does not necessarily mean that the stump site distal to the fracture will not be viable. The ability to perform the procedure in a timely manner, and being proactive about resuscitation, will give the remaining portion of the limb the best chance of viability and lead to the best patient outcomes.

KEY POINTS

- Field amputation is a life-over-limb, high-risk, low-frequency procedure. Training and simulation are essential to success.
- Preplanning with your trauma center is important. Develop a protocol, including indications, necessary personnel, and equipment, with your emergency medicine, surgical, and orthopedic colleagues.
- Forming a "go team" and having the necessary equipment prepackaged will result in a shorter response time to the entrapped patient.

BIBLIOGRAPHY

Bunyasaranand JC, Espino E, Rummings KA, Christiansen GM. Management of an entrapped patient with a field amputation. *J Emerg Med*. 2018;54(1):90-95.

Colella MR. Emergency medicine. Medical College of Wisconsin, 2019. www.mcw.edu/departments/emergency-medicine/education/section-of-ems-and-disaster-medicine/field-ems-physicians#.VLvVOC5GwZ4.

Kampen KE, Krohmer JR, Jones JS, Dougherty JM, Bonness RK. In-field extremity amputation: prevalence and protocols in emergency medical services. *Prehosp Disaster Med*. 1996;11(1):63-66.

Latimer A. Field amputation. Taming the SRU. April 30, 2015. www.tamingthesru.com/blog/procedural-education/field-amputation.

Leech C, Porter K. Man or machine? An experimental study of prehospital emergency amputation. *Emerg Med J*. 2016;33(9):641-644.

Macintyre A, Kramer EB, Petinaux B, Glass T, Tate CM. Extreme measures: field amputation on the living and dismemberment of the deceased to extricate individuals entrapped in collapsed structures. *Disaster Med Public Health Preparedness*. 2012;6(4):428-435.

McNicholas MJ, Robinson SJ, Polyzois I, Dunbar I, Payne AP, Forrest M. 'Time critical' rapid amputation using fire service hydraulic cutting equipment. *Injury*. 2011;42(11):1333-1335.

Porter KM. Prehospital amputation. *Emerg Med J*. 2010;27(12):940-942.

Way C, de Tar E, Isaacson S, Sincerbeaux C, Torgenson M, Wineinger D. Exclusive: field amputation difference between life and death. FireRescue1. February 8, 2017. www.firerescue1.com/rescue/articles/192121018-Exclusive-Field-amputation-difference-between-life-and-death/.

Yang C, Ross W, Peterson LM. Prehospital field amputation leads to improved patient outcome. *JEMS*. September 2, 2019. www.jems.com/articles/print/volume-43/issue-1/departments-columns/case-of-the-month/hand-entrapment.html.

CHAPTER 75

HEMORRHAGE CONTROL

Josh Knapp

QUESTIONS AND ANSWERS

Case: *You are dispatched to a call for "hemorrhage"; you arrive to find a woman who is pale and diaphoretic and looks to be in distress with a large pulsatile bleed from a left arm fistula site.*

1. How is massive or life-threatening hemorrhage defined?

   There is not a universally accepted definition of massive hemorrhage. It is bleeding that is rapid, large volume, and likely to result in shock with progression to death from exsanguination if not controlled. Examples include wounds associated with pulsatile arterial bleeding and wounds associated with other severe extremity trauma. It is important to recognize that large-volume bleeding is rapidly life threatening. Massive hemorrhage should be controlled even before airway management as it is futile to oxygenate and ventilate without a blood volume to circulate.

2. How common is hemorrhage as cause of death?

   Hemorrhage is one of the leading sources of preventable death on the battlefield. It is the second leading cause of death in civilian trauma cases.

3. What are the initial steps to effective control of a hemorrhage?

   For most wounds with active bleeding, the initial step should be firm direct pressure with an appropriate dressing if available. Pressure should be directed directly over the source of bleeding. In circumstances where direct pressure on a wound is not feasible or not successful, a tourniquet should be applied. In wounds that are felt to be immediately life threatening due to volume of bleeding or the presence of signs of hemorrhagic shock, tourniquet application as a first-line intervention is appropriate.

4. Have tourniquets been shown to be effective and improve mortality?

   In military use, tourniquets have been clearly shown to be effective in controlling hemorrhage. They are issued to every US servicemember in the battlefield setting. Kragh et al., in a landmark paper, showed decreased mortality in military prehospital use. Tourniquet use when shock was absent was associated strongly with increased survival. In cases where tourniquets were indicated but not applied, survival was 0%. This supports the practice of rapid use of tourniquets before significant amount of hemorrhage has occurred. In a civilian setting, tourniquet use has been associated with decreased need for blood products and higher systolic blood pressure (BP) on emergency department (ED) arrival supporting their use.

5. What is the process of tourniquet application?

   Current recommendations from military combat casualty care recommend that the tourniquet is applied several inches proximal to the bleeding site. If you cannot rapidly identify the site of bleeding, you should apply the tourniquet as high as possible into the groin or axilla. Tourniquets may be applied over clothes if necessary. Next, you will need to tighten the tourniquet sufficiently to occlude arterial flow. Each device is different and training and practice are important for correct application. In general, the strap must be applied around the extremity, as much slack as possible should be taken up to tighten the device, and then the windlass or other mechanical device should be tightened and secured to prevent loosening. Assess for effectiveness and record application time.

   The two broad categories that devices fall into are devices that use a windlass, pneumatic bladder or ratcheting mechanism to provide mechanical advantage and bungee or elastic-type tourniquets. Commercially available products are also recommended over any improvised device. The Committee on Tactical Combat Casualty Care (CoTCCC) publishes a list of recommended devices. Currently none of the bungee or elastic devices on the market today are recommended by CoTCCC. Fig. 75.1 shows several common devices approved by CoTCCC.

6. How is sufficient tightness of application determined?

   Both cessation of bleeding and loss of distal pulses are indicative of sufficient pressure.

7. Why is occlusion of arterial flow important?

   Insufficient pressure will not control bleeding from arterial sources without arterial occlusion. An insufficiently tight tourniquet can obstruct venous outflow but not prevent inflow of blood from arteries and lead to increased bleeding and possibly contribute to compartment syndrome.

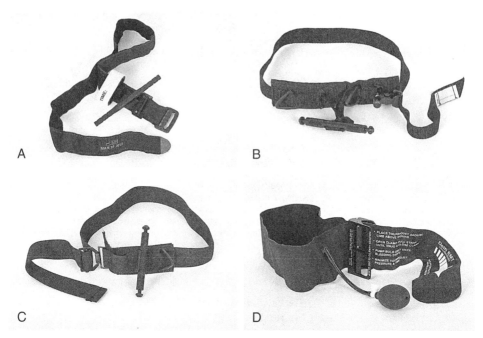

Fig. 75.1. (A) Combat action tourniquet. (B) Special operations forces tactical tourniquet. (C) Special operations forces tactical tourniquet—wide. (D) Emergency and military tourniquet. Note that (B) was removed from the most recent Committee on Tactical Combat Casualty Care recommendations as (C) has replaced it. *(From Drew B, Bennett BL, Littlejohn L. Application of current hemorrhage control techniques for backcountry care: part one, tourniquets and hemorrhage control adjuncts.* Wilderness Environ Med. *2015;26(2):236-245.)*

8. What are the next steps if the tourniquet does not seem to be effective?
   First, if there continues to be significant bleeding, apply a second tourniquet. This should be applied adjacent to the first tourniquet applied to your patient.
   Troubleshoot the suspected reason for failure to achieve hemorrhage control rapidly. Large or muscular individuals can make tourniquet application in the thigh challenging. Items in clothing or other obstructions can also cause tourniquet failure if not applied directly to skin. Bleeding from joints can also be difficult to control with tourniquets and a tourniquet should never be applied directly over a joint as it will be ineffective.
   Remember, you can use multiple methods such as direct pressure and wound packing in addition if needed. A properly applied tourniquet will be effective for most situations.

9. Are complications of tourniquet placements common? What are the complications?
   There are many potential complications of tourniquet placement. These include amputation, compartment syndromes, rhabdomyolysis, nerve injuries, and venous thromboembolism among other potential complications. Kragh et al. published about the military experience in Iraq with a series of papers; in one study, in over a total of 499 patients with tourniquets applied, less than 2% had nerve palsy and 0.4% had amputations. These amputations were not shown to be solely related to the placement of the tourniquet. Few patients, especially with application time under 2 hours, have been shown to suffer complications from application.

10. Should a tourniquet be discontinued in the field?
    In general, once a tourniquet has been placed prehospital, it should be remain in place until arrival in the ED, where more resources for bleeding control are available. In special circumstances, discuss any removal thought to be indicated with medical command. The wound must be completely exposed, adequate alternative supplies assembled, and a more proximal tourniquet should be placed first loosely in case of tourniquet failure if the need for reapplication is evident.

11. In locations not amenable to tourniquet application, what are other methods of bleeding control?
    Direct pressure will be the first method of control. If this is ineffective, there are other products and techniques that can be helpful. For deep wounds, wound packing can be an effective technique. This allows direct pressure to be applied directly to the site of bleeding. Any gauze material can be used for wound packing; there are specific products such as "Z" folded gauze that are relatively long and narrow, designed to be quickly packed into a

wound. The key to wound packing is to fully fill the wound cavity so that the dressing exerts as much pressure for control of the hemorrhage as possible.

12. What is a junctional hemorrhage?

A junctional hemorrhage is a wound in the groin or axilla that is at the meeting or junction of the abdomen or thorax and the extremity. These wounds can be more difficult to control because of the location not being easily amenable to the placement of the tourniquet and the presence of large vessels that can cause large volume bleeding. There have been specific junctional tourniquets developed that are designed to compress junctional hemorrhage and are CoTCCC approved. They are not yet widely carried in the civilian prehospital environment.

13. Name the locations that are appropriate for wound packing.

Primarily, the junctional areas of the pelvis and buttock, axilla, and neck, as well as the extremities. Wound packing is not appropriate in the torso.

14. What are hemostatic dressings and how to they work?

These are dressings that have additional materials that are designed to support clot formation. Several different types are available. Similar to tourniquets, there is a list of approved devices by the CoTCCC. In approved dressings, the active ingredient is either kaolin or chitosan. Kaolin is an inorganic mineral that functions by activating factor XII to XIIa to activate the clotting cascade. Chitosan is polysaccharide that is found in the shells of crustaceans. It functions to cross-link red blood cells (RBCs) in the wound to help form an additional barrier to bleeding.

15. Do hemostatic dressings still require direct pressure?

Yes, hemostatic dressings are effective only in conjunction with several minutes of direct pressure when applied.

16. What is TXA?

Tranexamic acid (TXA) is a medication that acts as an antifibrinolytic. It inhibits fibrin clot breakdown and has been used to assist in control of severe bleeding.

17. What are the current recommendations for use of TXA?

A large trial found that TXA may decrease mortality when given within 3 hours of injury. Current recommendations from CoTCCC are for use of TXA in patients predicted to require significant resuscitation with blood products. The use of TXA is also supported in advanced trauma life support (ATLS) guidelines.

KEY POINTS

- Massive hemorrhage is rapidly life-threatening and a leading cause of death.
- Tourniquet application in patients with massive hemorrhage is a life-saving intervention.
- A properly tightened tourniquet should occlude arterial flow.
- Complications from tourniquet use under 2 hours are rare.
- TXA has been shown to decrease mortality when given within 3 hours of injury.

BIBLIOGRAPHY

Bennett BL. Bleeding control using hemostatic dressings: lessons learned. *J Wilderness Environ Med.* 2017;28:S39-S49.
Drew B, Bennet BL, Littlejohn L. Application of current hemorrhage control techniques for backcountry care: part one, tourniquets and hemorrhage control adjuncts. *Wilderness Environ Med.* 2015;26:236-245.
Kragh Jr JF, Littrel ML, Jones JA, et al. Battle casualty survival with emergency tourniquet use to stop limb bleeding. *J Emerg Med.* 2011;41(6):590-597.
Kragh Jr JF, Walters TJ, Baer DG, et al. Practical use of emergency tourniquets to stop bleeding in major limb trauma. *J Trauma Inj Infect Crit Care.* 2008;64:2.
Kragh Jr JF, Walters TJ, Baer DG, et al. Survival with emergency tourniquet use to stop bleeding in major limb trauma. *Ann Surg.* 2009;249:1.
Roberts I, Shakur H, Coats T, et al. *The CRASH-2 trial: a randomized controlled trial and economic evaluation of the effects of tranexamic acid on death, vascular occlusive events and transfusion requirement in bleeding trauma patients. Lancet.* 2013 Mar;17(10):1-79.
Smith AA, Ochoa JE, Wong S, et al. Prehospital tourniquet use in penetrating extremity trauma: decreased blood transfusions and limb complications. *J Trauma Acute Care Surg.* 2019;86(1):43-51.

CHAPTER 76

INTRAVASCULAR/INTEROSSEOUS ACCESS AND FLUID RESUSCITATION

Josh Knapp

QUESTIONS AND ANSWERS

Case: *You arrive on scene to find an 80-year-old woman who appears to be in obvious distress. Family reports that she has had a fever for several days as well as a productive cough and shortness of breath. Vitals are blood pressure (BP) 80/40, heart rate (HR) 130, respiratory rate (RR) 26, and SPO$_2$ 91% on room air. You want to initiate a fluid bolus to treat hypotension associated with suspected septic shock. Unfortunately, after two attempts, you have been unable to place a peripheral IV.*

1. What is an alternative form of access that can be employed?

   Peripheral venous cannulation (PIV) and intraosseous (IO) access are the most common ways that access is established. Peripheral access is typically the primary form of venous access, with IO access being second line. Central venous access in the EMS setting is rare. In some cases, patients may have ports or preexisting central lines that can be accessed when an emergent need is present.

2. What are the flow rates that can be achieved by IO access?

   The EZ-IO manufactured by Teleflex is one IO access device that is in common use. Research has shown that the humeral mean flow rate is about 5 L per hour and tibial flow rate is about 1 L per hour. These flow rates were achieved using a pressure bag system. Using pressure infusion is key to achieving adequate flow using an intraosseous line. Per the manufacturer of the EZ-IO, a rapid flush is also needed to achieve high flow rates. This helps clear the marrow from around the insertion site.

3. What are the indications for IO access over PIV access?

   Indications for IO access include failed PIV access and/or the need for rapid access for resuscitation. Often, cardiac arrest can be an indication to use IO as a first-line option as it can often be faster to obtain than a PIV.

4. What are some contraindications to IO access?

   Contraindications to IO access include:
   - Acute fracture of the selected bone;
   - Overlying infection at the insertion site;
   - Any previous attempt in the same bone within 48 hours;
   - Inability to identify landmarks; and
   - Prosthetic bone or joint at insertion site.

       Contraindications at any one site do not preclude attempts at a different site. Osteoporosis or osteogenesis imperfecta and more proximal fractures are also relative contraindications.

5. Can all medications be given via the IO route?

   Yes, all medications that can be given via the intravenous route are appropriate for IO infusion, including vasopressors and blood products.

6. In alert patients, what can be used to provide analgesia for IO infusions? What is the recommended dose in children and adults?

   2% lidocaine can be infused via a slow push prior to the initial saline flush to provide analgesia. The dose in adults is 40 mg. In pediatric patients, 0.5 mg/kg with a maximum of 40 mg can be used. Only lidocaine that is designed for intravenous injection should be used.

7. What are the most common crystalloid solutions used in the prehospital setting?

   Isotonic crystalloid solutions are the most common solutions used in EMS. These include normal saline solution, lactated Ringer's (LR) solution, and Plasmalyte. In addition to isotonic fluids, hypotonic fluids such as D10 and hypertonic fluids such as 3% saline are sometimes carried for more limited applications.

8. What are the advantages to using saline as the initial choice of intravenous (IV) fluid in the EMS setting?
   Saline has been studied as a carrier fluid for most drugs and enjoys near universal drug compatibility. LR can cause precipitation of some drugs. Saline is also preferred over LR for patients with traumatic brain injury (TBI) as LR is slightly hypotonic and can decrease serum osmolarity, contributing to cerebral edema.

9. If giving blood products, what solution must not be used as a carrier fluid?
   LR is not compatible with blood products as it contains calcium that can lead to clotting of blood products. Both saline and Plasmalyte are compatible with blood.

10. What are the advantages to balanced crystalloid solutions?
    Balanced solutions include LR solution and Plasmalyte. These solutions more closely approximate blood plasma concentrations of potassium, chloride, and sodium compared to normal saline. Saline contains a much higher amount of chloride compared to blood plasma and can lead to a hyperchloremic acidosis. Saline has also been shown to contribute to kidney injury. Several trials have now been conducted comparing normal saline solution to balanced solutions. On the whole, these have pointed toward balanced solutions being the better choice.

11. In the prehospital setting, which patients should receive IV fluids?
    IV fluid should be used carefully like any other medication. Use of IV fluids should be guided by the presenting problem of the patient, with the goal of addressing a particular pathology. In general, IV fluids used prehospital are being used for volume expansion of a patient who has intravascular volume depletion. Examples include severe dehydration, sepsis, and trauma. Patients without signs of volume depletion do not require IV fluids.

Case: You are dispatched to respond to a motor vehicle accident. You find a patient with vitals of BP 85/30, HR 125, RR 24, and SPO$_2$ 96%. There is no external hemorrhage, but the patient has severe abdominal tenderness with a seatbelt sign. You want to obtain IV access to treat the patient.

12. What are the properties of the ideal catheter for volume infusion?
    Poiseuille's law describes the way IV fluids flow through a catheter.

$$\text{Volume flow rate} = \frac{\pi\,(\text{pressure difference})\,(\text{radius}^4)}{8\,(\text{viscosity})\,(\text{length})}$$

There are several important principles of the law applicable to everyday practice. Flow is proportional to the fourth power of the radius of the catheter. This means that if you double the diameter of the catheter, flow rate can be increased 16 times! Additionally, flow is directly proportional to pressure difference and inversely related to length.

Based on Poiseuille's law, if fluids need to be infused rapidly, a short, wide catheter under pressure is the ideal solution.

13. What are the current recommendations for IV fluid therapy in trauma patients?
    Advanced life support (ALS) trauma care traditionally involved large volume fluid resuscitation to restore blood pressure. More recently, evidence favors a more judicious use of IV fluids due to evidence of increased mortality in aggressively fluid resuscitated patients. This concept is called hypotensive resuscitation or damage control resuscitation.

    Using IV fluids to increase the BP back to normal ranges can be harmful due to the pressure effect on newly formed clot, increased bleeding with increased blood flow, the dilutional effect of crystalloid on the body's oxygen carrying capacity, dilution of coagulation factors, acidosis if saline is used, and contribution to hypothermia.

    The potential harms of crystalloid fluid must be balanced with the need to maintain some level of end organ perfusion. It is suggested to use small boluses of fluid to maintain radial pulses and a BP that is lower but adequate for perfusion.

    The National Association of State EMS Officials publishes model clinical guidelines. In adults, the recommended goal is to maintain a systolic pressure of 90 mm Hg. IV fluid is not needed in patients with a pressure of at least 90 mm Hg.

    The exception to the goal of 90 mm Hg systolic as an adequate pressure target for resuscitation is in a patient with TBI as reductions in mean arterial pressure (MAP) have been shown to increase mortality. Maintaining a BP of 110 mm Hg to 120 mm Hg systolic is recommended and is associated with better outcomes.

14. What is the role of EMS fluid resuscitation in nontrauma patients?
    Fluid resuscitation for patients with hypotension from medical causes such as septic shock is an important part of care for these patients. The presence of hypotension is a strong indication for the need for IV fluids. A recent paper showed a possible mortality benefit to patients with hypotension from sepsis being treated with fluids in the prehospital setting. In patients without hypotension, there was not a benefit shown to giving fluids.

Case: You are dispatched to the scene of a house fire. You encounter a patient who was burned in the fire. While initiating your transport to the burn center you want to initiate fluids and pain control.

15. What is the preferred fluid for burn patients?
    Burn patients often require large volumes of fluids for resuscitation. As such, hyperchloremic metabolic acidosis with normal saline can result if saline was used. To avoid this acidosis, LR is the preferred fluid for burn patients.

16. You calculate the total body surface area (BSA) burned as 25%. The patient weighs 80 kg. What is the formula used to estimate fluid requirements for the first 24 hours in a burn patient?
    The Parkland formula is used to estimate fluid needs. The formula is **4 mL × weight in kg × percentage BSA burned**. In our previous example, 4 mL × 80 kg × 25% BSA = 8000 mL in the first 24 hours.

17. How much fluid is given in the first 8 hours?
    By the Parkland formula, half is given in the first 8 hours and half is given over the next 16 hours. Prehospital fluids count toward this requirement so be sure to accurately relay the total fluids given to the next level of care.

KEY POINTS

- Humoral IO access allows much higher flow rates compared to the proximal tibia.
- Based on Poiseuille's law, if fluids need to be infused rapidly, a short, large-bore catheter using pressure is ideal.
- Targeted fluid resuscitation in trauma is preferred to large volume fluid resuscitation.
- The Parkland formula is commonly used to estimate fluid needs for burns for the first 24 hours. The formula is **4 mL × weight (kg) × percentage BSA burned**.
- Balanced crystalloid solutions have several advantages to saline.

BIBLIOGRAPHY

Barea-Mendoza J, Chico-Fernández M, Montejo-González JC. Balanced crystalloids versus saline in critically ill adults. *N Engl J Med.* 2018;378(20):1950-1951.

Brown JB, Cohen MJ, Minei JP, et al. Goal directed resuscitation in the prehospital setting: a propensity adjusted analysis. *J Trauma Acute Care Surg.* 2013 May;74(5):1207-1212.

Cotton BA, Jerome R, Collier BR. Guidelines for prehospital fluid resuscitation in the injured patient. *J Trauma Inj Infect Crit Care.* 2009;67(2):389-402.

Harris T, Rhys Thomas GO, Karim B. Early fluid resuscitation in severe trauma. *BMJ.* 2012;345:e5752.

Lane DJ, Wunsch H, Saskin R, et al. Association between early intravenous fluids provided by paramedics and subsequent in-hospital mortality among patients with sepsis. *JAMA Netw Open.* Published online December 14, 2018. https://jamanetwork.com/journals/jamanetworkopen/fullarticle/2718094.

National Association of State EMS Officials. National Model EMS Clinical Guidelines. Version 2.2. January 5, 2019. https://nasemso.org/wp-content/uploads/National-Model-EMS-Clinical-Guidelines-2017-PDF-Version-2.2.pdf.

Self WH, Semler MW, Wanderer JP, et al. Balanced crystalloids versus saline in noncritically ill adults. *N Engl J Med.* 2018;378(9):819-828.

Teleflex Global Research and Scientific Services, a Division of Clinical and Medical Affairs. The science and fundamentals of intraosseous vascular access, 2017. www.teleflex.com/en/usa/ezioeducation/documents/EZ-IO_Science_Fundamentals_MC-003266.pdf.

PERIMORTEM CAESARIAN SECTION

Jordan B. Schooler

CHAPTER 77

QUESTIONS AND ANSWERS

1. What is a perimortem caesarian section (PMCS)?

   PMCS is the delivery of a baby by means of a surgical incision into the uterus, in the event the mother is in cardiac arrest. The steps to perform a perimortem C-section are essentially the same as those done in a normal caesarian section. The main difference between PMCS and a normal caesarean section is simply the acuity, shifting the balance of risks and benefits in favor of allowing nonobstetricians to do the procedure in an attempt to save the mother and/or baby in extremis.

2. When was this first described?

   The Roman general Scipio Africanus was reported to have been delivered by perimortem C-section in 237 BC. There are reports of PMCS being performed in the late 19th and early 20th centuries for salvage of the fetus. It was during this time period that PMCS began to be viewed as a legitimate medical procedure.

3. Is a resuscitative hysterotomy different from PMCS?

   This is an alternate nomenclature for the same procedure. The term has been advocated to emphasize the fact that delivery has physiologic benefits for the mother, as well as the fetus.

4. Why is this procedure done?

   Delivery will reduce demand on maternal circulation, relieve aortocaval compression, and improve fetal oxygenation. Theoretically, this should improve the chances for both maternal and fetal survival. As much as 40% of the maternal cardiac output can go to the fetus, so delivery can reduce this load on the circulatory system. Aortocaval compression significantly reduces cardiac output in the supine pregnant woman and greatly reduces the efficacy of chest compressions to a large extent. Closed-chest cardiopulmonary resuscitation (CPR) delivers only 20%–30% of normal cardiac output, even under optimal conditions. This in turn will not be adequate to support fetal circulation, so delivery may improve fetal survival as well.

5. When is it indicated?

   A perimortem C-section should be considered in any pregnant woman in cardiac arrest with an estimated gestational age greater than 20 weeks, assuming appropriately trained personnel are available, and there is no other therapy being considered that may preclude this, such as extracorporeal cardiopulmonary resuscitation (ECPR). One may assume the gestational age is greater than 20 weeks if the uterine fundus is at or above the umbilicus.

6. Should you attempt any kind of fetal assessment before performing a PMCS?

   Very simply put, no. As stated earlier, delivery may have a significant physiologic benefit for the mother even if the fetus cannot survive. The procedure should therefore be performed regardless of viability. Additionally, assessment of fetal heart rate is likely to cause significant delay, which may lead to decreased survival of both the mother and the fetus.

7. What is the 4-minute rule?

   A 1986 review noted a few cases of fetal survival when PMCS was performed more than 5 minutes after arrest. The recommendation was then made that the decision ought to be made within 4 minutes, and the procedure completed within 5 minutes. This has been incorporated in American Heart Association (AHA) and American College of Obstetricians and Gynecologists (ACOG) guidelines. However, there are notable misconceptions about this rule. It is still reasonable to perform a perimortem C-section if more than 5 minutes have elapsed, as there are reports of maternal and fetal survival even after more than 30 minutes of CPR. It would also be reasonable to begin the procedure immediately if it were obvious that successful resuscitation of the mother were unlikely, for example, in the case of devastating head injury. Remember, even if the fetus does not survive, the procedure may improve the chances of the mother surviving.

8. What equipment is necessary?

   At minimum, personnel and apparatus for maternal and neonatal resuscitation, a scalpel, and scissors. Also helpful would be retractors, sterile gauze or lap pads for packing, a needle driver, and heavy suture for closing the uterus. Generally, if possible, you would want two teams of providers, one of which cares for the mother and the other cares for the baby you have delivered.

9. How is PMCS performed?

Optimal maternal resuscitation should be continued during the procedure as this will be beneficial for the mother and the unborn baby. While CPR is taking place, the uterus should be displaced laterally, or the mother tilted to the side, to relieve pressure on the aorta and vena cava. Quickly clean the abdomen from sternum to groin with Betadine or chlorhexidine/alcohol solution, but do not delay the procedure for this. Using the scalpel, make a midline incision from the xiphoid process to the symphysis pubis, down to the fascia and ideally going just around the umbilicus. Just superior to the symphysis pubis, deepen the incision until you enter the peritoneum, being careful of the bladder. Place two fingers of your nondominant hand into the peritoneum and use them to keep the uterus and intestines away from the abdominal wall as you extend the full-thickness incision to the xiphoid with your scissors. Using the scalpel, make a small vertical incision into the uterus. This should be low, toward the pelvis, and just large enough to get your fingers into the incision. Avoid cutting the fetus. As previously, use your fingers to elevate the uterine wall—and protect the fetus—as you complete the incision with scissors. At this point, you should be able to grasp the baby and remove it from the uterus, clamp and cut the umbilical cord, deliver the placenta, and continue resuscitation of both patients.

10. What should be done after the delivery?

Depending on the maternal hemodynamics, there may be bleeding from the uterine incision. This can be controlled by packing tightly with gauze or lap pads or by suturing the uterine wound. Resuscitation of the mother should continue in the usual manner. There will now be a second patient that must be resuscitated according to standard neonatal guidelines. If necessary, both patients, when stable, should be transported to a hospital capable of further management, ideally a trauma center.

11. What can go wrong?

Injury to maternal bowel and bladder as well as the fetus is easily possible. There is a high risk of infection given the nonsterile conditions generally present. Sharps injuries to medical personnel may be more likely in emergent procedures as well.

12. What results have been seen?

Maternal survival has been reported in case series to be 17%–59%, and fetal survival, 61%–80%. There is a paucity of data, most of which is in the form of case reports and case series with very high likelihood of bias. Most of this is from in-hospital arrests, limiting generalizability to the prehospital setting.

13. Can PMCS be done in the field?

Yes, and there have been multiple reported cases of prehospital PMCS. However, there are significant challenges. There have been only three cases of neurologically intact fetal survival, and there are no reported maternal survivors of prehospital perimortem C-section. All of the reports involved physician responders, who are rare in many parts of the world. If there are adequately trained personnel and the necessary equipment is available, it would be reasonable to perform this procedure in the field. However, if transport to the nearest facility can be accomplished within 4 or 5 minutes, this may be a reasonable alternative as well.

KEY POINTS

- PMCS can be done by nonobstetricians in a >20-week pregnant patient in cardiac arrest.
- PMCS increases maternal cardiac output and reduces circulatory demand and may improve the chance of survival for both the mother and fetus.
- PMCS should be done within 4 minutes of the presentation to physicians if possible, but survival has been reported even after more than 30 minutes.
- PMCS can be performed by prehospital physicians in the field, but it is logistically challenging.

BIBLIOGRAPHY

DePace NL, Betesh JS, Kotler MN. 'Postmortem' cesarean section with recovery of both mother and offspring. *JAMA*. 1982;248:971-973.
Einav S, Kaufman N, Sela HY. Maternal cardiac arrest and perimortem caesarean delivery: evidence or expert-based?. *Resuscitation*. 2012;83:1191-1200.
Jeejeebhoy FM, Zelop CM, Lipman S. Cardiac arrest in pregnancy: a scientific statement from the American Heart Association. *Circulation*. 2015;132:1747-1773.
Katz V, Balderston K, DeFreest M. Perimortem cesarean delivery: were our assumptions correct?. *Am J Obstet Gynecol*. 2005;192:1916-1920.
Rose CH, Faksh A, Traynor KD. Challenging the 4- to 5-minute rule: from perimortem cesarean to resuscitative hysterotomy. *AJOG*. 2015;213:653-656.
Tommila M, Pystynen M, Soukka H, Aydin F, Rantanen M. Two cases of low birth weight infant survival by prehospital emergency hysterotomy. *Scand J Trauma Resusc Emerg Med*. 2017;25(1):62.
Woods M. Prehospital perimortem caesarean section—a survivor. *Prehosp Emerg Care*. 2020; 24:595–599. doi: 10.1080/10903127.2019.1671563.
Zelop CM, Einav S, Mhyre JM, Martin S. Cardiac arrest during pregnancy: ongoing clinical conundrum. *AJOG*. 2018;219:52-61.

CHAPTER 78

EMS POINT-OF-CARE TESTING

Jeffrey S. Lubin

QUESTIONS AND ANSWERS

1. What is "point-of-care" testing?

   Point-of-care testing (POCT) is medical diagnostic testing done in a setting remote from a centralized laboratory facility. These tests are generally simple and can be performed at the bedside. This is in contrast to centralized laboratory facilities that perform a variety of testing in one location that does not perform patient care.

2. Which POCT has been performed in the prehospital environment?

   Blood glucose measurement was one of the first prehospital POCTs available. Some EMS systems have used handheld lactate analyzers, particularly with prehospital sepsis protocols. Other blood analyzer systems may be used for many different labs, such as troponin levels, blood gases, coagulation profiles, and electrolytes. These systems are most commonly seen in use by critical care transport or community paramedicine/mobile integrated healthcare programs rather than by 9-1-1 providers.

3. What are Clinical Laboratory Improvement Amendments (CLIA) regulations?

   CLIA regulations include federal standards applicable to all US sites that test human specimens for health assessment or to diagnose, prevent, or treat disease. In general terms, the CLIA regulations establish quality standards for laboratory testing performed on specimens from humans, such as blood, body fluid, and tissue, for the purpose of diagnosis, prevention, or treatment of disease or assessment of health. The CLIA program is administered by the Centers for Medicare & Medicaid Services (CMS) and is implemented through three federal agencies—CMS, the Centers for Disease Control and Prevention (CDC), and the Food and Drug Administration (FDA).

4. Can CLIA requirements be waived?

   All facilities in the US that perform laboratory testing on human specimens for health assessment or the diagnosis, prevention, or treatment of disease are regulated under CLIA. There are some waived tests that have been cleared by the FDA for home use and those tests approved for waiver under the CLIA criteria. CLIA requires that waived tests must be simple and have a low risk for erroneous results.

5. How are POCT and CLIA-waived testing different?

   CLIA waiver is a regulatory term and POCT refers to the location where the testing occurs. In other words, POCT means the testing is not happening in a central laboratory, but rather closer to the patient. Some POCTs are waived, whereas others can be designated as moderately complex or highly complex.

6. Which POCT is useful in the prehospital environment?

   Certain POCTs, such as glucometry and 12-lead electrocardiograms (EKGs), have clearly been shown in the literature to impact patient outcomes. However, in areas where patients receive rapid response to emergency calls with subsequent rapid transport, the value of POCT is questionable.

7. Is glucose measurement an advanced life support (ALS) or basic life support (BLS) skill?

   While previously considered an ALS skill, blood glucose monitoring was added to the list of emergency medical technician (EMT) skills in the 2018 National Highway Traffic Safety Administration (NHTSA) National EMS Scope of Practice Model. The abundant use of home glucometers seems to support the use of these devices even by people with no clinical training. There are, however, limited data that directly support the use of glucometers by basic EMTs.

8. What happened to blood glucose test strips?

   The development of a dry-reagent test strip for use with diabetic patients happened in 1957 when a stiff filter paper impregnated with glucose oxidase, peroxidase, and orthotolidine was used to qualitatively measure for urinary glucose measurements. In 1963, a research team adapted this technique to develop the first blood glucose test strip. The visually monitored strips became widely used in clinics, surgeries, and hospital wards, notably intensive care units. However, colors were prone to fade and there were highly significant visual variations in the assessment of colors across the range of glucose concentrations. These limitations became the trigger to develop an automatic, electronic glucose test strip reader to improve precision and give more quantitative blood glucose results.

9. What factors may affect the accuracy of prehospital blood glucose levels?

The FDA requires glucometers to produce measurements within 20% of the reference value at glucose concentrations above 75.68 mg/dL. Glucometer readings have been found to be both safe and accurate in the prehospital setting, providing that the glucose strips have been properly stored. Studies specifically looking at prehospital glucose testing have found the accuracy to be high. That said, most glucometers used in the prehospital setting measure the glucose in whole blood, while hospital lab tests generally measure glucose in plasma. As a result of this difference, lab results may be 10%–15% higher than the glucometer readings.

Other factors that may impact the accuracy of the measurement include:

- the quality of the glucometer;
- the quality and handling of the test strips;
- how the test is performed;
- the patient's hematocrit level;
- the presence of interfering substances in the sample; and
- environmental factors such as altitude, temperature, and humidity.

10. Does prehospital glucose testing change outcomes for patients?

Being able to definitively diagnose hypoglycemia as a cause for altered mental status, as opposed to head injury, intoxication, or other causes, clearly benefits the patient. In other cases, the benefit is less clear. Some trauma literature suggests that blood glucose measurements, in addition to common vital parameters, may help identify patients at risk for cardiopulmonary arrest and dysrhythmias. Conversely, some literature related to prehospital seizure patients suggests that rates of hypoglycemia are so low in patients treated by EMS for seizure that could create an unnecessary delay in benzodiazepine administration.

11. What is lactate?

Lactate is a normal end product of glycolysis, the process that converts glucose into pyruvate. Pyruvate is used to supply energy to cells through the Krebs cycle when oxygen is present. If oxygen is not present, some energy can be created by the fermentation of pyruvate to lactate. Therefore, blood lactate levels can be used to monitor tissue hypoxia because the utilization of pyruvate depends on the presence of oxygen.

12. How might lactate levels be important in the treatment of prehospital patients?

In the prehospital environment, measurement of lactate levels has generally been associated with screening for sepsis. Serum lactate is often used as an indicator of a septic patient's prognosis as well as a guide for determining the severity of the septic patient's illness and the effectiveness of treatment. However, the presence of lactate is not specific to sepsis. It can be increased in any condition that results in anaerobic metabolism such as hypoxia and shock from causes other than sepsis.

13. Does prehospital lactate measurement result in changes in patient care?

In some EMS systems, the measurement of prehospital lactate is included in the screening process for sepsis patients. More specifically, some systems are using the three vital sign parameters of systemic inflammatory response syndrome (SIRS) criteria (heart rate >90, respiratory rate >20, and temperature >38 °C or <36 °C), sometimes along with systolic blood pressure <90 mm Hg, mean arterial pressure <65 mm Hg, or a lactate level of > 4 mmol/L, to activate a prehospital sepsis alert.

There is some evidence that activation of a sepsis alert protocol utilizing point-of-care lactate levels may decrease mortality, but the literature is inconsistent. Some studies have found that EMS use of a combination of SIRS criteria, subjective assessment of infection, and blood lactate measurements did not achieve a level of diagnostic accuracy for sepsis that would warrant hospital prenotification and activation of committed resources at a receiving hospital. While the literature seems convincing that providing more education to EMS on sepsis can impact outcomes, the use of lactate measurement is not firmly supported.

14. What is troponin?

Troponin is an intracellular protein found in skeletal and cardiac muscle cells that is essential for muscle contraction. Both troponin T and troponin I are biomarkers of myocardial damage. Testing for troponin is considered positive when the manufacturer-specified threshold corresponding to a concentration above the 99th percentile is detected.

15. Can troponin be elevated in the absence of an acute coronary syndrome (ACS)?

Yes. Multiple other clinical conditions can result in an increased serum troponin. These include sepsis, stroke, chronic kidney disease, pulmonary disease, chemotherapy, heart failure, and stress cardiomyopathy. In some cases, the elevations can significantly confuse the clinical picture. Careful assessment, serial monitoring of troponin levels, and other supportive tests are typically necessary to tell whether troponin elevations are due to ACS or other causes.

16. What impact does prehospital troponin measurement have for patients?

There has been conflicting literature on this subject. In the "Providing Rapid Out of Hospital Acute Cardiovascular Treatment 3" (PROACT-3) trial, prehospital troponin testing did not shorten time from first medical contact to final disposition. However, the subsequent study (PROACT-4) did show a decrease in this time, with the greatest impact on patients discharged from the emergency department (ED). There was no difference in clinical outcomes.

Experts have speculated that the current POCT technology for troponin may not be analytically sensitive enough. However, a more sensitive prehospital troponin essay could benefit patients in rural areas where they might be directly routed to cardiac centers that offer immediate primary coronary interventional surgery.

17. Can other blood chemistry analyses be done in the prehospital environment?

Blood chemistry analysis is included in the NHTSA National EMS Scope of Practice Model at the paramedic level. There are several cartridge-based devices available on the market that can be used to assess parameters such as pH, blood gases, electrolytes, urea, creatinine, and international normalized ratio (INR). They are not commonly used in the 9-1-1 environment because they are expensive, require an affiliation with a CLIA-certified biomedical devices lab, and require frequent maintenance and calibration. They also tend to be sensitive to temperature extremes and vibration.

18. What nonblood POCT is commonly done in the prehospital environment?

Twelve-lead EKGs are often performed by EMS personnel and can be used to determine destination as well as activation of resources at the receiving hospital. End-tidal CO_2 monitoring can be used to confirm endotracheal tube placement, monitor breathing, and assist with certain diagnoses. The measurement of oxygen saturation by pulse oximetry has become commonplace; the measurement of carbon monoxide and methemoglobin levels by co-oximetry is also possible, but less common.

19. What is the status of prehospital ultrasound?

Point-of-care ultrasound by EMS personnel is an emerging technology that has not yet become universally accepted. It has the potential to aid in the diagnosis and management of a variety of critically ill and injured patients. The most commonly reported barriers to prehospital ultrasound implementation include, but are not limited to, cost, training, short transport times, concerns about delaying time to definitive care, lack of evidence, approval by EMS administration, buy-in by medical directors and ED staff, and acceptance by veteran EMS providers.

KEY POINTS

- POCT is medical diagnostic testing done that is generally simple and able to be performed at the bedside.
- Certain POCTs, including glucose measurement and 12-lead EKGs, have clearly been shown in the literature to impact patient outcomes.
- Other POCTs, such as lactate and troponin, have not definitively been proven to impact patient outcomes.

BIBLIOGRAPHY

Beskind DL, Rhodes SM, Stolz U, et al. When should you test for and treat hypoglycemia in prehospital seizure patients? *Prehosp Emerg Care*. 2014;18(3):433-441.

Blanchard IE, Kozicky R, Dalgarno D, et al. Community paramedic point of care testing: validity and usability of two commercially available devices. *BMC Emerg Med*. 2019;19(1):30.

Boland LL, Hokanson JS, Fernstrom K, et al. Prehospital lactate measurement by emergency medical services in patients meeting sepsis criteria. *West J Emerg Med*. 2016;17(5):648-655.

Clarke SF, Foster JR. A history of blood glucose meters and their role in self-monitoring of diabetes mellitus. *Br J Biomed Sci*. 2012;69(2):83-93.

Ezekowitz JA, Welsh RC, Weiss D, et al. Providing rapid out of hospital acute cardiovascular treatment 4 (PROACT-4). *J Am Heart Assoc*. 2015;4(12):e002859.

Guerra WF, Mayfield TR, Meyers MS, et al. Early detection and treatment of patients with severe sepsis by prehospital personnel. *J Emerg Med*. 2013;44(6):1116-1125.

Kreutziger J, Schmid S, Umlauf N, et al. Association between blood glucose and cardiac rhythms during pre-hospital care of trauma patients—a retrospective analysis. *Scand J Trauma Resusc Emerg Med*. 2018;26(1):58.

St John A, Price CP. Existing and emerging technologies for point-of-care testing. *Clin Biochem Rev*. 2014;35(3):155-167.

Venturini JM, Stake CE, Cichon ME. Prehospital point-of-care testing for troponin: are the results reliable? *Prehosp Emerg Care*. 2013;17(1):88-91.

CHAPTER 79

PROCEDURES IN THE TRAUMA PATIENT

Ethan J. Young

QUESTIONS AND ANSWERS

1. What is one of the most important things to remember before performing any prehospital procedures?
   The most important thing to remember in any patient encounter is your safety and health. The patients that you encounter in the prehospital environment could possibly have any number of communicable diseases. This means that for every patient encounter, proper BSI (body substance isolation) is required. At the bare minimum, gloves are required every time you touch a patient. For more invasive procedures with a possibility of exposure to bodily fluids, a mask and face shield are required.

2. What is the indication for a needle thoracostomy?
   A needle thoracostomy (needle decompression) should be performed when there is concern for a tension pneumothorax. There are a number of physical exam findings that can lead to the diagnosis of a tension pneumothorax. There will be decreased or absent breath sounds on the side of the pneumothorax. You can also see hypotension from the effects of the pneumothorax preventing proper filling of the heart. Jugular venous distention (JVD) can be seen but may not be present in a patient with significant blood loss. A late sign of a tension pneumothorax is tracheal deviation away from the affected lung.

3. Where should the needle be inserted during a needle thoracostomy?
   There are several sites that can be utilized by the prehospital provider to choose from (Fig. 79.1). The preferred site for a needle decompression is the 4th or 5th intercostal space in the anterior axillary line. The needle is inserted over the rib to avoid the nerves and blood vessels that run underneath every rib. A large angiocath (14 gauge) with a length of at least 3.5 cm should be used. The 4th/5th intercostal space in the anterior axillary line has the lowest average chest wall thickness and, therefore, the lowest failure rate.

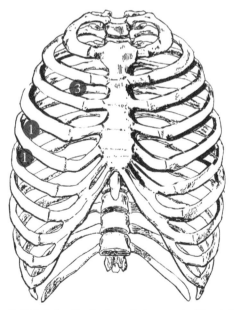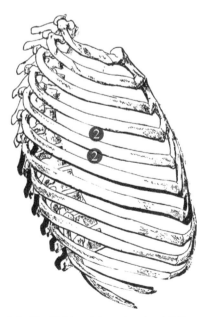

Fig. 79.1. Preferred location for needle decompression. The anterior axillary line in the 4th or 5th intercostal space is preferred *(1)*. The midaxillary line in the 4th or 5th intercostal space has the next lowest failure rate *(2)*. The midclavicular line in the 2nd intercostal space has the highest failure rate *(3)*.

		FAILURE RATE WITH 5-CM
Table 79.1. Preferred Site for Needle Thoracostomy		
PREFERENCE	**SITE**	**ANGIOCATHETER**
1	4th or 5th intercostal space—anterior axillary line	13%
2	4th or 5th intercostal space—midaxillary line	31%
3	2nd intercostal space—midclavicular line	38%

Alternative sites for a needle decompression include the 2nd intercostal space in the midclavicular line, the 4th intercostal space in the midaxillary line, or the 5th intercostal space in the midaxillary line. See Table 79.1 for needle thoracostomy sites by success rate.

4. What is a finger thoracostomy?

A finger thoracostomy is a procedure that is performed to rapidly relieve the cardiac dysfunction caused by either a tension pneumothorax or tension hemothorax. A scalpel, curved clamp, and gloved finger are all that are required. It is important to remember that this is a highly invasive procedure and there is a high risk of exposure to the patient's blood so proper BSI is essential.

5. How do you perform a finger thoracostomy?

A finger thoracostomy is performed by bringing the patient's arm away from their body and exposing their lateral chest on the side of the pneumothorax or hemothorax. The skin is then cleansed with alcohol or chloraprep. A 1–2-inch skin incision is made over the 4th or 5th rib in the anterior axillary line. A clam is then used in a spreading motion to get through the subcutaneous tissue, muscle, and pleura. A pop will be felt when the clamp enters the pleural cavity. Finally, a gloved finger is inserted through the tract that was created by the clamp and it is moved around within the pleural cavity to ensure there is no lung tissue adhering to the wall of the chest. After you have completed the procedure, an occlusive dressing should be applied.

6. What is an occlusive dressing?

An occlusive dressing is a dressing that is meant to be air and water tight. It is applied over an open or "sucking" chest wound and secured by tape. This allows the occlusive dressing to act as a one-way valve to allow air to escape the chest cavity but no air to reenter the chest cavity with inhalation.

7. How do you apply an occlusive dressing?

As stated previously, the occlusive dressing should be impermeable to air and water. The dressing should be applied over the entire chest wound. It is secured on three sides by tape, leaving the fourth side open to act as a one-way valve for air to escape the chest.

8. What are the most important considerations in regard to a fractured extremity?

Any exam of a fractured extremity should include an evaluation of distal pulses, sensation, and motor function. A close inspection of the fracture site is also important to evaluate for an open fracture or a fracture fragment that is close to exiting through the skin. This is also known as "skin tenting."

9. How do I splint a fractured joint?

There are many types of splinting material, but generally, the splint material will be flexible enough for the prehospital provider to mold it into the shape that is required, but rigid enough to provide support to the patient. An evaluation of pulses, sensation, and motor function is required before and after a splint application. The joint should be splinted in the position of comfort with the splint material extending to the long bones above and below the joint. The splint is then secured with gauze or an elastic bandage.

10. How do I splint a fractured long bone?

The principles of splinting a long bone fracture are similar to that of splinting a joint. The splint should include the joints above and below the fractured long bone.

11. What is a traction splint?

A traction splint is a device used to splint a midshaft femur fracture. The distal leg may be shortened or rotated compared to the unaffected leg. There are several brands, but the basic principle of the device is that it is anchored to the hip or pelvis and then to the ankle and mechanical traction is used to realign the leg. This is used to improve pain and to resolve issues with distal circulation caused by a misaligned femur fracture. Each device will have specific steps and instructions for proper application.

12. What is an open-book pelvic fracture?

   These are a specific subset of pelvic fractures that involve a fracture or disruption through the pubic symphysis. The pelvis will feel unstable with lateral compression during your physical exam. These fractures are important to recognize because there is a significant amount of blood loss that can occur from a pelvic fracture.

13. How do I apply a pelvic binder?

   It is important to know some basic pelvic anatomy in order to apply the pelvic binder appropriately. The pelvic binder should be applied at the level of the greater trochanters of the femur; this is the lateral bumps felt over the hips on either side. There are several devices designed for this purpose that each have their own instructions. If a premade device is unavailable, a bedsheet can be folded lengthwise into an approximately 18-inch-diameter sheet. This is rolled up and passed under the patient during a log roll maneuver, making sure that it remains at the level of the greater trochanters of the femurs. It is then twisted in the middle by passing the two ends of the sheet back and forth to a partner and finally secured with a hemostat or clamp (Fig. 79.2).

14. What are the indications for a cricothyrotomy?

   One of the most difficult things about the procedure is making the decision to perform it. A cricothyrotomy should be performed in the setting of a patient who is unable to be intubated and unable to be ventilated (no chest rise even with rescue devices such as bag valve mask (BVM) and supraglottic airway). This is most often in the setting of severe facial trauma. Early recognition of the need for a surgical airway is critical for patient survival.

15. How do I perform a cricothyrotomy?

   Proper landmark identification is key in the successful surgical airway. This is done by palpating the thyroid cartilage, which will be most superior, then the cricoid cartilage, which will be the next structure inferiorly. The appropriate area is the space between these two structures, the cricothyroid membrane. You will need at the minimum a scalpel, bougie, and endotracheal (ET) tube. The skin should be cleansed with alcohol or Betadine. A 3–4-cm vertical incision through the skin is made in the midline neck over the cricothyroid membrane. A small horizontal incision is then made through the membrane. A bougie should be passed through the incision into the trachea and tracheal rings should be felt. A cuffed 6.0 ET tube should then be passed over the bougie, the cuff inflated, and then secured. Standard airway confirmatory methods should be applied, including listening to breath sounds and evaluating capnography.

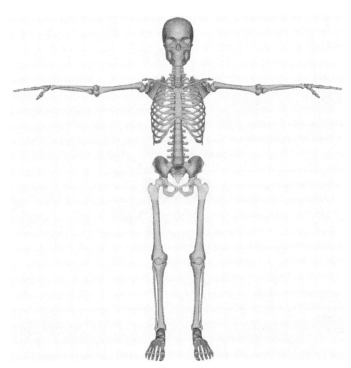

Fig. 79.2. Correct anatomic placement of a pelvic binder. The binder should be placed at the level of the greater trochanter of the femur.

- Perform procedures on trauma patients only when you can ensure your safety. This includes the safety of the scene itself and wearing appropriate personal protective equipment.
- A surgical airway is a critical skill in the management of a patient where a traditional oral or nasal management of an airway is not possible.
- Early recognition and treatment of a tension pneumothorax or hemothorax are essential in the management of a trauma patient.
- Splinting orthopedic injuries can provide pain relief during transportation.
- Recognition of an unstable pelvic injury and early application of a pelvic binder can prevent life-threatening internal blood loss.

BIBLIOGRAPHY

Carlson JN, Wang HE. Airway procedures. *Emergency Medical Services Clinical Practice and System Oversight*, Vol 1. UK: Wiley; 2009:30-42.

Escott ME, Gleisberg GR, Kimmel K, Karrer A, Cosper J, Monroe BJ. Simple thoracostomy: moving beyond needle decompression in traumatic cardiac arrest. *J Emerg Med Serv*. 2014;39(4):26-32.

Laan DV, Vu TD, Thiels CV, Pandian TK, Schiller Hj, Murad MH, et al. Chest wall thickness and decompression failure: a systematic review and meta-analysis comparing anatomic locations in needle thoracostomy. *Injury*. 2015;47(4):P797-804.

Stewart RM. *Thoracic Trauma. Advanced Trauma Life Support Student Course Manual*. In: Merrick C, ed. *Thoracic Trauma*. 10th ed. Chicago, IL: American College of Surgeons; 2018:62-81.

CHAPTER 80

TELEMEDICINE AND EMERGING TELECOMMUNICATIONS

Colby Redfield

QUESTIONS AND ANSWERS

Case: *You arrive on scene to a 55-year-old male with chest pain. While on scene, you take vitals, obtain a history, and perform a 12-lead electrocardiogram (EKG). The patient asks you how his EKG looks and after telling him that it looks ok, he does not want to go to the hospital. How might telemedicine influence your ability to treat and transport this patient?*

1. What is telemedicine?

   Telemedicine, sometimes also referred to as telehealth, is defined as the "use of medical information, exchanged from one site to another via electronic communications, to improve a patient's clinical health status." These exchanges may be voice, video, or data and may be one-way or two-way exchanges.

2. Are there different types of telemedicine?

   Telemedicine can generally be categorized into four types of interactions: Teleconsultation, telementoring, telemonitoring, and telesurgery are all types of telemedicine. Each of these involves an interaction, assisted by technology, occurring over a distance, with the goal of improving the health of the patient.

3. What is teleconsultation?

   Teleconsultation is the direct communication from EMS providers to a base station physician for advice and instructions while providing prehospital care. Traditionally, this has been done by voice over radio, but with increasing wireless expansion, video consultation is now possible in many areas. In some areas of the United States, EMS providers are able to obtain consultation with specialists, such as stroke neurologists, to assist in the examination of patients while in the field. The specialist is then able to assist in determining a transport mode and destination for patients who may benefit from being transported to a higher level of care, bypassing a local hospital.

   Another very common form of teleconsultation is the transmission of 12-lead EKGs for evaluation of ST elevation myocardial infarction (STEMI). Prehospital providers obtain the EKG and then transmit it to a facility for physician review. This is usually done in conjunction with a request for a cardiac catheterization lab activation. The prehospital transmission of the 12-lead EKG has been shown to shorten the time to cath lab activation and to improve outcomes for patients.

4. What other benefits have been shown for teleconsultation in the prehospital setting?

   Studies have demonstrated a reduction in patient refusals when they are able to speak to a physician during a prehospital encounter. Patients are much more likely to agree to transport if they are able to speak to a physician on the phone or by radio during the decision-making process. As patient refusals are an area of high medicolegal risk, reduction of refusals is desirable for risk reduction and improved patient care.

5. What is telementoring?

   Telementoring is a form of telemedicine where an experienced provider assists a less experienced provider in performing a procedure from a distance over a voice or video link. In the prehospital setting, this is typically an emergency medicine physician directing an EMT or paramedic in performance of a procedure in the prehospital setting. Some studies have shown that physicians are able to direct the intubation of patients by less experienced field providers in these high-risk, low-frequency events.

   Ultrasound is another area where telementoring may be helpful. The prehospital provider can be coached through image acquisition for the desired exam, such as an extended focused assessment with sonography in trauma (FAST) exam on a trauma patient, by a provider who is monitoring the process remotely. The images can then be interpreted the credentialed provider and appropriate transport mode and destination decisions can then be made for the patient.

6. What is telesurgery?

   Telesurgery is the ability of a surgeon to perform a procedure on a patient who is in another location. This requires wireless technology, a robotic surgery system, and a team of technicians to support the system. The first telesurgery was performed in 2001. A surgeon and team in New York performed a cholecystectomy on a patient in France without complication.

There are currently a number of limitations, technological, training related, funding and legal, that are inhibiting further development of these types of programs.

7. Besides traditional prehospital settings, where has telemedicine proven to be beneficial?

Telemedicine has been beneficial in battlefield settings and disaster medicine. Several telemedicine systems have been deployed with combat units. This allows physicians to see injuries and initiate treatments prior to the patient's arrival from the battlefield. Telemedicine has also been used in disaster settings such as Hurricanes Rita and Katrina. Physicians, using video technology in a specially equipped ambulance, were able to appropriately triage patients remotely using the enhanced technological capabilities installed in the vehicle.

8. What barriers exist with telemedicine currently?

Even though telemedicine has made leaps and bounds over the last 50 years, barriers still exist. One significant barrier is the lack of broadband cellular coverage in the most rural parts of the country. These are some of the areas in which telemedicine may be the most useful, but the limitations of technology hinder use.

Another barrier is the lack of a payment structure for nontransported patients in the prehospital setting. There may be less incentive for continued development of some of these technologies if there is no mechanism for EMS to be compensated for the service that is provided. An EMS service incurs various costs every time a unit is dispatched on a call regardless of whether the patient is transported or not. One can see the EMS may not have an incentive to incur expense to bring technology to the field that may reduce transports and their reimbursement.

9. What is ET3?

ET3 is the acronym for emergency triage, treat, and transport model. This is a joint project with the Centers for Medicare and Medicaid Services (CMS) and US Department of Health and Human Services (HHS), which will allow EMS to receive reimbursement for certain nontransport ambulance services and transport to alternate destinations. One area of focus for ET3 is the use of telemedicine to help determine the need for transport and appropriate destinations for patients who require transport. Instead of being transported to an emergency department, telemedicine may be able to help a clinician determine if a patient needs to be transported to a facility and if they may possibly be safely transported to another destination such as an urgent care center, psychiatric facility, or a clinic to receive care.

10. Has telemedicine shown to reduce cost to the healthcare system?

Telemedicine has been shown to reduce costs to the healthcare system in multiple settings. Of particular interest to EMS is a study showing savings resulting from a reduction of trips to the emergency department from nursing homes and rehab facilities. Another study showed a reduction in the use of helicopter transport for trauma patients when telemedicine was used to assess the patient and help determine a mode of transport. Additional research will be needed to assess the cost savings of these new telemedicine applications. It will also be crucial to demonstrate that patient outcomes are not worsened when they receive care mediated through a telehealth function.

KEY POINTS

- Telemedicine use has increased significantly over the last decades, and with increasing technological advancements, it will be a bigger part of medicine and prehospital care.
- ET3 will allow for EMS agencies to transport to alternative destinations with a component of telemedicine, while still allowing for payment to the EMS agency.
- The recent growth of wireless networks has allowed use of videoconference as a form of telemedicine.

BIBLIOGRAPHY

Burstein JL, Hollander JE, Delagi R, et al. Refusal of out-of-hospital medical care: effect of medical-control physician assertiveness on transport rate. *Acad Emerg Med.* 1998;5:4-8.

Ellis DG, Tanaka KP, Clemency BM. Telemedicine and emerging telecommunications. In: Cone D, Brice JH, Delbridge TR, Myers B, eds. *Emergency Medical Services: Clinical Practice and Systems Oversight.* Hoboken, NJ: John Wiley & Sons; 2015:392-397.

Emergency Triage, Treat, and Transport (ET3) Model. www.innovation.cms.gov/initiatives/et3/.

Norris JW. *Essentials of Telemedicine and Telecare.* West Sussex: John Wiley & Sons; 2002.

CHAPTER 81

TRANSPORT OF PATIENTS WITH HIGHLY HAZARDOUS COMMUNICABLE DISEASES

Lekshmi Kumar and Alexander P. Isakov

QUESTIONS AND ANSWERS

1. Your crew arrives on scene to a call dispatched as a "sick person." They find a 35-year-old male who recently returned from Saudi Arabia and is complaining of feeling unwell and has a cough. What measures can be taken by the crew to protect themselves and minimize exposure to others?

Emergency responders should adopt an **identify, isolate, and inform** strategy to ensure that they are aware of communicable disease hazards in their work environment and have a procedure to respond safely. To assist with identification of hazards, call centers can screen for travel history and signs and symptoms of highly hazardous communicable diseases (HHCD). Emergency responders can also screen patients. This strategy will help to identify patients at risk for having an HHCD. In this case, recent travel to the Arabian Peninsula, together with illness and cough, raises concern for Middle Eastern respiratory syndrome. Once this risk is **identified**, the patient should be **isolated,** meaning care should be taken to prevent unprotected exposure by other personnel. The patient should be asked to wear a surgical mask and responders who need to interact with the patient should don appropriate personal protective equipment (PPE). **Informing** supervisory personnel, the receiving facility, and local public health authorities will allow for safe transport of the patient to an appropriate facility and allow staff time to prepare for the patient's arrival.

2. You need to transport a patient who has screened positive for travel to a country with widespread transmission of Ebola virus disease. He has been having fever, nausea, vomiting, and diarrhea. What can you do to modify the ambulance to protect its environmental surfaces from contamination and the treatment team from unnecessary exposure?

When transporting a patient with confirmed or suspected HHCD, a hierarchy of controls must be implemented, which include environmental modifications, administrative policies and work practices, and appropriate use of safety equipment. The driver compartment of the ambulance should be isolated from the patient compartment to reduce likelihood of contamination. A positive-pressure environment can be created in the driver compartment using the ventilation system. The ventilation system in the driver compartment should be put in non-recirculating mode with the fan on high. The ventilation system in the back of the ambulance should not recirculate air and the exhaust fan should be set on high. This should maintain appropriate air exchange in the patient compartment.

The interior of the vehicle should be prepared to minimize exposure of environmental surfaces and equipment and to facilitate cleaning and disinfection following the mission. Various methods have been used to envelop the interior of the patient compartment with impervious barriers to protect against contamination of surfaces (Fig. 81.1). This is especially important for patients who pose a high risk for sharing infectious bodily fluids through active bleeding, vomiting, or diarrhea. The stretcher can be protected with an impervious sheet, and essential medical equipment can be placed in a clear plastic bag.

Patients may also be asked to wear a disposable undergarment to capture diarrhea and may be asked to wear a coverall to protect the healthcare worker from draining wounds or contaminated clothing. If they are unable to comply, impervious sheets may be used to envelop the patient during transport. A patient isolation unit may be employed as an environmental control if feasible.

3. Your agency is tasked to transport patients under investigation for HHCD from the airport to as assessment center. What guidelines do you put in place for the appropriate selection of PPE?

Selection of PPE should be based on standard and transmission-based precautions in accordance with Centers for Disease Control and Prevention (CDC) guidelines. PPE selection should consider the condition of the patient, the anticipated mission requirements, and the work environment.

Application of PPE in adherence with standard precautions should include using exam gloves during any patient contact, eye protection, simple face mask for any airway procedures (intubation, suctioning), and addition of a gown for any situations likely to generate splash/liquid exposures. Transmission-based precautions are added to standard precautions for conditions where it has been determined that standard precautions alone do not adequately prevent disease transmission. Implementation of contact precautions typically incudes a disposable

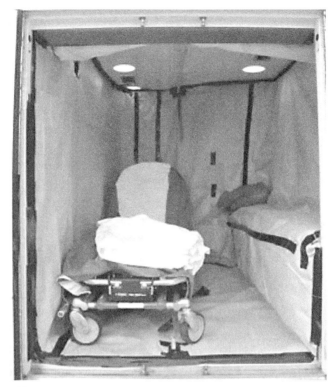

Fig. 81.1. The interior of the patient compartment with impervious barriers to protect against contamination of surfaces. The stretcher has been protected with an impervious sheet. Note that air supply and exhaust fans are not covered.

fluid-resistant gown that extends to at least midcalf or disposable fluid-resistant coveralls, along with disposable gloves. Droplet precautions require the use of a surgical face mask, and eye protection may also be advised. A surgical face mask should also be applied to the patient. Airborne precautions guard against inhalation of droplet nuclei or aerosols. PPE includes disposable National Institute for Occupational Safety and Health (NIOSH)–approved, fit-tested N95 respirators or powered air-purifying respirators (PAPRs) with full hood and high-efficiency particulate air (HEPA) filter. PAPRs should be considered for employees who cannot safely fit test on an N95 respirator. In cases of HHCDs like Ebola Virus Disease (EVD), Marburg virus, or Lassa fever, rigorous application of standard and transmission-based precautions is recommended. For stable "patients under investigation," PPE may be modified based on the presence or absence of symptoms.

On prolonged missions, PAPRs may be more comfortable when airborne precautions are required. Use of a hooded PAPR may also help avoid other challenges such as fogging of eyewear and risk of inadvertently touching the face. Exposure from splashing bodily fluids is also decreased. Consider work/rest cycles for personnel wearing PPE. Providers should be proficient with donning and doffing of PPE, which should be performed under the supervision of a trained observer. The CDC and the Assistant Secretary for Preparedness and Response (ASPR) have checklists available for donning and doffing procedures as well as training resources.

4. You are the operations director for a service tasked to transport patients who are under investigation for HHCDs. In addition to appropriate education and training, what policies and procedures would you consider? Other examples of work practices include preventing unprotected contact with the patient, prohibiting healthcare worker reentry into the driver compartment of the ambulance after making patient contact, limiting the number of healthcare workers exposed to the patient or contaminated waste, and utilization of trained observers and checklists for critical procedures and the donning and doffing of PPE. Standard clinical care guidelines may need to be modified for transport to enhance safety by avoiding invasive and aerosol-producing procedures when possible and eliminating exposure to sharps in a moving vehicle. Patients may require antiemetic or antidiarrheal medications to decrease the likelihood of these problems during transport. Healthcare workers must be familiar with procedures for managing a PPE breach. Medical consultation must be immediately available for decision

support. Procedures must be defined for patient handoff at the sending and receiving facilities. The patient should be transported to the designated location via the most direct path that limits exposure to unprotected staff, patients, and visitors. Facility security should be in place to secure the route and guide the transport personnel to the designated unit. The cleaning and disinfection of the route should be coordinated with environmental services. A postmission medical surveillance program should be implemented for the transport team to ensure early recognition of signs of illness.

5. In addition to standard EMS clinical care guidelines, specific protocols for transportation of patients under investigation for HHCDs are recommended. What topics should these cover?
   Plans for patient monitoring and treatment during transport must be considered, as should plans for resuscitation in case of clinical deterioration. The team should anticipate interventions and procedures that may be required during transport, including cardiac arrest resuscitation, intubation, or other invasive procedures, if warranted. Plans should consider patient condition, devices and medications, and length of transport time. Plans for resuscitation will require consideration of both provider safety and patient benefit and there may be value in having ethics and other experts included in the discussion.

   Ensure that plans are in place for transporting pediatric patients. Consider the developmental stage of the patient when addressing fears associated with PPE, and with not having family members present. Consider how patients with special healthcare needs will be managed. Consider plans for patients with functional or access needs (e.g., hearing, vision, limited mobility), device dependence, and limited English proficiency. Advance preparation with table-top, functional, and full-scale exercises will help prepare staff and refine procedures.

   The service medical director should be involved in the development of all guidelines to ensure quality patient care from initial patient contact to final destination. The medical director will assist in the development of clinical policies and procedures that are appropriate and within the EMS professional's scope of practice. The medical director should also be available for consultation during patient transport.

6. How do you best manage interpersonnel communications during a mission given the unique challenges?
   Communications can be challenging for the transport team, given the need for PPE and concerns about contaminating equipment. Communications can be facilitated by hands-free radios or devices, which are worn inside the protective ensemble. PAPRs can add significantly to ambient noise. Bone conduction earpieces may enable personnel wearing PPE to better hear communications. When communications are not encrypted, the transport team should be careful to protect privileged health information. Transport team supervisory personnel should ideally conduct the majority of the communication with external agencies like police, security, and the receiving facility to allow the clinical team to focus on patient care.

7. Following a mission, cleaning and disinfection of the ambulance and durable equipment are important. What are the key principles to be followed during this process?
   The ambulance cleaning and disinfection procedures, as well as the doffing of PPE, should be performed under supervision of qualified personnel. After cleaning, any visibly contaminated surfaces, the interior of the ambulance, the stretcher, and any exposed durable equipment should be disinfected with an Environmental Protection Agency–registered, hospital-grade disinfectant appropriate for the suspected or known pathogen. The risk for inadvertent or unrecognized exposure to infectious bodily fluids may be greatest during the doffing of potentially contaminated PPE.

   Once the ambulance and durable supplies are cleaned and disinfected, procedures are needed for waste handling that are in compliance with federal regulations and include waste packaging and transport to a disposal facility. It is common for EMS medical waste to be left with hospitals that will have a multidisciplinary team that includes environmental services, infection prevention and control, biosafety officers, and others with expertise in hazardous waste disposal.

8. Once your patient is transported and the mission is complete, what are the next steps to be considered?
   Once the transport is completed and the ambulance is cleaned and disinfected, the providers involved should be debriefed and postmission medical monitoring initiated. Appropriate public health, emergency management, and public safety authorities may need to be informed. The receiving facility should continue communications with the transporting agency regarding any further positive diagnostic tests on the patient that may impact the transport team.

9. Given public interest in patients with HHCD, how would you best manage public information?
   It is important to anticipate and prepare for public interest and media attention. Education of the community will help avoid misunderstanding and fear. Risk communications should be incorporated into the transport plan. Messaging should be proactive and short, using plain language while adhering to risk communication principles. Media relations and communications officers with experience in emergency risk communication should be identified in advance. They can also be used to provide communications guidance to the individuals or agencies involved in the transport.

KEY POINTS

- In order to increase awareness of highly hazardous communicable diseases and prevent unrecognized exposure, EMS personnel should adopt an **identify** (early screening and identification), **isolate** (prevention of unprotected exposure to others), and **inform** (prompt information transfer to receiving facility and public health) strategy.
- Implementation of a hierarchy of controls is necessary for management and transport of a patient suspected or confirmed to have a highly hazardous communicable disease.
- Donning and doffing of PPE should be performed under the supervision of a trained observer using checklists to lower the risk of to lower the risk of inadvertent exposure.
- Postmission medical surveillance programs should be implemented for the transport team to ensure early recognition of signs of illness in case of unrecognized exposure.

BIBLIOGRAPHY

American College of Emergency Physicians. Policy statement: medical direction of emergency medical services. http://www.acep.org/Content.aspx?id=29570.

Assistant Secretary for Preparedness and Response, Technical Resources, Assistance Center, and Information Exchange. EMS infectious disease playbook. https://asprtracie.hhs.gov/documents/aspr-tracie-transport-playbook-508.pdf.

Assistant Secretary for Preparedness and Response. Planning considerations when developing standard operating procedures for the transfer of an Ebola (or other highly infectious disease) patient from/to an air transport provider to/from a ground transport provider. https://www.phe.gov/Preparedness/responders/ebola/Pages/air-transport-factsheet.aspx.

Centers for Disease Control and Prevention. IV. Infection control for prehospital emergency medical services (EMS). http://www.cdc.gov/sars/guidance/i-infection/prehospital.html.

Centers for Disease Control and Prevention. Healthcare Infection Control Practices Advisory Committee (HICPAC). https://www.cdc.gov/infectioncontrol/guidelines/isolation/index.html. Accessed October 20, 2019.

Centers for Disease Control and Prevention. Guidance on personal protective equipment (PPE) to be used by healthcare workers during management of patients with confirmed Ebola or persons under investigation (PUIs) for Ebola who are clinically unstable of have bleeding, vomiting, or diarrhea in U.S. hospitals, including procedures for donning and doffing PPE. https://www.cdc.gov/vhf/ebola/healthcare-us/ppe/guidance.html.

Centers for Disease Control and Prevention. Transport of pediatric patients. https://www.cdc.gov/vhf/ebola/healthcare-us/emergency-services/transporting-pediatric-patients.html.

Isakov A, Miles W, Gibbs S, Lowe J, Jamison A, Swansiger R. Transport and management of patients with confirmed or suspected Ebola virus disease. *Ann Emerg Med*. 2015;66(3):297-305.

Lowe JJ, Jelden KC, Schenarts PJ, et al. Considerations for safe EMS transport of patients infected with Ebola virus. *Prehosp Emerg Care*. 2015;19(2):179-183.

INDEX

Pages followed by *b*, *t*, or *f* refer to boxes, tables, or figures, respectively.